SCHAUM'S
outlines
™

Nursing Laboratory and Diagnostic Tests

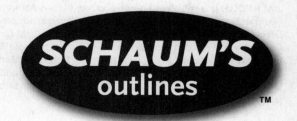

Nursing Laboratory and Diagnostic Tests

James Keogh, RN
Instructor, New York University

Schaum's Outline Series

New York   Chicago   San Francisco   Lisbon   London   Madrid
Mexico City   Milan   New Delhi   San Juan   Seoul
Singapore   Sydney   Toronto

JIM KEOGH is a registered nurse and has written books in the McGraw Hill's Nursing Demystified series. These include: *Pharmacology Demystified, Microbiology Demystified, Medical-Surgical Nursing Demystified, Medical Billing and Coding Demystified, Nursing Laboratory and Diagnostic Tests Demystified, Dosage Calculations Demystified, Medical Charting Demystified, Pediatric Nursing Demystified, and Nurse Management Demystified*. His books can be found in leading university libraries including Yale University School of Medicine, University of Pennsylvania Biomedical Library, Columbia University, Brown University, University of Medicine and Dentistry of New Jersey, Cambridge University, and Oxford University. Jim Keogh, RN, A.A.S., MBA, is a former member of the faculty at Columbia University and is a member of the faculty of New York University.

Schaum's Outline of
NURSING LABORATORY AND DIAGNOSTIC TESTS

1 2 3 4 5 6 7 8 9 ROV/ROV 9 8 7 6 5 4 3 2 1 0

ISBN: 978-0-07-173650-3
MHID: 0-07-173650-6

This publication is designed to provide accurate and authoritative information in regard to the subject matter covered. It is sold with the understanding that neither the author nor the publisher is engaged in rendering legal, accounting, securities trading, or other professional services. If legal advice or other expert assistance is required, the services of a competent professional person should be sought.

—From a Declaration of Principles Jointly Adopted by a Committee of the
American Bar Association and a Committee of Publishers and Associations

McGraw-Hill books are available at special quantity discounts to use as premiums and sales promotions, or for use in corporate training programs. To contact a representative please e-mail us at bulksales@mcgraw-hill.com.

Library of Congress Cataloging-in-Publication Data

Keogh, James Edward, 1948-
      Schaum's outline of nursing laboratory and diagnostic tests / James Keogh.
          p. ;   cm. — (Schaum's outline series)
      Other title: Outline of nursing laboratory and diagnostic tests
      ISBN 0-07-173650-6 (alk. paper)
      1. Diagnosis, Laboratory—Outlines, syllabi, etc. 2. Nursing diagnosis—Outlines,
      syllabi, etc. I. Title. II. Title: Outline of nursing laboratory and diagnostic tests.
      III. Series: Schaum's outline series.
      [DNLM: 1. Laboratory Techniques and Procedures—Examination Questions. 2. Laboratory Techniques
      and Procedures—Outlines. 3. Nursing Diagnosis—methods—Examination   Questions.
      4. Nursing Diagnosis—methods—Outlines. 5. Nursing Care—methods—Examination Questions.
      6. Nursing Care—methods—Outlines.

WY 18.2 K37s 2011]

*To Anne, Sandy, Joanne, Amber-Leigh Christine,
Shawn, and Eric, without whose help and support
this book couldn't have been written.*

Contents

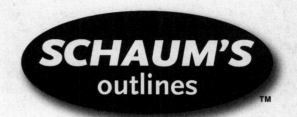

Nursing Laboratory and Diagnostic Tests

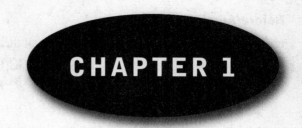

CHAPTER 1

Hematology Tests

1.1 Definition

Hematology clinical laboratory tests are used to examine blood and blood components to determine if they are within normal limits. Values outside normal limits might be signs of a hematological disorder.

Hematology tests count the number of white and red blood cells and platelets, measure the time necessary for blood to clot, measure the capability of blood to carry oxygen throughout the body, assess for inflammation, assess for infection and the type of infection, and assess the specific type and number of circulating white blood cells.

1.2 Blood Type Test

Blood is identified by an antigen on the surface of red blood cells. There are two major types of these antigens: (1) blood group antigens (ABO) and (2) Rh antigen. There are four types of blood group antigens that are determined by performing the ABO test:

1. **Type A**: has the A antigen and antibodies in plasma against B antigen (Type B)
2. **Type B**: has the B antigen and antibodies in plasma against A antigen (Type A)
3. **Type O**: has neither the A antigen nor the B antigen and antibodies in plasma against A antigen (Type A) and B antigen (Type B)
4. **Type AB**: has the A antigen and the B antigen and no antibodies in plasma against A antigen (Type A) and B antigen (Type B)

Red blood cells may have the Rh antigen—sometimes called the Rh factor—attached to it and is determined by the Rh test.

- Rh Positive (+): the Rh antigen is presented on the red blood cells.
- Rh Negative (−): the Rh antigen is not presented on the red blood cells.

A patient's *blood type* is described as a combination of blood group antigen and Rh antigen by using the blood type letter(s) followed by a plus (+) or minus (−) sign, indicating if the Rh antigen is present. For example, type A- means that the patient has the A antigen but does not have the Rh antigen attached to the red blood cells. The test also examines minor antigens that attach to red blood cells that can cause an adverse blood transfusion reaction.

Why the Test Is Performed

The test is performed to test for blood compatibility for a blood transfusion and organ transplant, and to test if a pregnant woman is Rh positive or negative.

Before Administering the Test

It is critical to assess if the patient has any one of the following factors that might affect the test result:

- The patient has taken methyldopa, levodopa, or cephalexin. These medications can cause a false Rh+ test result.
- Recent X-ray with contrast.
- Bone marrow transplant.
- A blood transfusion in the previous three months.
- Has or has had cancer or leukemia.

How the Test Is Performed

A sample of blood is taken from the patient's vein. The patient will experience a tight feeling when the tourniquet is tightened, a pinch or nothing at all when the needle is inserted into the vein, and pressure when a gauze pad is pressed against the insertion site to stop bleeding. It can take up to 10 minutes for bleeding to stop if the patient is taking anticoagulants (aspirin, coumadin). A small bruise might appear at the insertion site, which could become swollen following this test. This is called *phlebitis*. Applying a warm compress several times a day will reduce the swelling.

Teach the Patient

Prior to testing, explain to the patient that no special preparation is needed for the test, how the test is performed, and the conditions that can negatively affect the test results.

Understanding the Test Results

Test results are usually available in an hour. Table 1.1 lists blood type compatibility. Before any transfusion, a sample of the recipient's blood is cross matched (mixed) with the donor's blood in the laboratory to determine compatibility.

    Test results also determine if the patient is Rh positive or negative. If a mother is negative Rh factor and the father is positive Rh factor, then their baby might have a positive Rh factor. While in the womb, the baby's blood can enter the mother's vascular system, resulting in the mother's immune system producing antibodies against the baby's blood. The mother is typically administered an injection with Rh immunoglobulin (RhIg), which suppresses the mother's immune system to develop antibodies to the baby's blood.

TABLE **1.1** **Here are blood type compatibilities between a recipient (the patient) and a donor.**

Blood Transfusion Compatibility Chart

RECIPIENT	DONOR
A−	A−, O−
A+	A−, A+, O−, O+
B−	B−, O−
B+	B−, B+, O−, O+
AB−	AB−, O−
AB+	AB−, AB+, A−, A+, B−, B+, O−, O+
O−	O−
O+	O−, O+

1.3   Partial Thromboplastin Time (PTT)

When bleeding occurs, 12 blood clotting factors cause the blood to coagulate to stop the bleeding. Coagulation of blood is affected by blood clotting factors, which can be absent, decreased, or increased levels, or changes in the way blood clotting factors function. In addition, clotting inhibitors can reduce the effectiveness of clotting factors. The *partial thromboplastin time* (PTT) test measures the clotting time of blood.

Other blood clotting tests are *prothrombin time* (PT) and *activated partial thromboplastin time* (APTT). The *heparin neutralization assay* is performed to determine if substances other than heparin causes an increase in APTT.

Why the Test Is Performed

The test is performed to assess the blood's ability to clot prior to any invasive procedure, for hemophilia, for lupus anticoagulant syndrome, or antiphospholipid antibody syndrome—which is caused when the antibodies attack blood clotting factors—and the effectiveness of the dose of heparin administered to the patient (APPT test).

Before Administering the Test

It is important to assess:

- Prescription and nonprescription medications taken by the patient. Some medications such as aspirin and antihistamines affect the results of the test.
- Herbal and natural remedies taken by the patient, because these can affect the test results.

A patient with a high PTT or APTT value is at risk for bleeding and bruising. Pressure must be applied to the injection site longer than for a patient with a normal PTT or APTT value.

How the Test Is Performed

A sample of blood is taken from the patient's vein. The patient will experience a tight feeling when the tourniquet is tightened, a pinch or nothing at all when the needle is inserted into the vein, and pressure when a gauze pad is pressed against the insertion site to stop bleeding. It can take up to 10 minutes for bleeding to stop if the patient is taking anticoagulants (aspirin, coumadin). A small bruise might appear at the insertion site, which could become swollen following this test. This is called phlebitis. Applying a warm compress several times a day will reduce the swelling.

Teach the Patient

Prior to testing, explain to the patient why the blood sample is taken; that samples may be taken frequently until the healthcare provider determines the therapeutic dose of heparin for the patient, and that taking aspirin, antihistamines, and herbal and natural remedies may affect the test results.

Understanding the Test Results

Test results are usually available in an hour. The laboratory determines normal values based on calibration of testing equipment with a control test. Test results are reported as high, normal, or low based on the laboratory's control test. Patients who have inherited bleeding disorders may have normal PTT and APTT values.

Generally, normal range is:

- Partial thromboplastin time (PTT): 32 to 45 seconds
- Activated partial thromboplastin time (APTT): 10 to 14 seconds
- Proper heparin dose: PTT or APTT is 1.5 to 2.5 greater than the normal value

Longer times may indicate hemophilia, von Willebrand's disease, a blood clotting factor that is low or absent, nephrotic syndrome, cirrhosis, antiphospholipid antibody syndrome, lupus anticoagulant syndrome, factor XII deficiency, disseminated intravascular coagulation (DIC), that the patient has been administered heparin, or hypofibrinogenemia.

1.4 Total Serum Protein

The Total Serum Protein test assesses the levels of albumin, globulin, and total protein in a sample of blood. The result compares the ratio of albumin to globulin. Protein is not stored. It is continuously metabolized into amino acids, which are used to make enzymes, hormones, and new proteins.

Albumin is a protein produced by the liver that keeps blood from leaking out of the blood vessels. Albumin is also important for tissue growth and healing because it carries medicine to tissues. The level of albumin is also an indicator of the patient's nutritional status. *Globulin* is a group of proteins made by the liver and the immune system that binds with hemoglobin and transports iron and metals in the blood to help fight infection. Globulin is composed of three different proteins: (1) alpha, (2) beta, and (3) gamma. A test for total serum protein reports separate values for total protein, albumin, and globulin. The amounts of albumin and globulin are also compared (albumin/globulin ratio).

Why the Test Is Performed

The test is performed to screen for liver and kidney functions (albumin), malnutrition (albumin), cause of edema, ascites, pulmonary edema (albumin), risk of infection (globulin), multiple myeloma (globulin), and macroglobulinemia (globulin).

Before Administering the Test

Assess if the patient:

- Is taking adrogens (male sex hormones), estrogen, corticosteroids, insulin, and/or growth hormone, which can affect the test results
- Has a chronic illness that interferes with nutrition
- Has any recent injuries or infections
- Is pregnant
- Has been on extended bed rest

How the Test Is Performed

A sample of blood is taken from the patient's vein. The patient will experience a tight feeling when the tourniquet is tightened, a pinch or nothing at all when the needle is inserted into the vein, and pressure when a gauze pad is pressed against the insertion site to stop bleeding. It can take up to 10 minutes for bleeding to stop if the patient is taking anticoagulants (aspirin, coumadin). A small bruise might appear at the insertion site, which could become swollen following this test. This is called phlebitis. Applying a warm compress several times a day will reduce the swelling.

Teach the Patient

Prior to testing, explain to the patient why the blood sample is taken, the function of albumin and globulin, and the meaning of abnormal values.

Understanding the Test Results

Test results are available in 12 hours. The laboratory determines normal values based on calibration of testing equipment with a control test. Test results are reported as high, normal, or low based on the laboratory's control test. The healthcare provider is likely to order a serum protein electrophoresis if there is abnormal globulin levels. Liver damage reduces the protein level in blood, but this level may not be reduced for 2 weeks after the damage because protein stays in the blood for up to 18 days.

Generally the normal range is:

- Total protein: 5.5 to 9.0 g/dL
- Albumin: 3.5 to 5.5 g/dL
- Globulin: 2.0 to 3.5 g/dL
- Albumin/globulin ration: greater than 1.0
- A ratio less than 1 indicates abnormal function in the body.

High albumin levels may indicate severe dehydration.

High globulin levels may indicate liver disease, kidney disease, Hodgkin's lymphoma, leukemia, hemolytic anemia, macroglobulinemia, rheumatoid arthritis, lupus, sarcoidosis, autoimmune hepatitis, or tuberculosis.

Low albumin levels may indicate malnutrition, kidney disease, liver disease, uncontrolled diabetes, Hodgkin's lymphoma, severe burns, systemic lupus erythematosus (SLE), rheumatoid arthritis, heart failure, hyperthyroidism, Crohn's disease, or sprue disease.

1.5   Blood Alcohol

Large amounts of alcohol depress the central nervous system when it enters the blood. Alcohol is absorbed within a few minutes and peaks within an hour. Food decreases absorption of alcohol. Alcohol is mostly metabolized by the liver and excreted in urine and exhalation. The blood alcohol test measures the level of alcohol in the blood.

The patient's signed consent may be required before the test is administered because the result of the blood alcohol test can have legal repercussions for the patient. Consult the healthcare facility's policies regarding administering the blood alcohol test. A taximeter that measures alcohol levels in the patient's breath is another test to determine the level of alcohol consumed by the patient.

Why the Test Is Performed

The test is performed to screen for intoxication, the reason for altered mental status, and ingested alcohol.

Before Administering the Test

Assess if the patient (or check):

- Has taken sedatives, kava, ginseng, or antihistamines, since this can enhance the sedative effect of alcohol
- Has diabetic ketoacidosis
- Ingested methanol or isopropyl alcohol
- Vital signs, since alcohol ingestion can depress respiration and the central nervous system

Assess if the insertion site was cleaned using rubbing alcohol, since this can affect the test results. Take safety precautions since the patient may have an impaired reaction time and decreased vision.

The speed in which alcohol is metabolized is influenced by:

- *The proof of alcohol of each drink.* The higher the proof of alcohol, the higher the blood alcohol level.
- *The patient's weight.* Blood alcohol level decreases as weight increases, since additional weight represents increased water that dilutes the alcohol.
- *The number of drinks the patient ingested each hour.* It takes approximately an hour to metabolize a drink. The greater the number of drinks ingested per hour, the higher the blood alcohol level.
- *The patient's age.* The older patient will have a higher blood alcohol level than a young patient who consumed the same quantity of alcohol, because the older patient's metabolism is slow.
- *The amount of food ingested by the patient.* The higher the ingestion of food, the lower the blood alcohol level, since the food absorbs some alcohol.
- *Gender.* Women have a higher blood alcohol level than men because they have less water in their bodies than men.
- *Type of drink consumed.* The use of mixers such as club soda increases the absorption of alcohol, resulting in a higher blood alcohol level.

Quick Assessment:

- 0.03 to 0.059 blood alcohol level:
  - Talkativeness
  - Decreased inhibition
  - Decreased alertness, coordination, and concentration
- 0.06 to 0.1 blood alcohol level:
  - Decreased reflexes, peripheral vision, depth perception, reasoning
  - Blunted feelings
  - Impaired sexual pleasure

- 0.11 to 0.2 blood alcohol level:
  - Staggering
  - Slurred speech
  - Decreased reaction time
  - Emotional swings
  - Overexpression
- 0.21 to 0.29 blood alcohol level:
  - Blackout of memory
  - Stupor
  - Loss of consciousness
  - Impaired sensations
- 0.3 to 0.39 blood alcohol level:
  - Decreased breathing
  - Decreased heart rate
  - Severe depression
  - Unconsciousness
  - Risk of death
- Greater than .4 blood alcohol level:
  - Death

How the Test Is Performed

A sample of blood is taken from the patient's vein. The patient will experience a tight feeling when the tourniquet is tightened, a pinch or nothing at all when the needle is inserted into the vein, and pressure when a gauze pad is pressed against the insertion site to stop bleeding. It can take up to 10 minutes for bleeding to stop if the patient is taking anticoagulants (aspirin, coumadin). A small bruise might appear at the insertion site, which could become swollen following this test. This is called phlebitis. Applying a warm compress several times a day will reduce the swelling.

Teach the Patient

Explain to the patient why the blood sample is taken, that the patient's consent is needed to administer the test unless ordered by legal authorities (check your healthcare facility's policy), and the test result.

Understanding the Test Results

The result of the blood alcohol test represents the level of alcohol at the time the test was administered and cannot predict the amount of alcohol consumed by the patient, because alcohol continues to be metabolized by the liver. Test results are available quickly. The laboratory determines normal values based on calibration of testing equipment with a control test. Test results are reported as high, normal, or low based on the laboratory's control test.

- Normal range is: 0.0
- Abnormal level is: greater than 0.0
- Intoxicated (according to the National Highway Traffic Safety Administration): 0.08 or 80 mg/dL or 17 mmol/L

1.6   Lead

Lead affects growth and development if lead-tainted water, paint chips, food, or dust is ingested or if lead is in contact with the skin. Pregnant women can pass lead to the fetus or to the newborn through breast milk. Children who are in early development are at risk for permanent growth impairment if they ingest lead. The lead blood test measures the level of lead in the blood sample. The healthcare provider may order the urine aminolevulinic acid (ALA) test to determine the extent of load poisoning (not for children). The lead mobilization urine test is performed during chelation therapy to assess if the therapy is removing lead in urine.

Why the Test Is Performed

The test is performed to screen for lead poisoning and the treatment for lead poisoning.

Before Administering the Test

Assess if the patient is taking herbal medicine.

Quick assessment using the United States Centers for Disease Control and Prevention (CDC) classes:

- Learning problems: Class 1 or Class 2
- Slow growth: Class 2
- Hearing problems: Class 2
- Headache: Class 3
- Neurological problems: Class 3
- Weight loss: Class 3
- Anemia: Class 4
- Seizures: Class 4
- Brain damage: Class 5

How the Test Is Performed

A blood sample is taken from either a heel stick or from a finger stick.

Heel Stick: Several drops of blood are collected from the heel of a newborn or baby. The heel is cleaned using alcohol. A sterile lancet is used to puncture the heel. Several drops of blood are collected in a small test tube. A gauze pad is pressed over the site until bleeding stops. A small bandage is applied.

Finger Stick: Several drops of blood are collected from the finger. The finger is cleaned using alcohol. A sterile lancet is used to puncture the finger. Several drops of blood are collected in small test tube. A gauze pad is pressed over the site until bleeding stops. A small bandage is applied.

Teach the Patient

Prior to testing, explain to the patient why the blood sample is taken, that multiple samples may be taken, and why the healthcare provider must report certain results to the local health department.

Heel/Finger Stick: The patient may feel a pinch or nothing at all when the lancer punches the skin. A bandage will be on the puncher site for a short time period. A small bruise might appear at the site. If test results are positive, then a blood sample will have to be taken from a vein to verify the test results.

Understanding the Test Results

Test results are available in 1 week. The laboratory determines normal values based on calibration of testing equipment with a control test. Test results are reported as high, normal, or low based on the laboratory's control test.

- Normal range is: 0 mcg/dL
- Abnormal Class 1: 1 to 9 mcg/dL
- Abnormal Class 2A: 10 to 14 mcg/dL
- Abnormal Class 2B: 15 to 19 mcg/dL
- Abnormal Class 3: 20 to 44 mcg/dL
- Abnormal Class 4: 45 to 69 mcg/dL
- Abnormal Class 5: greater than 69 mcg/dL

Test results of 10 mcg/dL or above from a finger or heel stick requires blood to be drawn from a vein to confirm the results, since the blood sample might be contaminated from lead at the site of the stick.

Consult your healthcare institution's policy to determine if a positive test result must be reported to the local health department. Lead levels above 10 mcg/dL on two occasions typically must be reported so the source of the lead can be found. Tests are repeated within a few days or month following the initial test. Businesses whose employees work with lead and are required to test lead levels in their employees can provide the employee with documentation if the lead level in their blood is 40 mcg/dL or greater as required by the United States Occupational Safety and Health Administration (OSHA) regulation. Employees with a level higher than 60 mcg/dL should be seen by their healthcare providers.

1.7 Serum Osmolality

Serum osmolality is the number of particles of substances that are dissolved in the serum (liquid). These substances include glucose, chloride, sodium, proteins, and bicarbonate. Serum osmolality should be balanced between fluid and particles of substances.

Serum osmolality is controlled by adjusting the fluid output of the kidneys using the antidiuretic hormone (ADH) produced by the pituitary gland. ADH is a vasopressin that reduces fluid output from the kidneys when ADH is released into the blood stream, thereby increasing fluid in the blood. A decrease in ADH production increases fluid output by the kidneys and decreases fluid in the blood.

A decrease in fluid results in an increase in serum osmolality—less fluid in the blood. This signals the pituitary gland to release ADH, which stimulates the kidneys to retain fluid, thereby increasing fluid in the blood and decreasing serum osmolality—fluid level in the blood is restored.

An increase in fluid results in a decrease in serum osmolality—more fluid in the blood. This signals the pituitary gland to stop releasing ADH, which causes the kidneys to increase the output of fluid, and thereby decreasing fluid in the blood and increasing serum osmolality—fluid level in the blood is restored.

The serum osmolality test measures the amount of substances dissolved in blood. The healthcare provider may test urine osmolality. The result of the urine test is compared with the serum osmolality to estimate kidney function.

Why the Test Is Performed

The test is performed to screen for dehydration, overhydration, the quantity of poison ingested by the patient, the underlying cause of a seizure, the underlying cause of a coma, the function of the hypothalamus (the hypothalamus signals the pituitary gland to release ADH), and the presence of inappropriate antidiuretic hormone secretion (SIADH).

Before Administering the Test

Assess if the patient has ingested alcohol, since this can affect the test results, or has recently received a blood transfusion.

How the Test Is Performed

A sample of blood is taken from the patient's vein. The patient will experience a tight feeling when the tourniquet is tightened, a pinch or nothing at all when the needle is inserted into the vein, and pressure when a gauze pad is pressed against the insertion site to stop bleeding. It can take up to 10 minutes for bleeding to stop if the patient is taking anticoagulants (aspirin, coumadin). A small bruise might appear at the insertion site, which could become swollen following this test. This is called phlebitis. Applying a warm compress several times a day will reduce the swelling.

Teach the Patient

Prior to testing, explain to the patient why the blood sample is taken and not to ingest alcohol 12 hours before the test is administered.

Understanding the Test Results

Test results are available in 4 hours.

- Normal range is: 280 to 300 mOSm/kg of water.
- High values may indicate buildup of urea in the blood, poisoning, a high level of salt in the blood, diabetes insipidus, a high level of glucose in the blood, or dehydration.
- Low values may indicate lung cancer, overproduction of ADH, overhydration, or a low salt level in the blood.

1.8   Uric Acid in Blood

Uric acid is produced when purine, which is contained in some foods, is metabolized. Uric acid enters the blood and is then excreted by the kidneys in urine and a small amount in stool. The uric acid test measures the level of uric acid in blood. The healthcare provider may order a 24-hour uric acid urine test.

Uric crystals can form in joints, leading to gout even when uric acid levels are normal. A high level of uric acid does not mean that the patient has gout. Gout is diagnosed by testing fluid from the affected joint for uric acid crystals.

Why the Test Is Performed

The test is performed to screen for uric acid kidney stones, gout, adverse reaction of radiation therapy and chemotherapy, and to assess treatment for hyperuricemia.

Before Administering the Test

Assess if the patient:

- Shows signs of starvation
- Has performed strenuous exercise
- Has eaten a high protein diet, since these can raise the level of uric acid
- Has consumed liver, red meats, game meat, herring, sardines, scallops, or beer
- Is taking aspirin, theophylline, diuretics, niacin, caffeine, vitamin C, ascorbic acid, epinephrine, levodopa, warfarin, diazoxide, cisplatin, cyclosporine nicotinic acid, phenothiazines, tacrolimus, methyldopa, or ethambutol, which can affect the test results
- Is pregnant, since uric acid level can increase during pregnancy and assist the healthcare provider diagnose preeclampsia

Uric acid levels are higher in the morning and lower in the evening. Therefore, note the time that the test is administered.

How the Test Is Performed

A sample of blood is taken from the patient's vein. The patient will experience a tight feeling when the tourniquet is tightened, a pinch or nothing at all when the needle is inserted into the vein, and pressure when a gauze pad is pressed against the insertion site to stop bleeding. It can take up to 10 minutes for bleeding to stop if the patient is taking anticoagulants (aspirin, coumadin). A small bruise might appear at the insertion site, which could become swollen following this test. This is called phlebitis. Applying a warm compress several times a day will reduce the swelling.

Teach the Patient

Prior to testing, explain to the patient why the blood sample is taken; that the patient should avoid consuming liver, red meats, game meat, herring, sardines, scallops, and beer for 24 hours before the test is administered; and that the healthcare provider may ask the patient to stop taking aspirin, theophylline, diuretics, niacin, caffeine, vitamin C, ascorbic acid, epinephrine, levodopa, warfarin, diazoxide, cisplatin, cyclosporine nicotinic acid, phenothiazines, tacrolimus, methyldopa, or ethambutol for 2 weeks.

Understanding the Test Results

Test results are available in 2 days. The laboratory determines normal values based on calibration of testing equipment with a control test. Test results are reported as high, normal, or low based on the laboratory's control test.

Normal uric acid range is:

- Men: 3.4 to 7.0 mg/dL
- Women: 2.4 to 6.0 mg/dL
- Children: 2.5 to 5.5 mg/dL

High uric acid values may indicate kidney disease, multiple myeloma, lymphoma, hemolytic anemia, heart failure, leukemia, sickle cell anemia, preeclampsia, cirrhosis, alcohol abuse, hypoparathyroidism, hypothyroidism, starvation, lead poisoning, malnutrition, psoriasis, Lesch-Nyhan syndrome, obesity, or a high purine diet.

Low uric acid values may indicate a low protein diet, SIADH, Wilson's disease, cancer, liver disease, or that the patient is taking aloprim, zyloprim, benemid, probalan, sulfinpyrazone, or 1500 mg or more aspirin each day.

1.9   C-Reactive Protein (CRP)

C-reactive protein is produced as part of the inflammatory process and attaches to the invading microorganism or damaged cells, enhancing phagocytosis in the destruction of the microorganism or damaged cell. A high level of C-reactive protein indicates that there is inflammation. Other tests are then performed to identify the source of the inflammation. The high-sensitivity CRP test (hs-CRP) may also be ordered to determine if inflammation has damaged the inner lining of arteries, increasing the risk of a heart attack. Also, the total cholesterol test and HDL cholesterol test might be ordered with the C-reactive protein test to help determine if the patient is at risk for cardiac problems.

Why the Test Is Performed

The test is performed to screen for inflammation.

It assesses the treatment for inflammation, the treatment for diseases that cause inflammation, and the response to cancer treatment.

Before Administering the Test

Assess if the patient:

- Exercised immediately prior to administering the test
- Has taken NSAIDs, birth control pills, aspirin, hormone replacement therapy, pravastatin, or corticosteroids
- Has an intrauterine device (IUD)
- Is pregnant
- Is obese

How the Test Is Performed

A sample of blood is taken from the patient's vein. The patient will experience a tight feeling when the tourniquet is tightened, a pinch or nothing at all when the needle is inserted into the vein, and pressure when a gauze pad is pressed against the insertion site to stop bleeding. It can take up to 10 minutes for bleeding to stop if the patient is taking anticoagulants (aspirin, coumadin). A small bruise might appear at the insertion site, which could become swollen following this test. This is called phlebitis. Applying a warm compress several times a day will reduce the swelling.

Teach the Patient

Prior to testing, explain to the patient why the blood sample is taken, that the patient should not exercise before the test, and that the healthcare provider may ask the patient to stop taking NSAIDs, birth control pills, aspirin, hormone replacement therapy, pravastatin, or corticosteroids for 2 weeks.

Understanding the Test Results

Test results are available in 1 day. The laboratory determines normal values based on calibration of testing equipment with a control test. Test results are reported as high, normal, or low based on the laboratory's control test.

- Normal C-reactive protein range is: 0 to 1 mg/mL.
- High C-peptide values may indicate inflammation, infection, or risk for a heart attack.

The C-reactive protein level peaks 6 hours following surgery and decreases by the third day. Infection as a result of the surgery is suspected if the C-reactive protein level remains high after the third day. Elevated C-reactive protein level prior to surgery increases the risk of infection following surgery. The C-peptide level quickly rises then returns to normal if treatment for infection or cancer is successful.

1.10 Complete Blood Count (CBC)

The complete blood count (CBC) test with a differential, part of a routine blood screening, measures blood components to assess the patient for various disorders. The healthcare provider may also order the erythrocyte sedimentation rate (ESR) test to detect inflammation, and the reticulocyte count to identify the number of immature leukocytes.

Here are the blood components that are measured:

- **Leukocyte Count (WBC)**: Leukocytes increase when infection is present and can also increase in the absence of infection if the patient has leukemia.
- **Leukocyte Cell Type (WBC differential)**: There are five major types of leukocyte cells, each having a role in the immune process. These are (1) neutrophils, (2) lymphocytes, (3) monocytes, (4) eosinophils, and (5) basophils. The quantity of each leukocyte cell type provides important information in diagnosing the patient's condition.
- **Erythrocyte Count (RBC)**: Erythrocyte cells carry oxygen and carbon dioxide.
- **Erythrocyte Indices**:
  - *Mean corpuscular volume (MCV)*: This is the size of erythrocytes.
  - *Mean corpuscular hemoglobin (MCH)*: This is the amount of hemoglobin in an erythrocyte cell.
  - *Mean corpuscular hemoglobin concentration (MCHC)*: This is concentration of hemoglobin in an erythrocyte cell.
  - *Red cell distribution width (RDW)*: This shows the different sizes of erythrocyte cells.
- **Hematocrit (HCT, packed cell volume)**: The hematocrit test measures the volume in percentage taken up by erythrocytes in the patient's blood.
- **Hemoglobin (Hgb)**: The hemoglobin measures the amount of hemoglobin in blood. Hemoglobin is the part of erythrocyte that carries oxygen.
- **Thrombocyte Count (Platelet)**: Platelets form blood clots.
- **Reticulocyte count**: Identifies the number of immature leukocytes and is used to determine the cause of anemia.
- **Erythrocyte sedimentation rate (ESR)**: A high proportion of fibrinogen in blood causes red blood cells to attach to each other during the inflammatory process, forming stacks of red blood cells. These stacks of red blood cells settle faster than unattached red blood cells. This rate is used to detect inflammation.

Why the Test Is Performed

The test is performed to screen for anemia, infection, leukemia, risk for bleeding, asthma, allergies, the cause of bruising, the cause of fatigue polycythemia, and blood loss.

Before Administering the Test

Assess if the patient:

- Is taking antibiotics, steroids, Equanil, thiazide diuretics, Miltown, quinidine, meprospan or chemotherapy
- Has a high level of triglycerides, since this can affect the hemoglobin test
- Has an enlarged spleen, since this can reduce the platelet count
- Is pregnant
- Smokes
- Is stressed
- Has exercised before the test is administered

Be sure to document:

- How long the tourniquet was tightened when acquiring the blood sample
- If the blood sample clumps in the test tube, indicating that the sample is contaminated

How the Test Is Performed

A blood sample is taken from either a heel stick or from a vein.

Heel Stick: The heel is cleaned using alcohol. A sterile lancet is used to puncture the heel. Several drops of blood are collected in a small test tube. A gauze pad is pressed over the site until bleeding stops. A small bandage is applied.

Vein: The patient will experience a tight feeling when the tourniquet is tightened, a pinch or nothing at all when the needle is inserted into the vein, and pressure when a gauze pad is pressed against the insertion site to stop bleeding. It can take up to 10 minutes for bleeding to stop if the patient is taking anticoagulants (aspirin, coumadin). A small bruise might appear at the insertion site, which could become swollen following this test. This is called phlebitis. Applying a warm compress several times a day will reduce the swelling.

Teach the Patient

Prior to testing, explain to the patient why the blood sample is taken, that the patient should not exercise before the test is administered, that the patient should tell the healthcare provider if he or she smokes, and that the healthcare provider may request that the patient stop taking antibiotics, steroids, Equanil, thiazide diuretics, Miltown, quinidine, or meprospan for 2 weeks prior to the test.

Understanding the Test Results

Test results are available quickly. The laboratory determines normal values based on calibration of testing equipment with a control test. Test results are reported as high, normal, or low based on the laboratory's control test. Hematocrit and hemoglobin results indicate the same disorders as high and low erythrocyte (RBC) count. The mean corpuscular hemoglobin result indicates the same disorders as high and low mean corpuscular volume.

Normal leukocyte (WBC) count range is:

- Men: 5000 to 10,000 mcL^3
- Non-pregnant women: 4500 to 11,000 mcL^3
- Pregnant women:
  ○ First trimester: 6600 to 14,100 mcL^3
  ○ Second trimester: 6900 to 17,100 mcL^3
  ○ Third trimester: 5900 to 14,700 mcL^3
  ○ Postpartum: 9700 to 25,700 mcL^3

Normal leukocyte cell type (differential) range is:

- Neutrophils: 55% to 70%
- Band neutrophils: 0% to 3%
- Lymphocytes: 20% to 40%
- Monocytes: 2% to 8%
- Eosinophils: 1% to 4%
- Basophils: 0.5% to 1%

Normal erythrocyte (RBC) count range is:

- Men: 4.7 to 6.1 million mcL
- Women: 4.2 to 5.4 million mcL
- Children: 4.0 to 5.5 million mcL
- Newborns: 4.8 to 7.1 million mcL

Normal hematocrit range is:

- Men: 42% to 52%
- Women: 37% to 47%
- Pregnant women:
  - First trimester: 35% to 46%
  - Second trimester: 30% to 42%
  - Third trimester: 34% to 44%
  - Postpartum: 30% to 44%
- Children: 32% to 44%
- Newborns: 44% to 64%

Normal hemoglobin range is:

- Men: 14 to 18 g/dL
- Women: 12 to 16 g/dL
- Pregnant women:
  - First trimester: 11.4 to 15 g/dL
  - Second trimester: 10 to 14.3 g/dl
  - Third trimester: 10.2 to 14.4 g/dL
  - Postpartum: 10.4 to 18 g/dL
- Children: 9.5 to 15.5 g/dL
- Newborns: 14 to 24 g/dL

Normal erythrocyte indices range is:

- Mean corpuscular volume: 80 to 95 fL
- Mean corpuscular hemoglobin: 27 to 31 pg
- Mean corpuscular hemoglobin concentration: 32 to 36 g/dL

Normal red cell distribution width range is: 11% to 14.5%.
Normal thrombocyte count range is:

- Adults and children: 150,000 to 400,000 mm³
- Babies: 200,000 to 475,000 mm³
- Newborns: 150,000 to 300,000 mm³

High leukocyte (WBC) count might indicate inflammation, infection, leukemia, tissue damage, stress, malnutrition, burns, lupus, kidney failure, rheumatoid arthritis, tuberculosis, or thyroid gland problems.

High erythrocyte (RBC) count might indicate lung disease, alcoholism, polycythemia vera, smoking, kidney disease, dehydration, burns, sweating, vomiting, diarrhea, spurious polycythemia, carbon monoxide exposure, or that the patient is using diuretics.

High thrombocyte count might indicate that the patient is bleeding, has cancer, bone marrow disorder, or iron deficiency.

High mean corpuscular volume might indicate folate deficiency or vitamin B_{12} deficiency.

Low leukocyte (WBC) count might indicate alcoholism, lupus, Cushing's syndrome, AIDS, aplastic anemia, enlarged spleen, viral infection, or malaria.

The patient is undergoing chemotherapy.

Low erythrocyte count might indicate anemia, Addison's disease, sickle cell disease, inflammatory bowel disease, cancer, peptic ulcer, lead poisoning, removal of the spleen, pernicious anemia, or heavy menstrual bleeding.

Low thrombocyte count might indicate risk for bleeding, idiopathic thrombocytopenic purpura, pregnancy, or enlarged spleen.

Low mean corpuscular volume might indicate iron deficiency or thalassemia deficiency.

1.11　Chemistry Screen

A chemistry screen test examines blood components and is used to assess the patient's overall health. There are various types of chemistry screens including chem–20, chem–12, and chem–7. The number represents the number of blood components examined in the test.

A chemistry screen test is also called sequential multichannel analysis (CMA) or sequential multichannel analysis with computer (CMAC), followed by the number of components being examined.

The following tests are included in a chemistry screen: albumin, alkaline phosphatase, alanine aminotransferase (ALT), aspartate aminotransferase (AST), bilirubin, blood glucose, blood urea nitrogen, calcium (Ca) in blood, carbon dioxide, chloride (CL), cholesterol and triglycerides tests, creatinine and creatinine clearance, lactic acid, phosphate in blood, potassium (K) in blood, sodium (NA) in blood, total serum protein, and uric acid in blood. Refer to each test for details.

1.12　Vitamin B$_{12}$

Vitamin B$_{12}$ is required for cell growth and metabolism and is stored in the liver. The vitamin B$_{12}$ test measures the level of vitamin B$_{12}$ in a blood sample. It is not unusual for the healthcare provider to order the folic acid test along with the vitamin B$_{12}$ test and the Schilling test to assess the patient's ability to absorb vitamin B$_{12}$ if pernicious anemia is suspected.

Why the Test Is Performed

The test is performed to screen for the underlying cause of anemia, peripheral neuropathy, dementia, and vitamin B$_{12}$ deficiency.

Before Administering the Test

Assess if the patient:

- Has eaten or drunk 12 hours before the test is administered
- Has taken vitamin C
- Is pregnant
- Is breastfeeding
- Has pernicious anemia
- Has undergone dye testing less than a week prior to the test
- Has taken birth control pills, Prilosec, neopmycin, Dilantin, Protonix, Glucophage, Prevacid, colchicines, para-aminosalicylic acid, rabeprazole, triamterene, or methotrexate

How the Test Is Performed

A sample of blood is taken from the patient's vein. The patient will experience a tight feeling when the tourniquet is tightened, a pinch or nothing at all when the needle is inserted into the vein, and pressure when a gauze pad is pressed against the insertion site to stop bleeding. It can take up to 10 minutes for bleeding to stop if the patient is taking anticoagulants (aspirin, coumadin). A small bruise might appear at the insertion site, which could become swollen following this test. This is called phlebitis. Applying a warm compress several times a day will reduce the swelling.

Teach the Patient

Prior to testing, explain to the patient why the blood sample is taken, not to eat or drink 12 hours before the test, and that the healthcare provider may request that the patient stop taking birth control pills, Prilosec, neopmycin, Dilantin, Protonix, glucophage, Prevacid, colchicines, para-aminosalicylic acid, rabeprazole, triamterene, vitamin C, or methotrexate for 2 weeks prior to the test.

Understanding the Test Results

Test results are available quickly. The laboratory determines normal values based on calibration of testing equipment with a control test. Test results are reported as high, normal, or low based on the laboratory's control test.

- Normal vitamin B_{12} range is: 160 to 950 pg/mL
- High values of vitamin B_{12} may indicate hepatitis, cirrhosis, or leukemia.
- Low values of vitamin B_{12} may indicate folic acid deficiency anemia, pernicious anemia, hyperthyroidism, fish tapeworm infection, or multiple myeloma.

1.13   Cold Agglutinins

Agglutinins are antibodies that cause red blood cells to form a clump called *rouleaux formation* at low temperatures. This is an immune reaction to an infection. High levels of agglutinins can impede blood flow to the extremities when exposed to cold, resulting in tissue damage. It can cause hemolytic anemia. The cold agglutinins test measures the level of agglutinins in a blood sample.

Why the Test Is Performed

The test is performed to screen for hemolytic anemia and the underlying cause for pneumonia.

Before Administering the Test

Assess if the patient has:

- Taken penicillin or cephalosporins
- Measles, malaria, congenital syphilis, pneumonia, chickenpox, anemia, infectious mononucleosis, cirrhosis, or multiple myeloma, since these can produce a false positive test result

How the Test Is Performed

A sample of blood is taken from the patient's vein. The patient will experience a tight feeling when the tourniquet is tightened, a pinch or nothing at all when the needle is inserted into the vein, and pressure when a gauze pad is pressed against the insertion site to stop bleeding. It can take up to 10 minutes for bleeding to stop if the patient is taking anticoagulants (aspirin, coumadin). A small bruise might appear at the insertion site, which could become swollen following this test. This is called phlebitis. Applying a warm compress several times a day will reduce the swelling.

Teach the Patient

Prior to testing, explain to the patient why the blood sample is taken and that the healthcare provider may request the patient stop taking penicillin or cephalosporins for 2 weeks prior to the test.

Understanding the Test Results

Test results are available quickly. The laboratory determines normal values based on calibration of testing equipment with a control test. Test results are reported as high, normal, or low based on the laboratory's control test.

Results are reported as a *titer*. A titer specifies how much of the sample of blood is diluted with saline before antibodies are no longer detected. The titer is reported as a ratio of parts of the blood sample and saline. The higher the second number of the ratio, the greater the number of antibodies in the blood sample.

Normal cold agglutinins titer range is below 1 to 40 (1:40). A high cold agglutinins titer may indicate pneumonia, hepatitis C, cirrhosis, infectious mononucleosis, rheumatoid arthritis, malaria, hemolytic anemia, multiple myeloma, lymphoma, cytomegalovirus, scleroderma, or risk for thromboses.

1.14 Toxicology Tests (Tox Screen)

A *toxin* is a substance that disrupts the body's function and includes prescription medication, nonprescription medication, and illegal medication. Toxicology tests measure the levels of one or a series of toxins in a blood sample. The healthcare provider may order a urine toxicology test (because traces of toxins can remain in urine longer than in blood) and a saliva toxicology test.

Why the Test Is Performed

The test is performed to screen for the underlying cause of the patient's unusual behavior, the underlying cause why the patient is unconscious, and use of medication (toxin).

Before Administering the Test

Assess if the patient has:

- Taken cough medicine in the previous 4 days
- Eaten poppy seeds in the previous 4 days
- Signed a consent form before administering the test, unless the patient is incapacitated to provide written consent
- Listed medications, vitamins, and herbal supplements that have been taken in the previous 4 days

The chain of custody must be adhered to if the patient is suspected of drug abuse. Each person who handles the blood sample must sign the chain of custody document. The chain of custody document must be attached to the test result.

Note on the specimen the time that the blood sample was taken.

How the Test Is Performed

A sample of blood is taken from the patient's vein. The patient will experience a tight feeling when the tourniquet is tightened, a pinch or nothing at all when the needle is inserted into the vein, and pressure when a gauze pad is pressed against the insertion site to stop bleeding. It can take up to 10 minutes for bleeding to stop if the patient is taking anticoagulants (aspirin, coumadin). A small bruise might appear at the insertion site, which could become swollen following this test. This is called phlebitis. Applying a warm compress several times a day will reduce the swelling.

Teach the Patient

Prior to testing, explain to the patient why the blood sample is taken, that the patient must provide written consent—otherwise the toxicology test cannot be administered unless the patient is incapacitated to provide written consent—and that the patient should identify any medication, vitamins, herbal supplement, cough medicine, and poppy seeds that have been ingested in the previous 4 days.

Understanding the Test Results

Test results are available quickly. A positive test result must be confirmed by two or more testing methods to rule out a false positive result. The healthcare provider may order a quantitative toxicology test to determine the level of toxin in the blood sample if the toxicology test is positive.

- Normal toxin range: 0 except for therapeutic levels of medication taken by the patient.
- Abnormal toxin range: Greater than 0 or higher than the therapeutic levels of medication taken by the patient.

1.15 Folic Acid

Folic acid, a type of vitamin B, is necessary for cell development and maintenance. Women who plan to become pregnant should increase the intake of folic acid to reduce the risk of spina bifida and cleft lip and palate. The folic acid test measures the level of folic acid in blood. The healthcare provider may order a vitamin B_{12} blood test along with the folic acid blood test.

Why the Test Is Performed

The test is performed to screen for malnutrition, anemia, malabsorption, sufficient level of folic acid to reduce the risk of birth defects, and treatment for folic acid deficiency.

Before Administering the Test

Assess if the patient has:

- Eaten or drunk anything other than water for 8 hours before the test
- Vitamin B_{12} anemia
- Iron deficiency anemia
- Taken Dyrenium, Proloprim, Dilantin, pentamidine, phenobartial mysoline, or methotrexate, since these may affect the test result

How the Test Is Performed

The patient must refrain from eating and drinking anything other than water for 8 hours before the test. A sample of blood is taken from the patient's vein. The patient will experience a tight feeling when the tourniquet is tightened, a pinch or nothing at all when the needle is inserted into the vein, and pressure when a gauze pad is pressed against the insertion site to stop bleeding. It can take up to 10 minutes for bleeding to stop if the patient is taking anticoagulants (aspirin, coumadin). A small bruise might appear at the insertion site, which could become swollen following this test. This is called phlebitis. Applying a warm compress several times a day will reduce the swelling.

Teach the Patient

Prior to testing, explain to the patient why the blood sample is taken, that the patient must not eat or drink anything except water for 8 hours before the test, and that the healthcare provider may ask the patient to stop taking Dyrenium, Proloprim, Dilantin, pentamidine, phenobartial mysoline, or methotrexate for 2 weeks prior to the test.

Understanding the Test Results

Folic acid test results are available quickly. The laboratory determines normal values based on calibration of testing equipment with a control test. Test results are reported as high, normal, or low based on the laboratory's control test.

Normal Folate range is:

- In plasma:
  - Adult: 2 to 20 ng/mL
  - Children: 5 to 21 ng/mL
- In red blood cells:
  - Adult: 140 to 628 ng/mL
  - Children: greater than 160 ng/mL

High folic acid may indicate increased dietary folic acid, supplements, or vitamin B_{12} deficiency.

Low folic acid may indicate alcohol abuse, anorexia nervosa, Crohn's disease, cirrhosis, celiac disease, sprue, hemolytic anemia, kidney disease, or cancer.

1.16   Gastrin

Gastrin is a hormone produced by the G cells of the stomach lining when food enters the stomach. Gastrin stimulates the parietal cells in the stomach to secrete hydrochloric acid (HCl) that is used in digestion and stimulates the product of *pepsin*, which is a digestive enzyme. The gastrin test measures the level of gastrin in the blood. The healthcare provider may order an intravenous secretin test, where *secretin*, a digestive hormone, is injected into a vein and blood samples are taken immediately, then every 5 minutes for 15 minutes, and then at 30 minutes.

Why the Test Is Performed

The test is performed to screen for Zollinger-Ellison syndrome, pernicious anemia, pancreatic tumor, and G-cell hyperplasia.

Before Administering the Test

Assess if the patient has:

- Refrained from:
  - Drinking alcohol 1 day before the test is administered
  - Eating and drinking anything except water 12 hours before the test
  - Smoking for 4 hours before the test
  - Drinking water 1 hour before the test
- Rested 30 minutes before the test is administered
- Taken a calcium supplement or medication containing calcium, tricyclic antidepressants, Urised, Lomotil, or Motofed Rolaids, Prilosec, Pepcid, Zantac, or Tums 12 hours before the test
- Hypoglycemia
- Cirrhosis, kidney failure, or rheumatoid arthritis
- Undergone small bowel resection or peptic ulcer surgery

How the Test Is Performed

- Refrain from drinking alcohol 1 day before the test is administered and from eating and drinking anything except water 12 hours before the test
- No smoking 4 hours before the test
- Refrain from drinking water 1 hour before the test
- Refrain from taking a calcium supplement or medication containing calcium, tricyclic antidepressants, Urised, Lomotil, or Motofed Rolaids, Prilosec, Pepcid, Zantac, or Tums 12 hours before the test
- Rest 30 minutes before the test is administered

A sample of blood is taken from the patient's vein. The patient will experience a tight feeling when the tourniquet is tightened, a pinch or nothing at all when the needle is inserted into the vein, and pressure when a gauze pad is pressed against the insertion site to stop bleeding. It can take up to 10 minutes for bleeding to stop if the patient is taking anticoagulants (aspirin, coumadin). A small bruise might appear at the insertion site, which could become swollen following this test. This is called phlebitis. Applying a warm compress several times a day will reduce the swelling.

Teach the Patient

Prior to testing, explain to the patient why the blood sample is taken and that the healthcare provider may want the patient to stop taking tricyclic antidepressants, Urised, Lomotil, calcium supplements, or Motofed for 2 weeks before the test.

The patient must refrain from:

- Drinking alcohol 1 day before the test is administeredf
- Eating and drinking anything except water 12 hours before the test
- Smoking 4 hours before the test
- Drinking water 1 hour before the test
- Taking Rolaids, Prilosec, Pepcid, Zantac, or Tums 12 hours before the test

The patient should rest 30 minutes before the test is administered.

Understanding the Test Results

Gastrin test results are available in 2 days. The laboratory determines normal values based on calibration of testing equipment with a control test. Test results are reported as high, normal, or low based on the laboratory's control test.

Normal gastrin range is:

- Adult: less than 200 pg/mL
- Children: less than 125 pg/mL

A high gastrin level may indicate kidney failure, pernicious anemia, Zollinger-Ellison syndrome, hypercalcemia, peptic ulcers, G-cell hyperplasia, hyperparathyroidism, stomach cancer, sarcoidosis, or small bowel resection. A low gastrin level may indicate hypothyroidism.

1.17   Ferritin

Ferritin is a protein found in bone marrow, liver, skeletal muscles, and the spleen. It binds to iron. The ferritin test measures the level of ferritin in blood to determine the amount of iron in the body. Blood should contain a small amount of ferritin, since most ferritin is bound to iron.

Why the Test Is Performed

The test is performed to screen for hemochromatosis (excess iron), iron deficiency anemia, treatment of hemochromatosis and iron deficiency anemia, and inflammation.

Before Administering the Test

Assess if the patient has:

- A diet high in red meat
- Had a radioactive scan three days prior to the test
- Taken birth control pills or antithyroid medication
- Had a blood transfusion four months prior to the test
- Inflammation (since inflammation increases ferritin levels)
- Had recent changes in her menstrual cycle

Note the age of the patient, since ferritin levels increase with age.

How the Test Is Performed

A sample of blood is taken from the patient's vein. The patient will experience a tight feeling when the tourniquet is tightened, a pinch or nothing at all when the needle is inserted into the vein, and pressure when a gauze pad is pressed against the insertion site to stop bleeding. It can take up to 10 minutes for bleeding to stop if the patient is taking anticoagulants (aspirin, coumadin). A small bruise might appear at the insertion site, which could become swollen following this test. This is called phlebitis. Applying a warm compress several times a day will reduce the swelling.

Teach the Patient

Prior to testing, explain to the patient why the test is performed.

Understanding the Test Results

The ferritin test results are available quickly. The laboratory determines normal values based on calibration of testing equipment with a control test. Test results are reported as high, normal, or low based on the laboratory's control test.

Normal ferritin test results:

- Men: 12 to 300 ng/mL
- Women: 10 to 150 ng/mL
- Infants and children 6 months to 15 years: 7 to 142 ng/mL
- Infants 2 months to 5 months: 50 to 200 ng/mL

- Infants 1 month: 200 to 600 ng/mL
- Newborns: 25 to 200 ng/mL

A high ferritin level may indicate hemochromatosis, thalassemia, alcoholism, iron deficiency anemia, hepatitis, cirrhosis, Hodgkin's disease, arthritis, leukemia, lupus, or excess dietary iron.

A low ferritin level may indicate iron deficiency, excessive menstrual bleeding, bleeding, colon cancer, ulcers, colon polyps, pregnancy, or insufficient dietary iron.

1.18   Lactic Acid

Muscle cells convert glucose into lactic acid and use lactic acid for energy when oxygen levels are low during strain of heart failure, exercise, shock, and sepsis. Lactic acid is not used for energy when there is a normal oxygen level in the blood. Lactic acid is metabolized by the liver. Liver disorders can result in lactic acidosis due to a high level of lactic acid in the blood. The lactic acid test measures the level of lactic acid in blood. The healthcare provider may order an arterial blood gas test to measure lactic acid in blood.

Why the Test Is Performed

The test is performed to screen for L acidosis, the underlying cause of acidosis and tissue oxygenation.

Before Administering the Test

Assess if the patient:

- Exercised 12 hours prior to the test
- Ate or drank 10 hours before the test
- Clenched his or her fist when the blood sample is drawn since a clenched fist may increase the lactic acid level
- Has taken alcohol, Glucophage, isoniazid, epinephrine, or Tylenol 12 hours prior to the test
- Has an infection

Note the time the tourniquet was in place when the blood sample was drawn, since there is a risk of increased lactic acid level the longer the tourniquet is in place.

How the Test Is Performed

The patient should avoid eating or drinking 10 hours before the test, exercising 12 hours before the test, and clenching his or her fist during the test.

A sample of blood is taken from the patient's vein. The patient will experience a tight feeling when the tourniquet is tightened, a pinch or nothing at all when the needle is inserted into the vein, and pressure when a gauze pad is pressed against the insertion site to stop bleeding. It can take up to 10 minutes for bleeding to stop if the patient is taking anticoagulants (aspirin, coumadin). A small bruise might appear at the insertion site, which could become swollen following this test. This is called phlebitis. Applying a warm compress several times a day will reduce the swelling.

Teach the Patient

Prior to testing, explain to the patient why the sample is taken and that the healthcare provider may ask the patient to refrain from taking alcohol, Glucophage, isoniazid, epinephrine, or Tylenol 12 hours prior to the test.

Inform the patient to avoid eating or drinking 10 hours before the test, exercising 12 hours before the test, and clenching his or her fist during the test.

Understanding the Test Results

The lactic acid test results are available in 1 day. The laboratory determines normal values based on calibration of testing equipment with a control test. Test results are reported as high, normal, or low based on the laboratory's control test.

Normal lactic acid test results are 5 to 20 mg/dL.

A high lactic acid level may indicate lactic acidosis, heart failure, pulmonary embolism, anemia, dehydration, leukemia, cirrhosis, disruption of blood flow, alcohol poisoning, that the patient exercised prior to the test, that the patient has taken Glucophage or isoniazid prior to the test, or excess dietary iron.

1.19 Prothrombin Time

There are 12 factors that must be present to coagulate (clot) blood. *Prothrombin* is clotting factor II, synthesized by the liver with the assistance of vitamin K. When a blood vessel is injured, prothrombin is converted to thrombin, a protein that forms a blood clot with other proteins to stop the bleeding. The prothrombin time (PT) test is the time necessary for plasma to clot. The healthcare provider orders the prothrombin time test to assess the patient's risk for bleeding and to assess the therapeutic effect of anticoagulate medication.

The healthcare provider is likely to order the International Normalized Ratio (INR) test, which was established by the World Health Organization as a standard for measuring blood coagulation. Also, the healthcare provider is likely to order the Partial Thromboplastin Time (PTT) test to measure blood coagulation, and the complete blood count to measure the platelet count.

Why the Test Is Performed

The test is performed to screen for risk for bleeding, therapeutic level of coumadin, bleeding disorders, vitamin K deficiency, and liver function.

Before Administering the Test

Assess if the patient:

- Is vomiting or having diarrhea
- Abuses alcohol
- Has eaten pork liver, broccoli, beef liver, soybean, chickpeas, turnip greens, or kale
- Is taking vitamin K, Tagamet, birth control pills, aspirin, antibiotics, hormone replacement therapy, or coumadin
- Has taken laxatives

How the Test Is Performed

The sample must be taken at the same time each day. A sample of blood is taken from the patient's vein. The patient will experience a tight feeling when the tourniquet is tightened, a pinch or nothing at all when the needle is inserted into the vein, and pressure when a gauze pad is pressed against the insertion site to stop bleeding. It can take up to 10 minutes for bleeding to stop if the patient is taking anticoagulants (aspirin, coumadin). A small bruise might appear at the insertion site, which could become swollen following this test. This is called phlebitis. Applying a warm compress several times a day will reduce the swelling.

Teach the Patient

Prior to testing, explain to the patient why the sample is taken and that several samples may be taken at the same time each day to assess the therapeutic level of coumadin, if the patient is taking this medication.

Understanding the Test Results

The prothrombin time test results are available quickly. The laboratory determines normal values based on calibration of testing equipment with a control test. Test results are reported as high, normal, or low based on the laboratory's control test.

Normal test results:

- Prothrombin time: 10 to 13 seconds
- INR: 1 to 1.4 seconds

- Coumadin prothrombin time: 1.5 to 2.5 times normal prothrombin time
- Coumadin INR time: 2 to 3 times normal prothrombin time

A longer prothrombin time may indicate cirrhosis, risk for bleeding, vitamin K deficiency, disseminated intravascular coagulation (DIC), or too much coumadin or heparin.

A low coumadin prothrombin time may indicate not enough coumadin.

1.20 Reticulocyte Count

Reticulocyte is an immature red blood cell that is released by bone marrow and develops into a mature red blood cell in two days. The reticulocyte count test determines the amount of reticulocyte in a blood sample. The healthcare provider may order the reticulocyte index (RI).

Why the Test Is Performed

The test is performed to screen for anemia and assess the treatment of anemia.

Before Administering the Test

Assess if the patient:

- Is undergoing radiation therapy
- Is pregnant
- Has had a blood transfusion in the previous week
- Has undergone a prostate biopsy in the past eight weeks
- Is taking Bactrim, Septra, corticotrophin, Imuran, levodopa, Chloromycetin, methotrexate, or Cosmegen

How the Test Is Performed

A sample of blood is taken from the patient's vein. The patient will experience a tight feeling when the tourniquet is tightened, a pinch or nothing at all when the needle is inserted into the vein, and pressure when a gauze pad is pressed against the insertion site to stop bleeding. It can take up to 10 minutes for bleeding to stop if the patient is taking anticoagulants (aspirin, coumadin). A small bruise might appear at the insertion site, which could become swollen following this test. This is called phlebitis. Applying a warm compress several times a day will reduce the swelling.

Teach the Patient

Prior to testing, explain to the patient why the sample is taken and that the healthcare provider may ask the patient to avoid taking Bactrim, Septra, corticotrophin, Imuran, levodopa, Chloromycetin, methotrexate, or Cosmegen before the test.

Understanding the Test Results

The reticulocyte test results are available in 1 day. The laboratory determines normal values based on calibration of testing equipment with a control test. Test results are reported as high, normal, or low based on the laboratory's control test.

Normal test results are 0.5% to 2.5%.

Higher levels may indicate hemolysis, anemia, that the patient is being treated for anemia, that the patient is in a high altitude location, or that the patient has been hemorrhaging.

Low levels may indicate aplastic anemia, iron deficiency anemia, folic acid deficiency, vitamin B_{12} deficiency, radiation exposure, or bone marrow cancer.

1.21   Schilling Test

Adequate absorption of vitamin B_{12} is central to cell metabolism and energy production. Vitamin B_{12} attaches to the intrinsic factor produced by the parietal cells in the stomach. The intrinsic factor protects vitamin B_{12} from intestinal bacteria and enables absorption of vitamin B_{12} by the intestines. The Schilling test measures the absorption of vitamin B_{12}. There are two parts to the Schilling test.

Part 1: The patient ingests vitamin B_{12} that is radioactively tagged. A 24-hour urine sample is examined for the presence of vitamin B_{12}. Up to 25% of the ingested vitamin B_{12} will normally be detected in the 24-hour urine sample. Little or no vitamin B_{12} detected is a sign of vitamin B_{12} malabsorption.

Part 2: If part 1 is abnormal, then the healthcare provider may order part 2. The patient ingests vitamin B_{12} that is radioactively tagged, and the intrinsic factor. A 24-hour urine sample is examined for the presence of vitamin B_{12}. Detection of vitamin B_{12} is a sign that the patient has pernicious anemia. Absence of vitamin B_{12} is a sign of an intestinal absorption problem.

The Schilling Test is not performed on a pregnant woman or a woman who is breast-feeding. The healthcare provider may order a 48 or 72 hour urine sample if the patient has kidney disease. The healthcare provider may also order the methylmalonic acid (MMA) test and the homocysteine test.

Why the Test Is Performed

The test is performed to screen for absorption of vitamin B_{12} and production of the intrinsic factor.

Before Administering the Test

Assess if the patient:

- Is pregnant
- Has properly collected the 24-hour urine sample
- Is taking Mycitracin, Dilantin, or colchicine
- Has kidney disease
- Used a laxative prior to administering the test
- Has had a radioactive scan two weeks prior to the test

How the Test Is Performed

Part 1:

- Avoid eating or drinking anything except water for 12 hours before the test is administered.
- Avoid taking vitamin B_{12} supplements for 3 days before the test is administered.
- Avoid taking laxatives for 24 hours before the test is administered.
- The patient will swallow a small capsule containing radioactively tagged vitamin B_{12}.
- The patient receives an IM injection of nonradioactive vitamin B_{12} 2 hours after ingesting the capsule. This prevents the radioactively tagged vitamin B_{12} from binding with tissues.
- Collect a 24-hour urine sample.

Part 2 (within 7 days of Part 1):

- Avoid eating or drinking anything except water for 12 hours before the test is administered.
- Avoid taking vitamin B_{12} supplements for 3 days before the test is administered.
- Avoid taking laxatives for 24 hours before the test is administered.
- The patient with swallow a small capsule containing radioactively tagged vitamin B_{12} and the intrinsic factor,
- The patient receives an IM injection of nonradioactive vitamin B_{12} 2 hours after ingesting the capsule. This prevents the radioactively tagged vitamin B_{12} from binding with tissues.
- Collect a 24-hour urine sample.

The patient may have an allergic reaction to radioactive B_{12}, but this is rare. The amount of radioactivity in the radioactive B_{12} capsule is very low and poses no risk.

Teach the Patient

Prior to testing, explain to the patient why the sample is taken, that the patient will not feel any discomfort when ingesting the capsule, that the radioactivity in the radioactive vitamin B_{12} is low and not dangerous, and that the healthcare provider may ask the patient to refrain from taking Mycitracin, Dilantin, or colchicines prior to the test. Demonstrate how to take a 24-hour urine sample.

Understanding the Test Results

The Schilling test results are available quickly. The laboratory determines normal values based on calibration of testing equipment with a control test. Test results are reported as high, normal, or low based on the laboratory's control test.

Normal test resultsare 8% to 10% of vitamin B_{12} found in urine.

Lower levels may indicate:

- Part 1: pernicious anemia, sprue, celiac disease, hypothyroidism, cirrhosis, or hepatitis
- Part 2: sprue, celiac disease, hypothyroidism, cirrhosis, or hepatitis

1.22   Sedimentation Rate (SED)

An increase in fibrinogen in blood during the inflammatory process causes erythrocytes (RBC) to adhere to each other, forming a stack called *rouleaux*. The sedimentation rate test measures how many millimeters per hour erythrocytes settle to the bottom of a test tube. Rouleaux settle quicker than erythrocytes. Therefore, the increased sedimentation rate indicates that the patient has inflammation. Not all inflammation increases the sedimentation rate. Therefore, a normal sedimentation rate does not rule out inflammation. The healthcare provider might order other tests in addition to the sedimentation rate to diagnosis inflammation. The healthcare provider might order the C-reactive protein (CRP) test to determine if the patient has inflammation.

Why the Test Is Performed

The test is performed to screen for inflammation and to assess treatment for inflammation.

Before Administering the Test

Assess if the patient:

- Is pregnant
- Has her menstrual period
- Has anemia

Note the patient's age, since sedimentation rate increases with age.

How the Test Is Performed

A sample of blood is taken from the patient's vein. The patient will experience a tight feeling when the tourniquet is tightened, a pinch or nothing at all when the needle is inserted into the vein, and pressure when a gauze pad is pressed against the insertion site to stop bleeding. It can take up to 10 minutes for bleeding to stop if the patient is taking anticoagulants (aspirin, coumadin). A small bruise might appear at the insertion site, which could become swollen following this test. This is called phlebitis. Applying a warm compress several times a day will reduce the swelling.

Teach the Patient

Prior to testing, explain to the patient why the sample is taken, that additional tests are necessary to diagnose inflammation, and that normal results does not rule out inflammation.

Understanding the Test Results

The sedimentation rate test results are available quickly. The laboratory determines normal values based on calibration of testing equipment with a control test. Test results are reported as high, normal, or low based on the laboratory's control test.

Normal test results:

- Men: 0 to 15 mm/hr
- Women: 0 to 20 mm/hr
- Children: 0 to 10 mm/hr
- Newborns: 0 to 2 mm/hr

Higher levels may indicate inflammation, rheumatoid arthritis, Systemic lupus erythematosus, appendicitis, pneumonia, chronic kidney disease, lymphoma, pelvic inflammatory disease, Graves' disease, giant cell arteritis, polymalgia rheumatical, or toxemia of pregnancy.

Lower levels may indicate sickle cell disease, hyperglycemia, or polycythemia.

1.23 Iron (Fe)

Iron is a mineral in food that is needed for cell growth. Once metabolized, iron binds to the transferrin protein, which transports iron to bone marrow and other tissues. The iron tests measure the amount of iron that is bound to transferrin.

There are three iron tests:

- *Total Iron Binding Capacity (TIBC) test*: This test measures the capacity of the blood to carry iron by determining the amount of iron needed to bind to all the available transferring protein.
- *Serum Iron Test*: This test measures the amount of circulate iron in blood.
- *Transferrin Saturation Test*: This is the percentage of serum iron of total iron binding capacity.

The healthcare provider may order the ferritin test, the siderocyte stain test, and a complete blood count (CBC), along with the iron tests.

Why the Test Is Performed

The test is performed to screen for the nutritional status of the patient, iron deficiency anemia, and hemochromatosis. It also assesses treatment for iron deficiency anemia.

Before Administering the Test

Assess if the patient:

- Has taken iron supplements 12 hours before the test is administered
- Has taken vitamin B_{12} supplements two days before the test
- Is sleep deprived
- Is stressed
- Has received a blood transfusion four months prior to the test
- Is taking estrogen, birth control pills, chloromycetin, aspirin, corticotrophin, and St. John's Wort

Document if the sample was taken in the morning.

How the Test Is Performed

- Avoid taking iron supplements 12 hours before the test is administered.
- Avoid taking vitamin B_{12} supplements two days before the test.
- Draw the sample in the morning to assure the highest level of iron.

A sample of blood is taken from the patient's vein. The patient will experience a tight feeling when the tourniquet is tightened, a pinch or nothing at all when the needle is inserted into the vein, and pressure when a gauze pad is pressed against the insertion site to stop bleeding. It can take up to 10 minutes for bleeding to stop if the patient is taking anticoagulants (aspirin, coumadin). A small bruise might appear at the insertion site, which could become swollen following this test. This is called phlebitis. Applying a warm compress several times a day will reduce the swelling.

Teach the Patient

Prior to testing, explain to the patient why the sample is taken, that the sample must be taken in the morning, and that the healthcare provider may ask the patient to refrain from taking iron supplements, vitamin B_{12} supplements, estrogen, birth control pills, chloromycetin, aspirin, corticotrophin, and St. John's Wort prior to the test.

Understanding the Test Results

The iron test results are available quickly. The laboratory determines normal values based on calibration of testing equipment with a control test. Test results are reported as high, normal, or low based on the laboratory's control test.
    Normal test results:

- Serum Iron:
  - Men: 80 to 180 mcg/dL
  - Women: 60 to 160 mcg/dL
  - Children: 50 to 120 mcg/dL
- Total iron binding capacity (TIBC): 250 to 450 mcg/dL
- Transferrin saturation:
  - Men: 20% to 50%
  - Women: 15% to 50%

A high level may indicate hemochromatosis, kidney disease, cirrhosis, or lead poisoning.
    A low level may indicate iron deficiency anemia, an iron deficient diet, bleeding, pregnancy, or rapid growth.

1.24   Serum Protein Electrophoresis (SPE)

Blood serum contains two groups of proteins. These are albumin and globulin. Serum protein electrophoresis separates albumin and globulin into five groups by placing the sample of blood serum on an agarose gel and then exposing the gel to an electric current.
    These groups are:

- Albumin
- Alpha-1 globulin
- Alpha-2 globulin
- Beta globulin
- Gamma globulin (antibodies)

Serum protein electrophoresis is not used to diagnose liver disorders, kidney disorders, or rheumatoid arthritis, although an abnormal protein level may be associated with these disorders. The healthcare provider may order urine protein electrophoresis. The healthcare provider may also order the total serum protein test along with the serum protein electrophoresis.

Why the Test Is Performed

The test is performed to screen for the underlying cause of hypogammaglobulinema (HGG), amyloidosis, multiple myeloma, and macroglobulinemia.

Before Administering the Test

Assess if the patient:

- Has hyperlipidemia
- Is pregnant

- Has taken birth control pills, chlorpromazine, corticosteroids, aspirin, sulfonamides, Neomycin, or isoniazid
- Is undergoing chemotherapy

How the Test Is Performed

A sample of blood is taken from the patient's vein. The patient will experience a tight feeling when the tourniquet is tightened, a pinch or nothing at all when the needle is inserted into the vein, and pressure when a gauze pad is pressed against the insertion site to stop bleeding. It can take up to 10 minutes for bleeding to stop if the patient is taking anticoagulants (aspirin, coumadin). A small bruise might appear at the insertion site, which could become swollen following this test. This is called phlebitis. Applying a warm compress several times a day will reduce the swelling.

Teach the Patient

Prior to testing, explain to the patient why the sample is taken, that the sample must be taken in the morning, and that the healthcare provider may ask the patient to refrain from taking birth control pills, chlorpromazine, corticosteroids, aspirin, sulfonamides, Neomycin, or isoniazid prior to the test.

Understanding the Test Results

The serum protein electrophoresis results are available in three days. The laboratory determines normal values based on calibration of testing equipment with a control test. Test results are reported as high, normal, or low based on the laboratory's control test.

Normal test results:

- Albumin: 58% to 74%
- Alpha-1 globulin: 2% to 3.5%
- Alpha-2 globulin: 5.4% to 10.6%
- Beta globulin: 7% to 14%
- Gamma globulin: 8% to 18%

A high level may indicate leukemia, multiple myeloma, lymphoma, rheumatoid arthritis, liver disease, systemic lupus erythematosus, pregnancy, dehydration, infection, kidney disease, or heart disease.

A low level may indicate leukemia, multiple myeloma, lymphoma, rheumatoid arthritis, liver disease, systemic lupus erythematosus, pregnancy, dehydration, infection, kidney disease, heart disease, hypothyroidism, burns, emphysema, spruce, Crohn's disease, and malnutrition.

Solved Problems

Blood Type Test

1.1   What does Rh positive/negative mean?

Rh Positive (+Z): The Rh antigen is presented on the red blood cells. Rh Negative (−): The Rh antigen is not presented on the red blood cells.

1.2   What should you tell the patient before administering the blood type test?

No special preparation is needed for the test. Explain how the test is performed and that the patient may feel a pinch or nothing at all when the needle is inserted and that there might be a small bruise at the needle insertion site.

1.3   What should be done if the insertion site is swollen following the blood type test?

This is called phlebitis and is treated by applying a warm compress several times a day on the site to reduce the swelling.

Blood Alcohol

1.4   Why should the patient sign a consent form prior to administering the blood alcohol test?

The patient's signed consent may be required before the test is administered because the result of the blood alcohol test can have legal repercussions for the patient.

1.5   What are three reasons for administering the blood alcohol test?

To screen the patient for alcohol intoxication, for ingestion of alcohol, and for the reason for altered mental status.

1.6   How does the patient's age affect the metabolism of alcohol?

The older patient will have a higher blood alcohol level than a young patient who consumed the same quantity of alcohol, because the older patient's metabolism is slow.

Lead

1.7   What should be expected if the results of a finger stick lead test reveal high levels of lead in the blood?

The healthcare provider is likely to order a blood sample be taken from a vein and tested for lead to confirm the original result.

1.8   How are normal values determined in a blood lead test?

The laboratory determines normal values based on calibration of testing equipment with a control test. Test results are reported as high, normal, or low based on the laboratory's control test.

1.9   What happens when lead levels above 10 mcg/dL are discovered on two occasions with the same patient?

Lead levels above 10 mcg/dL on two occasions typically must be reported to the local health department so the source of the lead can be found.

C-Reactive Protein

1.10   Why is the C-reactive protein test ordered?

The test is performed to screen for inflammation. It is also administered to assess treatment for inflammation and treatment for the underlying disease that is causing the inflammation. The test is also ordered as part of treatment for cancer.

1.11   What must be considered before administering the C-reactive protein test?

Assess if the patient:
- Has exercised immediately prior to administering the test
- Has taken NSAIDs, birth control pills, aspirin, hormone replacement therapy, pravastatin or corticosteroids
- Has an intrauterine device (IUD)
- Is pregnant

1.12   What might happen if the patient is taking birth control pills?

The healthcare provider may ask the patient to stop taking birth control pills and other medications for 2 weeks prior to the C-reactive protein test.

1.13   How are the results of the C-reactive protein test interspersed if the test is administered following surgery on the patient?

The C-reactive protein level peaks 6 hours following surgery and decreases by the third day. Infection as a result of the surgery is suspected if the C-reactive protein level remains high after the third day. Elevated C-reactive protein level prior to surgery increases the risk of infection following surgery.

1.14   What might a high C-reactive protein level infer?

Inflammation, infection, and risk of a heart attack.

1.15   What might a healthcare provider order if there is a high C-reactive protein level?

The healthcare provider will likely order tests to identify the source of the inflammation.

1.16   What is the function of the C-reactive protein?

C-reactive protein is produced as part of the inflammatory process and attaches to the invading microorganism or damaged cells, enhancing phagocytosis in the destruction of the microorganism or damaged cell.

1.17   Why should the patient not exercise before administering the C-reactive protein test?

Rigorous exercise might increase C-reactive protein in the blood, resulting in a false-positive test result.

Complete Blood Count

1.18   Why are leukocytes counted?

Leukocytes increase when infection is present and can also increase in the absence of infection if the patient has leukemia.

1.19   Why is hemoglobin counted?

The amount of hemoglobin in blood determines the capability of the blood to carry oxygen.

1.20   Why is there a thrombocyte count?

Thrombocytes are platelets that form blood clots. A low thrombocyte count might indicate that the blood has a diminished capability of forming blood clots.

1.21   Why is a patient administered the complete blood count test?

The test is performed to screen for anemia, infection, leukemia, risk for bleeding, asthma, allergies, the cause of bruising, the cause of fatigue, for polycythemia, and blood loss.

1.22   What should be done if blood samples clump in the test tube after the blood sample is drawn from the patient?

Take a new blood sample, since this blood sample is contaminated.

1.23   What instructions should the patient receive if the patient is taking antibiotics?

Stop taking antibiotics for two weeks prior to the test or postpone the test until 2 weeks after the patient is no longer taking antibiotics.

1.24   What might a high thrombocyte count infer?

The patient is bleeding, has cancer, has bone marrow disorder, or has iron deficiency.

1.25   What CBC results would you expect to find if the patient is dehydrated?

The patient might have a high erythrocyte count.

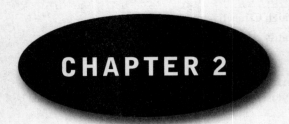

CHAPTER 2

Electrolytes

2.1 Definition

Electrolytes are salts that are electrically charged ions used to maintain voltage across cell membranes and carry electrical impulses within the body. The concentration of electrolytes within the body is constantly changing. The kidneys make adjustments to balance electrolytes. Electrolytes must be in balance to assure proper physiology.

Six key electrolytes are monitored by clinical laboratory tests:

1. Calcium
2. Magnesium
3. Phosphate
4. Potassium
5. Sodium
6. Chloride

Electrolyte Tests

Electrolyte tests are referred to as:

- *An electrolyte panel*: Measures only the electrolytes in a sample of blood
- *Basic metabolic panel*: Measures electrolytes and other components
- *Comprehensive metabolic panel*: Measures electrolytes and other components

2.2 Calcium (Ca)

Calcium is required for bone and teeth growth, muscle contraction, and blood clotting. Calcium in the body is stored in bone with a minimum amount in blood. Calcium has a homeostasis relationship with phosphate. As calcium increases in blood, phosphate decreases, and when phosphate increases in blood, calcium decreases.

The parathyroid keeps calcium and phosphate balanced in this way:

- When there is too much phosphate (too little calcium) in blood, the parathyroid releases the parathyroid hormone (PTH) that stimulates osteoclast, breaking down bone to increase the calcium level in blood.
- Too much calcium in the blood causes the thyroid gland to release calcitonin, which moves calcium from blood to bone.

PTH also activates vitamin D to increase absorption of calcium in the GI tract. Vitamin D is necessary for calcium absorption. The kidneys retain calcium.

There are two kinds of calcium blood tests:

- The *nonionized calcium test* measures calcium attached to albumin in the blood and is affected by the amount of albumin in the blood.
- The *ionized calcium test* measures calcium not attached to albumin in the blood, and therefore is not affected by the amount of albumin in the blood.

Calcium is also measured in urine.

Why the Test Is Performed

The test is performed to screen for parathyroid gland function, kidney function, kidney stones, pancreatitis, and bone disease. The test is also performed to screen for the cause of:

- Muscle spasms, depression, confusion, tingling around the mouth and fingers, muscle cramping and twitching caused by a low calcium level in blood
- An abnormal electrocardiogram
- Nausea, vomiting, bone pain, lack of appetite, weakness, abdominal pain, and constipation and increased urination caused by a high calcium level in blood

These symptoms appear only when calcium levels are very high or very low.

The blood calcium test is not used to diagnose osteoporosis. The bone mineral density test is used to diagnose osteoporosis.

Before Administering the Test

Assess if the patient has:

- Taken milk, antacid, calcium salt, or calcium supplements 8 hours before administering the test, since this will affect the test result
- Eaten or drunk 12 hours before the test is administered
- Taken Diamox, estrogen, albuterol, corticosteroids, vitamin D, lithium, laxatives, aspirin, theophylline or birth control pills, since these can affect the test result
- Had a blood transfusion recently

How the Test Is Performed

A sample of blood is taken from the patient's vein. The patient will experience a tight feeling when the tourniquet is tightened, a pinch or nothing at all when the needle is inserted into the vein, and pressure when a gauze pad is pressed against the insertion site to stop bleeding. It can take up to 10 minutes for bleeding to stop if the patient is taking anticoagulants (aspirin, coumadin). A small bruise might appear at the insertion site, which could become swollen following this test. This is called phlebitis. Applying a warm compress several times a day will reduce the swelling.

Teach the Patient

Explain why the blood sample is taken, that the patient should not eat or drink 12 hours before the test is administered, and that the healthcare provider may ask the patient to stop taking Diamox, estrogen, albuterol, corticosteroids, vitamin D, lithium, laxatives, aspirin, theophylline, or birth control pills 2 weeks before the test is administered, since these can affect the test result.

Understanding the Test Results

Test results are available quickly. The laboratory determines normal values based on calibration of testing equipment with a control test. Test results are reported as high, normal, or low based on the laboratory's control test.

- Normal range is:
  - ○ Nonionized calcium, adult: 9.0 to 10.5 mg/dL or 2.25 to 2.75 mmol/L
  - ○ Nonionized calcium, children: 7.6 to 10.8 mg/dL or 1.9 to 2.7 mmol/L
  - ○ Ionized calcium, adult: 4.65 to 5.28 mg/dL

High level values may indicate hyperparathyroidism, cancer metastasized to the bone, kidney disease, that the patient has been on bed rest for a long period, tuberculosis, sarcoidosis, Addison's disease, dehydration, hyperthyroidism, Paget's disease, chronic liver problems, that the patient has ingested too much calcium, vitamin D, or vitamin A, or decreased phosphate blood level.

Low level values may indicate hypoparathyroidism, malabsorption syndrome, pancreatitis, hypoalbuminemia, low magnesium, kidney disease, and an increased phosphate blood level.

Special Considerations

- Calcium values are high in children who are growing.
- Calcium values are low in older men and pregnant women.
- If calcium levels in blood are abnormal, the healthcare provider may order additional tests for the parathyroid hormone, vitamin D, alkaline phosphatase, acid phosphatase, and chloride, which can affect the calcium levels in blood.

2.3   Magnesium (Mg)

Magnesium is found mostly in bones and inside cells. Magnesium is used to transfer potassium and sodium in and out of cells and is used to activate nerves, muscles, and enzymes. The magnesium blood test measures the level of magnesium in a blood sample and is tested along with other electrolytes. Levels of calcium and magnesium have an inverse relationship.

Why the Test Is Performed

The test screens for the underlying cause of:

- Muscle weakness, muscle twitches, and muscle irritability
- Arrhythmia
- The source of nausea, vomiting, low blood pressure, muscle weakness, and dizziness

The test also screens for the effects of medication that causes changes in the level of magnesium and the therapeutic treatment for high or low levels of magnesium.

Before Administering the Test

Assess if the patient:

- Has taken antacids, laxatives, Milk of Magnesia, diuretics, Epsom salts, or magnesium supplements 3 days before administering the test, since these can affect the test result
- Has taken insulin, antibiotics, or received IV fluids before the test is administered
- Is in the second or third trimester of pregnancy, since magnesium levels are normally low at this stage

How the Test Is Performed

A sample of blood is taken from the patient's vein. The patient will experience a tight feeling when the tourniquet is tightened, a pinch or nothing at all when the needle is inserted into the vein, and pressure when a gauze pad is pressed against the insertion site to stop bleeding. It can take up to 10 minutes for bleeding to stop if the patient is taking anticoagulants (aspirin, coumadin). A small bruise might appear at the insertion site, which could become swollen following this test. This is called phlebitis. Applying a warm compress several times a day will reduce the swelling.

Teach the Patient

Explain why the blood sample is taken and that the patient should not take antacids, laxatives, Milk of Magnesia, diuretics, Epsom salts, or magnesium supplements 3 days before administering the test, since these can affect the test result.

Understanding the Test Results

Test results are available quickly. The laboratory determines normal values based on calibration of testing equipment with a control test. Test results are reported as high, normal, or low based on the laboratory's control test.

- Normal range is:
  - Adult: 1.3 to 2.1 mEq/L
  - Children: 1.4 to 1.7 mEq/L
  - Newborns: 1.4 to 2 mEq/L

High values may indicate hyperparathyroidism, Addison's disease, hypothyroidism, dehydration, kidney failure, or overmedication with antacids and laxatives that contain magnesium.

Low values may indicate diabetic ketoacidosis, pancreatitis, hypercalcemia, kidney disease, alcohol abuse, alcohol withdrawal, sprue, preeclamsia, hyperthyroidism, hypoparathyroidism, burns, starvation, insufficient ingestion of magnesium, or diarrhea.

2.4 Phosphate

Phosphorus is a mineral that contains a particle called phosphate, which is necessary for the growth of bone and teeth and for contracting muscles. Most phosphate is in bone. Phosphate and calcium have an inverse relationship. The phosphate test measures the level of phosphate in blood. Phosphate is measured along with other electrolytes.

Why the Test Is Performed

The test screens for bone disease, kidney disease, and parathyroid gland function.

Before Administering the Test

Assess if the patient has:

- Ingested alcohol, since this can affect the test results
- Taken vitamin D supplements, antacids, insulin, epinephrine, acetazolamide, anabolic steroids, or a phosphate-based enema
- Has diabetes insipidus
- Has lymphoma
- Has Type 2 diabetes

How the Test Is Performed

A sample of blood is taken from the patient's vein. The patient will experience a tight feeling when the tourniquet is tightened, a pinch or nothing at all when the needle is inserted into the vein, and pressure when a gauze pad is pressed against the insertion site to stop bleeding. It can take up to 10 minutes for bleeding to stop if the patient is taking anticoagulants (aspirin, coumadin). A small bruise might appear at the insertion site, which could become swollen following this test. This is called phlebitis. Applying a warm compress several times a day will reduce the swelling.

Heel Stick: Several drops of blood are collected from the heel of a newborn or baby. The heel is cleaned using alcohol. A sterile lancet is used to puncture the heel. Several drops of blood are collected in a small test tube. A gauze pad is pressed over the site until bleeding stops. A small bandage is applied.

Teach the Patient

Explain why the blood sample is taken, not to ingest alcohol 12 hours before the test is administered, and that the healthcare provider may ask the patient to stop taking vitamin D supplements, antacids, epinephrine, acetazolamide, anabolic steroids, or a phosphate-based enema 2 weeks prior to the test.

Understanding the Test Results

Test results are available in 2 hours. The laboratory determines normal values based on calibration of testing equipment with a control test. Test results are reported as high, normal, or low based on the laboratory's control test.

- Normal range is:
  - Adult: 3.0 to 4.5 mg/dL or 0.97 to 1.45 mmol/L
  - Children: 4.5 to 6.5 mg/dL or 1.45 to 2.1 mmol/L
  - Children under 1 year of age: 4.3 to 9.3 mg/dL or 1.4 to 3 mmol/L

High values may indicate pregnancy, acromegaly, hypoparathyroidism, kidney disease, diabetic ketoacidosis, bone fracture that is healing, excess vitamin D, or low level of magnesium.

Low values may indicate osteomalacia, malnutrition, hyperparathyroidism, low level of vitamin D, liver disease, sprue, alcohol abuse, high level of calcium, and burns.

2.5   Potassium (K)

Potassium is a mineral stored inside the cell. Potassium has multiple functions including, muscle contractions, neural transmission, and fluid balance. Potassium is excreted by the kidneys and regulated by the hormone aldosterone, which is released by the adrenal glands. Potassium and sodium have an inverse relationship. The potassium test measures the level of potassium in blood. Potassium is measured along with other electrolytes. The healthcare provider may order a urine analysis to determine the level of potassium that is being excreted by the kidneys.

Why the Test Is Performed

The test screens for cell lysis syndrome and assesses the effects of total parenteral nutrition (TPN) being administered to the patient, adverse effect of diuretics which can decrease potassium levels, the source of high blood pressure, and the effect of kidney dialysis.

Before Administering the Test

Assess if the patient has:

- Taken potassium supplements
- Taken heparin, glucose, NSAIDs, antibiotics that contain potassium, natural licorice, corticosteroids, ACE inhibitors, or insulin
- Experienced severe vomiting
- Improperly used laxatives

How the Test Is Performed

A sample of blood is taken from the patient's vein. The patient will experience a tight feeling when the tourniquet is tightened, a pinch or nothing at all when the needle is inserted into the vein, and pressure when a gauze pad is pressed against the insertion site to stop bleeding. It can take up to 10 minutes for bleeding to stop if the patient is taking anticoagulants (aspirin, coumadin). A small bruise might appear at the insertion site, which could become swollen following this test. This is called phlebitis. Applying a warm compress several times a day will reduce the swelling.

Teach the Patient

Explain why the blood sample is taken and that the healthcare provide may ask the patient to stop taking heparin, glucose, NSAIDs, antibiotics that contain potassium, natural licorice, corticosteroids, or ACE inhibitors for two weeks.

Understanding the Test Results

Test results are available quickly. The laboratory determines normal values based on calibration of testing equipment with a control test. Test results are reported as high, normal, or low based on the laboratory's control test.

- Normal range is:
  - Adult: 3.5 to 5.0 mEq/L
  - Children: 3.4 to 4.7 mEq/L
  - Children under 1 year of age: 3.9 to 5.3 mEq/L

High values may indicate heart attack, ingestion of too many potassium supplements, ingestion of ACE inhibitors, diabetic ketoacidosis, or kidney damage.

Low values may indicate alcoholism, cystic fibrosis, diarrhea, hyperaldosteronism, use of diuretics, Bartter's syndrome, vomiting, burns, malnutrition, or dehydration.

2.6   Sodium (Na)

Sodium is a mineral stored outside the cell in blood and lymph fluid. Sodium has multiple functions, including muscle contractions, neural transmission, and fluid balance. Sodium is excreted by the kidneys and regulated by the hormone aldosterone, which is released by the adrenal glands. Sodium and potassium have an inverse relationship. The sodium test measures the level of sodium in blood. Sodium is measured along with other electrolytes. The healthcare provider may order fractional excretion of sodium (FENa) urine test to determine the amount of sodium and creatinine in the urine.

Why the Test Is Performed

The test screens for adrenal gland diseases, electrolyte balance, water balance, and kidney disease.

Before Administering the Test

Assess if the patient has:

- Elevated protein levels
- Received IV fluid containing sodium
- High triglyceride levels
- Taken Heparin, birth control pills, NSAIDs, antibiotics, tricyclic antidepressants, corticosteroids, lithium, or estrogen

How the Test Is Performed

A sample of blood is taken from the patient's vein. The patient will experience a tight feeling when the tourniquet is tightened, a pinch or nothing at all when the needle is inserted into the vein, and pressure when a gauze pad is pressed against the insertion site to stop bleeding. It can take up to 10 minutes for bleeding to stop if the patient is taking anticoagulants (aspirin, coumadin). A small bruise might appear at the insertion site, which could become swollen following this test. This is called phlebitis. Applying a warm compress several times a day will reduce the swelling.

Teach the Patient

Explain why the blood sample is taken and that the healthcare provider may ask the patient to stop taking heparin, birth control pills, NSAIDs, antibiotics, tricyclic antidepressants, corticosteroids, lithium, or estrogen for 2 weeks.

Understanding the Test Results

Test results are available quickly. The laboratory determines normal values based on calibration of testing equipment with a control test. Test results are reported as high, normal, or low based on the laboratory's control test.

- Normal range is: 136 to 145 mEq/L

High values may indicate diabetic ketoacidosis, Cushing's syndrome, dehydration, kidney disease, diabetes insipidus, high sodium intake, vomiting, diarrhea, or hyperaldosteronism.

Low values may indicate psychogenic polydipsia (drinking too much water), heart failure, vomiting, diarrhea, burns, SIADH, Cirrhosis malnutrition, or kidney disease.

2.7   Chloride (Cl)

Chloride is an electrolyte found outside the cell. Chloride is involved in fluid balance. The chloride test measures the level of chloride in blood. The healthcare provider may order a chloride urine test or a skin sweat test. The healthcare provider will likely order the chloride test along with tests for other electrolytes.

Why the Test Is Performed

The test screens for the underlying cause of confusion, muscle spasms, muscle weakness, difficulty breathing, metabolic alkalosis, kidney disorder, and adrenal gland disorder.

Before Administering the Test

Assess if the patient:

- Is pregnant
- Has taken coumadin, aspirin, NSAIDs, corticosteroids, cholestyramine, diuretics, androgens, or estrogens
- Is dehydrated or overhydrated

How the Test Is Performed

A sample of blood is taken from the patient's vein. The patient will experience a tight feeling when the tourniquet is tightened, a pinch or nothing at all when the needle is inserted into the vein, and pressure when a gauze pad is pressed against the insertion site to stop bleeding. It can take up to 10 minutes for bleeding to stop if the patient is taking anticoagulants (aspirin, coumadin). A small bruise might appear at the insertion site, which could become swollen following this test. This is called phlebitis. Applying a warm compress several times a day will reduce the swelling.

Teach the Patient

Explain why the sample is taken and that the healthcare provider may ask the patient to refrain from taking coumadin, aspirin, NSAIDs, corticosteroids, cholestyramine, diuretics, androgens, or estrogens prior to the test.

Understanding the Test Results

The chloride test results are available quickly. The laboratory determines normal values based on calibration of testing equipment with a control test. Test results are reported as high, normal, or low based on the laboratory's control test.

- Normal test results:
  - Adults: 98 to 106 mEq/L
  - Children: 90 to 110 mEq/L
  - Newborns: 96 to 106 mEq/L
  - Premature infants: 95 to 110 mEq/L

Higher levels may indicate dehydration, anemia, kidney disease, hyperparathyroidism, or ingestion of salt.

Lower levels may indicate kidney failure, burns, Cushing's syndrome, heart failure, vomiting, diabetic ketoacidosis, or SIADH.

Solved Problems

Electrolytes

2.1   What is an electrolyte?

Electrolytes are salts that are electrically charged ions used to maintain voltage across cell membranes. They carry electrical impulses within the body.

2.2   Name three electrolyte tests.

An electrolyte panel, basic metabolic panel, and comprehensive metabolic panel.

2.3   What electrolyte test measures only electrolytes in a sample of blood?

An electrolyte panel.

Calcium

2.4   Where is calcium stored in the body?

Calcium in the body is stored in bone with a minimum amount in blood.

2.5   What happens when there is too little calcium in the blood?

When there is too much phosphate (too little calcium) in blood, the parathyroid releases the parathyroid hormone (PTH) that stimulates osteoclast, breaking down bone to increase the calcium level in blood.

2.6   Name and describe two types of calcium tests.

The nonionized calcium test measures calcium attached to albumin in the blood and is affected by the amount of albumin in the blood. The ionized calcium test measures calcium not attached to albumin in the blood, and therefore is not affected by the amount of albumin in the blood.

2.7   What symptoms can be caused by either very high or very low calcium levels in the body?

Very high calcium levels in the blood can cause nausea, vomiting, bone pain, lack of appetite, weakness, abdominal pain, constipation, and increased urination. Very low calcium levels in the blood can cause muscle spasms, depression, confusion, tingling around the mouth and fingers, and muscle cramping and twitching.

2.8   What should you assess in the patient before testing the patient's calcium?

You should assess if the patient has:
- Taken milk, antacid, calcium salt, or calcium supplements 8 hours before administering the test, since this will affect the test result
- Eaten or drunk 12 hours before the test is administered
- Taken Diamox, estrogen, albuterol, corticosteroids, vitamin D, lithium, laxatives, aspirin, theophylline, or birth control pills, since these can affect the test result
- Had a blood transfusion recently

2.9   How are calcium test results reported?

Test results are reported as high, normal, or low based on the laboratory's control test.

Magnesium

2.10   How does the body use magnesium?

Magnesium is used to transfer potassium and sodium in and out of cells and to activate nerves, muscles, and enzymes.

2.11 Why is the test for magnesium given?

The magnesium test screens for the underlying cause of muscle weakness, muscle twitches, muscle irritability, arrhythmia, and the source of nausea, vomiting, low blood pressure, muscle weakness, and dizziness. The test also screens the effects of medication that causes changes in the level of magnesium and the therapeutic treatment for high or low levels of magnesium.

2.12 What should the patient avoid taking prior to the magnesium test?

Explain not to take antacids, laxatives, Milk of Magnesia, diuretics, Epsom salts, or magnesium supplements three days before administering the test, since these can affect the test results.

Potassium

2.13 How does the body use potassium?

Potassium has multiple functions, including muscle contractions, neural transmission, and fluid balance.

2.14 What regulates potassium?

Potassium is excreted by the kidneys, which is regulated by the hormone aldosterone that is released by the adrenal glands.

2.15 Why is the potassium test ordered by the healthcare provider?

The potassium test screens for cell lysis syndrome. It also assesses the effects of total parenteral nutrition (TPN) being administered to the patient, adverse effect of diuretics, which can decrease potassium levels, the source of high blood pressure, and the effect of kidney dialysis.

2.16 What should you assess in the patient who is taking the potassium test?

Assess if the patient has:
- Taken potassium supplements
- Taken heparin, glucose, NSAIDs, antibiotics that contain potassium, natural licorice, corticosteroids, ACE inhibitors or insulin
- Experienced severe vomiting
- Improperly used laxatives

2.17 What might a high potassium value indicate?

A high potassium value might indicate heart attack, ingestion of too many potassium supplements, ingestion of ACE inhibitors, diabetic ketoacidosis, or kidney damage.

Sodium

2.18 What electrolyte has an inverse relationship with sodium?
Potassium.

2.19 Where is sodium stored in the body?
Sodium is a mineral stored outside the cell in blood and lymph fluid.

2.20 What regulates sodium in the body?
Aldosterone released by the adrenal glands.

2.21 Besides the electrolyte test, what other test might be ordered to measure sodium?
The healthcare provider may order a fractional excretion of sodium (FENa) urine test to determine the amount of sodium and creatinine in the urine.

2.22 What should be assessed before administering the sodium test?
Assess if the patient has:
- Elevated protein levels
- Received IV fluid containing sodium

- High triglyceride levels
- Taken heparin, birth control pills, NSAIDs, antibiotics, tricyclic antidepressants, corticosteroids, lithium, or estrogen

2.23 Why would a healthcare provider order a sodium test?

A sodium test screens for adrenal gland diseases, electrolyte balance, water balance, and kidney disease.

2.24 What might a low sodium value indicate?

A low sodium value might indicate psychogenic polydipsia (drinking too much water), heart failure, vomiting, diarrhea, burns, SIADH, cirrhosis, malnutrition, and kidney disease.

2.25 Why would the sodium test be used to screen for kidney disease?

Sodium is excreted by the kidneys. Therefore, high sodium levels would be expected in kidney disease because the kidneys are not adequately excreting sodium.

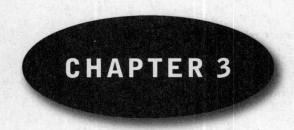

CHAPTER 3

Arterial Blood Gas Tests

3.1 Definition

Blood taken from an artery is analyzed to identify the concentration of oxygen, carbon dioxide, and bicarbonate in arterial blood. The arterial blood gases test indicates how well the patient's lungs transfer oxygen and carbon dioxide to and from blood, and determines the pH value of the blood sample. Blood concentration is altered, depending on the patient's condition. The body compensates for these changes by adjusting the levels of acid and bicarbonate in the blood.

3.2 Arterial Blood Gases

Blood contains oxygen and carbon dioxide. Measuring the partial pressure of these gases indicates how well lungs are exchanging oxygen and carbon dioxide. Measuring the oxygen saturation of the blood indicates the amount of hemoglobin-carrying oxygen, and measuring the oxygen content of blood indicates the amount of oxygen in the blood. Blood must be within acidity range. Acidity is measured using the pH scale, which measures the hydrogen ions (H+).

- The pH of blood must be between 7.35 and 7.45 pH.
- If it is less than 7.35, blood is considered too acidic.
- If it is greater than 7.45, the blood is too alkaline (basic).

Bicarbonate (HCO_3) is a chemical in the blood that ensures that the blood remains within the acceptable pH range. If blood becomes too acidic, the amount of bicarbonate is increased by increasing the absorption of bicarbonate by the kidneys.

Why the Test Is Performed

The test screens gas exchange capabilities of the lungs, the effectiveness of treatment for lung disease, the blood acidity level, the effectiveness of treatment for an imbalance of blood acidity, and kidney function.

Before Administering the Test

Assess if the patient:

- Has been taking anticoagulants (aspirin, coumadin, NSAIDs)
- Has been taking over-the-counter medications, since some contain aspirin. If so, the test can still be performed. However, coagulation time following the test may be longer than 10 minutes.
- Has allergies, especially to anesthetics

- Conditions that might affect the test:
  - Anemia
  - Polycytemia
  - Exposure to smoke (including second-hand smoke), paint removers, or carbon monoxide
  - Abnormally high or low body temperature
- Discontinued oxygen therapy 20 minutes before the test unless the patient is unable to breathe without oxygen therapy. This assures that gas exchange measurement is based on room air without supplemental oxygen.

How the Test Is Performed

Blood is drawn from an artery before blood enters body tissues so that use of oxygen by tissues does not interfere with the measurement. The artery can be:

- Radial artery (inside of the wrist) (typical)
- Femoral artery (groin)
- Brachial artery (above crease in the elbow)

Do not use a site that is infected, inflamed, or used for dialysis.

An arterial catheter (thin tube) is placed in the artery if blood samples are collected at regular intervals. This increases patient comfort since an indwelling catheter eliminates having another needle stick.

1. Seat the patient with the arm extended and the wrist resting on a small pillow.
2. Administer a local anesthetic, if prescribed. Collecting blood from an artery is more painful than collecting blood from a vein.
3. Perform the Allen test to ensure that there is normal blood flow.
   a. Stop the blood flow to both arteries to the hand until the hand becomes pale.
   b. Release and allow blood to flow through the arteries.
   c. The hand should regain normal color quickly, indicating injury to an artery. The Arterial Blood Gas test will not block blood flow to the hand.
   d. If normal color is slow to return, then perform the Allen test on the other wrist. If color to this hand is also slow to return, then use an alternative site for the Arterial Blood Gas test.
4. Clean the puncture site with alcohol.
5. Instruct the patient to breathe normally.
6. Insert the needle into the artery.
7. Attach a test tube to the needle. Allow the blood to fill the test tube.
8. Place a gauze pad over the site while withdrawing the needle.
9. Apply firm pressure to the site for 10 minutes or longer until bleeding has stopped.

Teach the Patient

Explain why the blood sample is taken. Inform the patient that arteries are narrower and deeper than veins and are protected by nerves, making them sensitive to pain. Therefore, there is more pain experienced when collecting blood from an artery than collecting blood from a vein. Ask the patient if he/she wishes to have a local anesthetic. The patient may feel a brief pinch as the needle enters the skin, and there are risks of nerve damage and a blockage of the artery as a result of the test, although incidents are rare. After the test, the patient may see a small bruise at the site. The patient may feel dizzy, lightheaded, and nauseated during the test, and should not lift or carry objects or exercise for 24 hours following the test.

Explain the function of blood gases and the meaning of abnormal values. Firm pressure may be applied to the site for 10 minutes or more, especially if the patient is taking anticoagulants. Explain that oxygen therapy will be discontinued for 20 minutes before the test unless the patient is unable to breathe without oxygen therapy.

Understanding the Test Results

Results are available quickly. The laboratory determines normal values based on calibration of testing equipment with a control test. Test results are reported as high, normal, or low based on the laboratory's control test.

- Generally, normal ranges are:
  - Partial pressure of oxygen (PaO_2) = 75 to 100 mm Hg
  - Partial pressure of carbon dioxide ($PaCO_2$) = 34 to 45 mm Hg
  - Oxygen saturation (O_2Sat) = 95% to 100% (means 95 to 100 mL per 100 mL of blood)
  - Oxygen content (O_2CT) = 15% to 22% (means 15 to 22 mL per 100 mL of blood)
  - Blood pH = 7.35 to 7.45 pH
  - Bicarbonate (HCO_3) = 20 to 29 mEq/L or mmol/L

High values can be a sign of COPD, pulmonary edema, Cushing's disease, Conn's syndrome, kidney failure, sepsis, dehydration, drug overdose, diabetes, or that the patient is taking hydrocortisone, prednisone, or diuretics.

Low values can indicate liver disease (low bicarbonate), aspirin overdose (low bicarbonate), alcohol overdose (low bicarbonate), severe malnutrition (low bicarbonate), diarrhea (low bicarbonate), dehydration (low bicarbonate), hyperventilation (low bicarbonate), kidney disease (low bicarbonate), hyperthyroidism (low bicarbonate), shock (low bicarbonate), or severe burns (low bicarbonate).

3.3　Total Carbon Dioxide

Blood contains three forms of carbon dioxide. These are bicarbonate (HCO_3), carbonic acid (H_2CO_3), and dissolved carbon dioxide (CO_2). Carbon dioxide is a gaseous byproduct of metabolism that is transported to the lungs where carbon dioxide is exhaled. Most of the carbon dioxide is in the form of bicarbonate. Levels of these types of carbon dioxide are balanced by the lungs and kidneys. The total carbon dioxide test measures the level of all three types of carbon dioxide and is administered at the same time the arterial blood gas is administered. The total carbon dioxide test is part of the chemistry screen.

Why the Test Is Performed

The test assesses lung function and kidney function.

Before Administering the Test

Assess if the patient:

- Has taken corticosteroids, antibiotics, antacids, diuretics, aspirin, sodium bicarbonate, or barbiturates
- Has hyperthermia

How the Test Is Performed

A sample of blood is taken from the patient's vein. The patient will experience a tight feeling when the tourniquet is tightened, a pinch or nothing at all when the needle is inserted into the vein, and pressure when a gauze pad is pressed against the insertion site to stop bleeding. It can take up to 10 minutes for bleeding to stop if the patient is taking anticoagulants (aspirin, coumadin). A small bruise might appear at the insertion site, which could become swollen following this test. This is called phlebitis. Applying a warm compress several times a day will reduce the swelling.

Teach the Patient

Explain why the blood sample is taken and that the healthcare provider may ask the patient to stop taking corticosteroids, antibiotics, antacids, diuretics, aspirin, sodium bicarbonate, or barbiturates for 2 weeks prior to the test.

Understanding the Test Results

Test results are available quickly. The laboratory determines normal values based on calibration of testing equipment with a control test. Test results are reported as high, normal, or low based on the laboratory's control test.

- Normal range is:
  - Adult: 23 to 29 mmol/L
  - Children: 20 to 28 mmol/L
  - Under 1 year old: 13 to 22 mmol/L

High level values may indicate vomiting, pneumonia (respiratory acidosis), COPD (respiratory acidosis), Conn's syndrome (metabolic acidosis), alcoholism (metabolic acidosis), or Cushing's syndrome (metabolic acidosis).

Low level values may indicate hyperventilation (respiratory alkalosis), cirrhosis (respiratory alkalosis), liver failure (respiratory alkalosis), pneumonia (respiratory alkalosis), diabetes (metabolic alkalosis), aspirin overdose (metabolic alkalosis), diarrhea (metabolic alkalosis), heart failure (metabolic alkalosis), kidney failure (metabolic alkalosis), chronic starvation (metabolic alkalosis), ingestion of antifreeze (metabolic alkalosis), or ingestion of methanol (metabolic alkalosis).

3.4   Carbon Monoxide (CO)

Carbon monoxide (CO) is a colorless, odorless gas that replaces oxygen attached to the hemoglobin red blood cells, creating a compound called *carboxyhemoglobin*. Carboxyhemoglobin decreases oxygenation of blood and can result in death. The carbon monoxide blood test measures the level of carboxyhemoglobin in blood.

Quick Assessment is used to determine the level of carboxyhemoglobin in a patient's blood based on the following signs and symptoms. The percentage is the estimated level of carboxyhemoglobin.

- 20% to 30%
  - Nausea, vomiting, headache, poor judgment
- 30% to 40%
  - Vision problems, dizziness, confusion, increased heart rate, increased respiratory function, muscle weakness
- 50% to 60%
  - Loss of consciousness
- Greater than 60%
  - Seizures, risk of death

Why the Test Is Performed

The test screens for exposure to breathing carbon monoxide and the underlying cause of headache, dizziness, vision problems, muscle weakness, confusion, extreme sleepiness, and nausea or vomiting.

Before Administering the Test

Assess if the patient:

- Has smoked before administering the test
- Has been exposed to carbon monoxide from automobiles and gas burning machines such as an old heating system

How the Test Is Performed

A sample of blood is taken from the patient's vein. The patient will experience a tight feeling when the tourniquet is tightened, a pinch or nothing at all when the needle is inserted into the vein, and pressure when a gauze pad is pressed against the insertion site to stop bleeding. It can take up to 10 minutes for bleeding to stop if the patient is taking anticoagulants (aspirin, coumadin). A small bruise might appear at the insertion site, which could become swollen following this test. This is called phlebitis. Applying a warm compress several times a day will reduce the swelling.

Teach the Patient

Explain why the blood sample is taken and that the patient must stop smoking before the test is administered.

Understanding the Test Results

Test results are available right away. The laboratory determines normal values based on calibration of testing equipment with a control test. Test results are reported as high, normal, or low based on the laboratory's control test.

- Normal range is:
  - Nonsmoker: less than 3% of total hemoglobin
  - Smoker: 2% to 10% of total hemoglobin

High level values may indicate carbon monoxide poisoning. Patients exposed to automobile traffic have normal carbon monoxide levels of 8% to 12%. A patient with 20% carbon monoxide level will show no symptoms of carbon monoxide poisoning. Women and children have fewer red blood cells than men and therefore have more severe symptoms at lower carbon monoxide levels. The healthcare provider will likely order an arterial blood gases and complete blood count tests if carbon monoxide levels are high.

Solved Problems

Carbon Dioxide

3.1   What are the three forms of carbon dioxide?

Bicarbonate (HCO_3), carbonic acid (H_2CO_3), and dissolved carbon dioxide (CO_2).

3.2   What is the most common form of carbon dioxide?

Most of the carbon dioxide is in the form of bicarbonate.

3.3   What balances types of carbon dioxide?

Levels of these types of carbon dioxide are balanced by the lungs and kidneys.

3.4   Why is the carbon dioxide test administered?

The carbon dioxide test is administered to assess lung and kidney functions.

3.5   What should you assess in the patient before administering the carbon dioxide test?

You should assess if the patient has taken corticosteroids, antibiotics, antacids, diuretics, aspirin, sodium bicarbonate, or barbiturates or has hyperthermia.

3.6   What would a high level of carbon dioxide indicate?

A high level of carbon dioxide indicates vomiting, pneumonia (respiratory acidosis), COPD (respiratory acidosis), Conn's syndrome (metabolic acidosis), alcoholism (metabolic acidosis), or Cushing's syndrome (metabolic acidosis).

Arterial Blood Gases

3.7   What does an arterial blood gas test measure?

An arterial blood gas test measures the partial pressure of oxygen and carbon dioxide.

3.8   What is the acidity of blood?

Acidity is measured using the pH scale, which measures the hydrogen ions (H+).

3.9   What is the purpose of bicarbonate?

Bicarbonate (HCO_3) is a chemical in the blood that ensures that the blood remains within the acceptable pH range.

3.10   What happens when blood is too acidic?

If blood becomes too acidic, the amount of bicarbonate is increased by increasing the absorption of bicarbonate by the kidneys.

3.11   What is the acceptable pH range of blood?

The pH of blood must be between 7.35 and 7.45 pH.

3.12   What is the purpose of measuring the oxygen saturation of blood?

Measuring the oxygen saturation of the blood indicates the amount of oxygen that hemoglobin is carrying.

3.13   What does it mean when blood has a pH greater than 7.45?

When it is greater than 7.45, the blood is too alkaline (basic).

3.14   Why is the arterial blood gas test ordered?

The arterial blood gas test screens gas exchange capabilities of the lungs, effectiveness of treatment for lung disease, blood acidity level, effectiveness of treatment for an imbalance of blood acidity, and kidney function.

3.15   What must you assess in the patient before administering the arterial blood gas test?

Assess if the patient:
- Has been taking anticoagulants (aspirin, coumadin, NSAIDs)
- Has taken any over-the-counter medications, since some contain aspirin. The test can still be performed. However, coagulation time following the test may be longer than 10 minutes.
- Has allergies, especially to anesthetics
- Has been exposed to conditions that might affect the test: anemia, polycytemia, exposure to smoke (including second-hand smoke), paint removers, or carbon monoxide
- Has abnormally high or low body temperature

3.16   What should you do if a patient is on oxygen therapy and requires an arterial blood gas test?

Discontinue oxygen therapy 20 minutes before the test unless the patient is unable to breathe without oxygen therapy. This assures that gas exchange measurement is based on room air without supplemental oxygen.

3.17   Why is there a risk of nerve damage as a result of administering the arterial blood gas?

Arteries are narrower and deeper than veins and are protected by nerves, making them sensitive to pain. Therefore, there is more pain experience collecting blood from an artery than collecting blood from a vein.

Carbon Monoxide

3.18   What is carboxyhemoglobin?

Carbon monoxide (CO) is a colorless, odorless gas that replaces oxygen attached to the hemoglobin red blood cells, creating a compound called carboxyhemoglobin.

3.19   What is the effect of carboxyhemoglobin?

Carboxyhemoglobin decreases oxygenation of blood and can result in death.

3.20   What does the carbon monoxide blood test measure?

The carbon monoxide blood test measures the level of carboxyhemoglobin in blood.

3.21   What is the purpose of the Quick Assessment test?

Quick Assessment is used to determine the level of carboxyhemoglobin in a patient's blood based on signs and symptoms.

3.22   What should be assessed in the patient before administering the carbon monoxide test?

Before administering the test, assess if the patient has smoked, and if the patient has been exposed to carbon monoxide from automobiles and gas burning machines such as an old heating system.

3.23   What can affect the normal range of the carbon monoxide test result?

Whether or not the patient is a smoker.

3.24   Why would women and children have more severe symptoms of carbon monoxide at lower carbon monoxide levels?

Women and children have fewer red blood cells than men and therefore have more severe symptoms at lower carbon monoxide levels.

3.25   How is the carbon monoxide test results reported?

High, normal, or low.

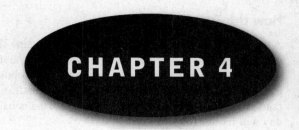

CHAPTER 4

Liver Tests

4.1 Definition

The liver:

- Synthesizes albumin, which maintains blood volume and clotting factors.
- Synthesizes, stores, and metabolizes fatty acids and cholesterol. Fatty acids are used for energy by the body.
- Stores and metabolizes carbohydrates. Carbohydrates are converted into glucose for energy.
- Forms and secretes bile. Bile contains acids that help the intestines absorb fats and vitamins A, D, E, and K, which are fat-soluble vitamins.
- Clears the body of medication and harmful chemicals such as bilirubin, which is the result of the metabolism of aged red blood cells, and ammonia, which is the result of metabolism of proteins.
- Transforms these chemicals into components that are easily excreted by the body in urine or stool.

4.2 Hepatitis A Virus Test

The hepatitis A virus test determines if the patient has hepatitis A antibodies. A patient who is or has been infected with the hepatitis A virus (HAV) has hepatitis A antibodies in his or her blood. A patient who received the hepatitis A virus vaccine will also have these antibodies.

- There are two types of antibodies:
  1. *IgM anti-HAV*: Presence of this antibody indicates that the patient was recently infected. This antibody is detectable 2 weeks after being infected and remains in the blood for 3 to 12 months.
  2. *IgG anti-HAV*: Presence of this antibody indicates that the patient has at some point been infected. This antibody is detectable between 8 and 12 weeks following the infection and remains in the blood.

Why the Test Is Performed

The test screens for hepatitis A virus infection. The test assesses the effectiveness of the hepatitis A vaccine, if the patient is protected against the hepatitis A vaccine, and if the infection from hepatitis A is the source of abnormal liver function tests.

Before Administering the Test

Consult the state's regulations to determine if cases of hepatitis A infection must be reported to the health department.
Assess if the patient has:

- Been taking anticoagulants (aspirin, coumadin, NSAIDs). Ask the patient if any over-the-counter medications have been taken, since some contain aspirin. The test can still be performed. However, coagulation time following the test may be longer than 10 minutes. If the vein is swollen after the test (phlebitis), apply a warm compress several times a day.

How the Test Is Performed

A sample of blood is taken from the patient's vein. The patient will experience a tight feeling when the tourniquet is tightened, a pinch or nothing at all when the needle is inserted into the vein, and pressure when a gauze pad is pressed against the insertion site to stop bleeding. It can take up to 10 minutes for bleeding to stop if the patient is taking anticoagulants (aspirin, coumadin). A small bruise might appear at the insertion site, which could become swollen following this test. This is called phlebitis. Applying a warm compress several times a day will reduce the swelling.

Teach the Patient

Explain why the test is administered and that a negative test result does not mean that the patient is infection-free. It takes 2 weeks or more to develop antibodies. A positive test result indicates the presence of antibodies and not the presences of the hepatitis A virus.

Understanding the Test Results

Results are available in 5 to 7 days and reported as positive (the presences of the antibody), or negative (the antibody was not found in the blood sample).

A negative test result does not mean that the patient is not infected with the hepatitis A virus. It can take 2 weeks or more before the antibodies are detectable. This is referred to as a false-negative.

A positive test result in the absence of the patient previously receiving the hepatitis A vaccine may be followed with liver function tests.

4.3 Hepatitis B Virus (HBV) Tests

The hepatitis B virus test determines if the patient has hepatitis B antibodies. Hepatitis B is a virus that can cause an infection. There are several hepatitis B virus tests used to determine if blood has signs of a hepatitis B virus (HBV).

There are three signs:

1. **HBV antibodies**: HBV antibodies are produced as part of the immune response to the presence of the HBV in the patient and may remain in the patient's blood long after the HBV is destroyed.
2. **HBV antigens**: HBV antigens are markers created by the HBV when the HBV infects the patient.
3. **HBV DNA**: HBV DNA is present when HBV infects the patient.

There are seven types of HBV tests. They are:

1. **Hepatitis B surface antigen (HBsAg)**: This is the first test that detects HBV antigen even before symptoms are present. It is also used to detect if the patient will be an HBV carrier and if the HBsAg level is elevated for more than 6 months.
2. **Hepatitis B surface Antibody (HBsAb)**: This test detects HBV antibodies, which are elevated 4 weeks after HBsAg is no longer detectable, and is used to determine if the patient requires an HBV vaccination.
3. **Hepatitis B e-antigen (HBeAg)**: This test detects the HBeAg antigen, which is present if the patient is currently infected and is used to monitor HBV treatment.
4. **Hepatitis DNA test**: This test determines the level of HBV DNA in the patient's blood, and is used to monitor treatment for chronic HBV infection.
5. **Hepatitis B core Antibody (HBcAb)**: This test detects the HBcAb antibody a month after the HBV infection and is used to screen the transfused blood for hepatitis B.
6. **Hepatitis B core antibody IgM (HBcAbIgM)**: This test detects the HBcAbIgM antibody within 6 months of the patient becoming infected with HBV.
7. **Hepatitis B e-antibody (HBeAb)**: This test detects the HBeAb antibody, indicating that the patient has almost recovered from an acute HBV infection.

The healthcare provider may also order the following liver function tests: alanine aminotransferase (ALT), alkaline phosphatase, bilirubin, and aspartate aminotransferase (AST).

Why the Test Is Performed

The test assesses for hepatitis B virus infection (if transfused blood is or was infected with the hepatitis B virus), the effect of the hepatitis B vaccination, and the treatment of the hepatitis B virus.

Before Administering the Test

A negative test result does not rule out HBV, since signs of HBV can take weeks to develop. A patient who received an HBV vaccination may have HBsAb antibodies. A patient who received an HBV vaccination is protected against hepatitis D infection.

How the Test Is Performed

A sample of blood is taken from the patient's vein. The patient will experience a tight feeling when the tourniquet is tightened, a pinch or nothing at all when the needle is inserted into the vein, and pressure when a gauze pad is pressed against the insertion site to stop bleeding. It can take up to 10 minutes for bleeding to stop if the patient is taking anticoagulants (aspirin, coumadin). A small bruise might appear at the insertion site, which could become swollen following this test. This is called phlebitis. Applying a warm compress several times a day will reduce the swelling.

Teach the Patient

Explain why the sample is taken.

Understanding the Test Results

The HBV test results are available quickly.

- Normal HBV level is negative: No antigens, antibodies, or DNA
- Abnormal HBV level is positive: Antigens, antibodies, or DNA is present in a patient who has not received immunization

Consult your local laws to determine if HBV infections must be reported to the health department.

4.4   Alanine Aminotransferase (ALT)

The alanine aminotransferase test determines if the patient has alanine aminotransferase enzyme in the blood. *Alanine aminotransferase* (ALT), formerly called serum glutamic pyruvic transaminase (SGPT), is an enzyme mainly found in the liver, but is also in the heart, pancreas, muscles, and kidneys in small amounts. Damage to the liver caused by injury or disease results in the release of ALT in the blood. The alanine aminotransferase test measures the level of ALT in the blood as a way to detect liver disease. The alanine aminotransferase test is typically performed with the aspartate aminotransferase (AST) test to detect liver damage. Other tests that detect liver problems are the lactate dehydrogenase (LDH) test and the bilirubin test.

Why the Test Is Performed

The test screens for liver disorders and assesses the effects of medications that can cause liver damage, and for the underlying cause of jaundice.

Before Administering the Test

Assess if the patient:

- Has performed strenuous exercise before the test is administered. Strenuous exercise can affect the test results.
- Is pregnant. This can affect the test results.

- Has taken Echinacea or valerian and other herbal and natural treatments. If so, the patient should refrain from taking these for several days before the test, since they can affect the test results.
- Is allergic to any medications.
- Recently received any IM injections, injured a muscle, had cardiac catheterization or surgery. These can release ALT from injured muscle and affect the results of the test.
- Has taken prescription and non-prescription medications. Medications such as narcotics, barbiturates, antibiotics, chemotherapy, and statins affect the test results and should be stopped several days before taking the test.

How the Test Is Performed

A sample of blood is taken from the patient's vein. The patient will experience a tight feeling when the tourniquet is tightened, a pinch or nothing at all when the needle is inserted into the vein, and pressure when a gauze pad is pressed against the insertion site to stop bleeding. It can take up to 10 minutes for bleeding to stop if the patient is taking anticoagulants (aspirin, coumadin). A small bruise might appear at the insertion site, which could become swollen following this test. This is called phlebitis. Applying a warm compress several times a day will reduce the swelling.

Teach the Patient

Explain why the blood sample is taken. ALT testing is part of routine blood screening. Inform the patient that the ALT enzyme can be abnormal for a number of reasons, and therefore other testing is necessary to confirm an abnormal ALT test result. The patient should make it known before the test is performed if he or she:

- Performed strenuous exercise
- Has taken narcotics, barbiturates, antibiotics, chemotherapy, and statins
- Takes Echinacea or valerian and other herbal and natural treatments
- Experienced anything that could cause a muscle injury such as IM injections, injured a muscle, cardiac catheterization, or surgery

Understanding the Test Results

Test results are available in 12 hours. The laboratory determines normal values based on calibration of testing equipment with a control test. Test results are reported as high, normal, or low based on the laboratory's control test.

- Generally the normal range is: 4 to 36 U/L or 0.07 to 0.62 microKat/L

Slightly high levels may indicate chronic diseases that affect the liver, cirrhosis, fat deposits in the liver, or medications such as narcotics, barbiturates, antibiotics, chemotherapy, and statins.

Moderately high levels may indicate excessive amounts of acetaminophen, alcohol abuse, mononucleosis, hepatitis, or that the young child is growing quickly.

Very high levels may indicate necrosis, lead poisoning, shock, carbon tetrachloride exposure, reaction to medication, severe liver damage, recent liver damage, viral hepatitis, or rapid progression of acute lymphocytic leukemia (ALL) in a child.

4.5 Alkaline Phosphatase (ALP)

The alkaline phosphatase test determines if the patient has alkaline phosphatase enzyme in the blood. *Alkaline phosphatase* (ALP) is an enzyme produced mainly in the liver and is also produced by bones, kidneys, intestines, and placenta. The alkaline phosphatase test measures the level of ALP in blood. An alkaline phosphatase isoenzymes test is likely to be ordered if the ALP level is high. If the ALP level is high, the healthcare provider might order an ultrasound or CT scan, the gamma glutamyl transferase (GGT) test, the 5-nucleotidase, or the gamma glutamyl transpeptidase test to differentiate between bone ALP and liver ALP.

Why the Test Is Performed

The test screens for liver disease, medication damage to the liver, rickets, osteomalacia, Paget's disease, or bone tumors. The test also assesses treatment for Paget's disease, rickets, and osteomalacia, and the underlying cause of a high calcium level in blood.

Before Administering the Test

There is no special preparation required for this test.

If ALP is high, the healthcare provider orders a second test and asks the patient to refrain from eating or drinking 10 hours before the test. ALP increases after eating.

Assess if the patient:

- Has taken antibiotics, birth control pills, oral diabetes medication, or aspirin therapy
- Is pregnant, and the gestation age of the fetus. The placenta produces ALP in the third trimester.
- Is postmenopausal. The patient will have a high level of ALP.
- Is a child, since rapid bone growth increases ALP levels
- Uses alcohol, since this affects the test result

How the Test Is Performed

A sample of blood is taken from the patient's vein. The patient will experience a tight feeling when the tourniquet is tightened, a pinch or nothing at all when the needle is inserted into the vein, and pressure when a gauze pad is pressed against the insertion site to stop bleeding. It can take up to 10 minutes for bleeding to stop if the patient is taking anticoagulants (aspirin, coumadin). A small bruise might appear at the insertion site, which could become swollen following this test. This is called phlebitis. Applying a warm compress several times a day will reduce the swelling.

Teach the Patient

Explain why the blood sample is taken, the function of alkaline phosphatase, and the meaning of abnormal values. State that the patient may be asked to take the alkaline phosphatase test a second time if the test result indicates a high level of ALP. For the second test, the patient will be asked to refrain from eating or drinking 10 hours before the test. ALP increases after eating.

Understanding the Test Results

Test results are available in 2 to 5 days. The laboratory determines normal values based on calibration of testing equipment with a control test. Test results are reported as high, normal, or low based on the laboratory's control test.

- Generally, the normal range is:
  ○ Adult: 30 to 126 U/L or 0.5 to 2.0 microkat/L
  ○ Children: 30 to 300 U/L or 0.5 to 5.0 microkat/L

A high level may indicate:

- *Very high level*: gallstones, hepatitis, obstructive jaundice, cancer metastasized to the liver, liver disease
- *High level*: rickets, Paget's disease, osteomalacia, cancer metastasized to the bone, bone tumors, hyperparathyroidism, mononucleosis, kidney cancer, heart failure, heart attack, sepsis, bone healing
- *Low level*: malnutrition, scurvy, celiac disease

It is normal for a pregnant woman in the third trimester to have increased ALP because the placenta makes ALP. It is normal for a child who is experiencing rapid bone growth to have increased ALP.

4.6 Ammonia

The ammonia test measures the ammonia level in blood. Ammonia is formed when bacteria in the intestines breaks down protein. Ammonia is then converted into urea by the liver, which is excreted by the kidney in urine. If the liver is unable to convert ammonia to urea, ammonia levels in blood increase, indicating that there may be a liver function problem.

Why the Test Is Performed

The test screens for liver function, Reye's syndrome, hyperalimentation, cirrhosis, and acute liver failure. The test also assesses treatment of liver disease.

Before Administering the Test

Assess if the patient:

- Has eaten or drunk anything other than water 8 hours before the test
- Smoked 8 hours before the test
- Performed strenuous exercise before the test
- Is constipated
- Has eaten a high or low protein diet
- Is taking furosemide, heparin, valproic acid, acetazolamide, neomycin, tetracycline, lactuolse, Marplan, nardil, diphenhydramine, or Parnate. The patient will be asked to refrain from taking these medications several days before the test.
- Has confusion, sleepiness, hand tremors or coma, which could be signs of high ammonia levels

How the Test Is Performed

A sample of blood is taken from the patient's vein. The patient will experience a tight feeling when the tourniquet is tightened, a pinch or nothing at all when the needle is inserted into the vein, and pressure when a gauze pad is pressed against the insertion site to stop bleeding. It can take up to 10 minutes for bleeding to stop if the patient is taking anticoagulants (aspirin, coumadin). A small bruise might appear at the insertion site, which could become swollen following this test. This is called phlebitis. Applying a warm compress several times a day will reduce the swelling.

Teach the Patient

Explain why the blood sample is taken, the function of ammonia, and the meaning of abnormal values. Inform that patient that he/she must refrain from smoking, eating, or drinking anything except water for 8 hours and avoid strenuous exercise before the test. The patient should consult with the healthcare provider about whether he or she should stop taking furosemide, heparin, valproic acid, acetazolamide, neomycin, tetracycline, lactulose, Marplan, nardil, diphenhydramine, or Parnate several days before the test.

Understanding the Test Results

Test results are available in 12 hours. The laboratory determines normal values based on calibration of testing equipment with a control test. Test results are reported as high, normal, or low based on the laboratory's control test.

- Generally the normal range is:
  - Adults: 15 to 45 mcg/dL or 11 to 32 mcmol/L
  - Children: 40 to 80 mcg/dL or 28 to 57 mcmol/L
  - Newborns: 90 to 150 mcg/dL or 64 to 107 mcmol/L

A high level may indicate cirrhosis, hepatitis, Reye's syndrome, heart failure, bleeding from intestines or stomach, hemolytic disease of the newborn (incompatible blood types of mother and fetus), or kidney failure.

Lactulose is a laxative that reduces the intestinal bacteria's production of ammonia. Ammonia levels might be slightly elevated in a patient who has severe cirrhosis. Newborns normally have high levels of ammonia which is temporary.

4.7   Aspartate Aminotransferase (AST)

The Aspartate aminotransferase test measures the Aspartate aminotransferase enzyme level in blood. *Aspartate aminotransferase* (AST), previously known as serum glutamic oxaloacetic transaminase (SGOT), is an enzyme in the liver, heart, pancreas, kidneys, red blood cells, and muscle tissues. When these tissues or cells are damaged there is an increase of AST in the blood 6 to 10 hours after the damage, and it remains for four days. The healthcare provider orders tests to measure AST and ALT in a normal screen for liver damage and liver disease. The AST test is more effective in detecting liver damage caused by alcohol abuse than the ALT test. As the patient recovers from tissue damage, the AST level in the blood decreases.

Why the Test Is Performed

The test screens for liver damage, hepatitis, and cirrhosis. The test also assesses the treatment for liver disease, the underlying cause of jaundice, and if a medication is causing liver damage.

Before Administering the Test

Assess if the patient:

- Performed strenuous exercise before administering the test, since this can affect the test result
- Is taking Echinacea, valerian, or other herbs, since this can affect the test result. The patient may be required to stop taking these for several days before the test is administered.
- Is pregnant
- Takes mega doses of vitamin A
- Has had surgery, cardiac catheterization, recent IM injections or injury to muscle, since these can cause an increase in AST level in blood
- Has recently taken antibiotics, narcotics, statins, and barbiturates, or is undergoing chemotherapy

How the Test Is Performed

A sample of blood is taken from the patient's vein. The patient will experience a tight feeling when the tourniquet is tightened, a pinch or nothing at all when the needle is inserted into the vein, and pressure when a gauze pad is pressed against the insertion site to stop bleeding. It can take up to 10 minutes for bleeding to stop if the patient is taking anticoagulants (aspirin, coumadin). A small bruise might appear at the insertion site, which could become swollen following this test. This is called phlebitis. Applying a warm compress several times a day will reduce the swelling.

Teach the Patient

Explain why the blood sample is taken, the function of AST, and the meaning of abnormal values. Inform the patient that he/she must refrain from taking Echinacea, valerian, and vitamin A, and that the patient must notify the healthcare provider if the patient is taking antibiotics, narcotics, statins, and barbiturates, or is undergoing chemotherapy.

Understanding the Test Results

Test results are available within 12 hours. The laboratory determines normal values based on calibration of testing equipment with a control test. Test results are reported as high, normal, or low based on the laboratory's control test.

- Generally, the normal range is: 8 to 35 U/L or 0.14 to 0.58 microKat/L

A slightly high level may indicate fatty deposits in the liver, alcohol abuse, excessive acetaminophen, or that the patient has taken antibiotics, narcotics, statins, barbiturates, or is undergoing chemotherapy.

A moderately high level may indicate cirrhosis, chronic disease that directly or indirectly affects the liver, kidney damage, lung damage, Duchenne muscular dystrophy, mega dose of vitamin A, heart attack, heart failure, mononucleosis, cancer, myositis, or alcohol abuse.

A very high level may indicate viral hepatitis, necrosis, shock, drug reaction, burns, pulmonary embolism, trauma, heatstroke, or poison.

4.8 Bilirubin

The bilirubin test measures the bilirubin level in blood. The liver breaks down old red blood cells into bilirubin, which becomes the brownish yellow component of bile. Bilirubin is excreted through feces. Bilirubin gives feces their brown color. Indirect (unconjugated) bilirubin, which is insoluble in water, is carried by the blood to the liver, where indirect bilirubin is transformed into direct bilirubin. Direct bilirubin is soluble in water. The bilirubin test measures the total bilirubin level in the blood and the direct bilirubin level in the blood. Indirect bilirubin is measured by subtracting the direct bilirubin level from the total bilirubin level. Bilirubin can also be measured in urine.

Why the Test Is Performed

The test screens for liver function, hepatitis, cirrhosis, blocked bile duct from gallstones or pancreatic tumor, hemolytic anemia, hemolytic disease, neonatal jaundice, and liver damage caused by medication.

Before Administering the Test

Assess if the patient:

- Has eaten or drunk 4 hours before the test
- Has taken aspirin or coumadin
- Is pregnant
- Has taken caffeine. This can lower bilirubin levels.
- Has fasted for a long period. This increases indirect bilirubin levels
- Has taken dilantin, valium, indocin, birth control pills, or Dalmane, since these medications can increase bilirubin levels
- Has taken theophylline, phenobarbital, or ascorbic acid (Vitamin C), since these can lower bilirubin levels

How the Test Is Performed

A sample of blood is taken from the patient's vein or a heel stick is used.

Heel Stick: The heel is cleaned using alcohol. A sterile lancet is used to puncture the heel. Several drops of blood are collected in a small test tube. A gauze pad is pressed over the site until bleeding stops. A small bandage is applied.

A transcutaneous bilirubin meter may be used to measure the bilirubin level in a newborn. This handheld meter is placed against the skin. The skin is not punctured. If the bilirubin level is high, then the heel stick test is used to collect a blood sample from the newborn.

Vein: A sample of blood is taken from the patient's vein. The patient will experience a tight feeling when the tourniquet is tightened, a pinch or nothing at all when the needle is inserted into the vein, and pressure when a gauze pad is pressed against the insertion site to stop bleeding. It can take up to 10 minutes for bleeding to stop if the patient is taking anticoagulants (aspirin, coumadin). A small bruise might appear at the insertion site, which could become swollen following this test. This is called phlebitis. Applying a warm compress several times a day will reduce the swelling.

Teach the Patient

Explain why the blood sample is taken, the function of bilirubin, and the meaning of abnormal values. The patient must refrain from eating echinacea, valerian, or other herbs, and should also refrain from eating or drinking anything for 4 hours before the test is administered. The healthcare provider may want the patient to stop taking aspirin, coumadin, dilantin, valium, indocin, birth control pills, Dalmane, theophylline, phenobarbital, or ascorbic acid and caffeine several days before the test is administered.

Understanding the Test Results

Test results are available in 2 hours. The laboratory determines normal values based on calibration of testing equipment with a control test. Test results are reported as high, normal, or low based on the laboratory's control test.

- Normal range is:
  - Total bilirubin: 0.3 to 1.0 mg/dL or 5.1 to 17.0 mmol/L
  - Direct bilirubin: 0.1 to 0.3 mg/dL or 1.0 to 5.1 mmol/L
  - Indirect bilirubin: 0.2 to 0.7 mg/dL or 3.4 to 11.9 mmol/L
- Normal range for newborns:
  - Less than 24 hours old:
    - Full-term: Less than 6.0 mg/dL or less than 103 mmol/L
    - Premature: Less than 8.0 mg/dL or less than 137 mmol/L
  - Less than 48 hours old:
    - Full-term: Less than 10.0 mg/dL or less than 170 mmol/L
    - Premature: Less than 12.0 mg/dL or less than 205 mmol/L
  - 3 days to 5 days old:
    - Full-term: Less than 12.0 mg/dL or less than 205 mmol/L
    - Premature: Less than 15.0 mg/dL or less than 256 mmol/L
  - 7 days or older:
    - Full-term: Less than 10.0 mg/dL or less than 170 mmol/L
    - Premature: Less than 15.0 mg/dL or less than 256 mmol/L

A high level may indicate cholecystitis, infected gallbladder, hepatitis, cirrhosis, mononucleosis, blocked bile duct, gallstones, pancreatic cancer, Gilbert's syndrome, sickle cell disease, transfusion reaction, or that the patient has taken dilantin, valium, indocin, birth control pills, or Dalmane.

- High levels for newborns:
  - 24 hours old or less: More than 10 mg/dL or more than 170 mmol/L
  - 25 hours to 48 hours old: More than 15 mg/dL or more than 255 mmol/L
  - 49 hours to 72 hours old: More than 18 mg/dL or more than 205 mmol/L
  - More than 72 hours old: More than 20 mg/dL or more than 340 mmol/L

A low level may indicate that the patient has taken theophylline, phenobarbital, or ascorbic acid.

Newborns can experience physiologic jaundice between 1 and 3 days old because the newborn is unable to break down red blood cells. This usually resolves in a week. The healthcare provider may order phototherapy to prevent collateral problems from developing.

Solved Problems

Hepatitis A Virus

4.1   What are the two types of hepatitis A virus antibodies?

IgM anti-HAV antibodies indicate that the patient was recently infected. This antibody is detectable 2 weeks after being infected, and remains in the blood for 3 to 12 months. *IgG anti-HAV* antibodies indicate that the patient has been infected at some point. This antibody is detectable between 8 and 12 weeks following the infection, and remains in the blood.

4.2   What should you assess in the patient before administering the hepatitis A virus test?

Assess whether the patient has been taking anticoagulants (aspirin, coumadin, NSAIDs). Ask the patient if any over-the-counter medications have been taken, since some contain aspirin. The test can still be performed. However, coagulation time following the test may be longer than 10 minutes. If the vein is swollen after the test (phlebitis), apply a warm compress several times a day.

4.3 Does a negative test result mean that the patient is free of infection?

A negative test result does not mean that the patient is free of infection. It takes two weeks or more to develop antibodies.

4.4 Does a positive test result mean that the patient has the virus?

A positive test result indicates the presence of antibodies and not the presence of the hepatitis A virus.

Hepatitis B Virus

4.5 What are the three signs of the hepatitis B virus?

HBV antibodies are produced as part of the immune response to the presence of the HBV in the patient and may remain in the patient's blood long after the HBV is destroyed. *HBV antigens* are markers created by the HBV when the HBV infects the patient. *HBV DNA* is present when HBV infects the patient.

4.6 What does the hepatitis B surface antigen test detect?

This is the first test that detects the HBV antigen even before symptoms are present. It is also used to detect if the patient will be an HBV carrier if the HBsAg level is elevated for more than 6 months.

4.7 What does the hepatitis DNA test detect?

This test determines the level of HBV DNA in the patient's blood and is used to monitor treatment for chronic HBV infection.

4.8 What does the hepatitis B e-antibody test detect?

This test detects the HBeAb antibody, indicating that the patient has almost recovered from an acute HBV infection.

4.9 What should you teach the patient about the hepatitis B virus tests?

A negative test result does not rule out HBV, since signs of HBV can take weeks to develop. A patient who received an HBV vaccination may have HBsAb antibodies. A patient who received an HBV vaccination is protected against hepatitis D infection.

Alanine Aminotransferase

4.10 Why is the alanine aminotransferase test ordered?

The alanine aminotransferase test screens for liver disorders and assesses the effects of medications that can cause liver damage and the underlying cause of jaundice.

4.11 What must be assessed before administering the alanine aminotransferase test?

Assess if the patient:
- Has performed strenuous exercise before the test is administered. Strenuous exercise can affect the test results.
- Is pregnant. This can affect the test results.
- Has taken Echinacea or valerian and other herbal and natural treatments. If so, the patient should refrain from taking these for several days before the test, since they can affect the test results
- Is allergic to any medications
- Recently received any IM injections, injured a muscle, had cardiac catheterization, or surgery. These can release ALT from the injured muscle and affect the results of the test.

Identify prescription and nonprescription medications taken by the patient. Medications such as narcotics, barbiturates, antibiotics, chemotherapy, and statins affect the test results and should be stopped several days before taking the test.

4.12 What might a slightly high level of alanine aminotransferase indicate?

A slightly high level of alanine aminotransferase might indicate chronic diseases that affect the liver such as cirrhosis, fat deposits in the liver, or medications such as narcotics, barbiturates, antibiotics, chemotherapy, and statins.

4.13   What might a very high level of alanine aminotransferase indicate?

A very high level of alanine aminotransferase might indicate necrosis, lead poisoning, shock, carbon tetrachloride exposure, reaction to medication, severe liver damage, recent liver damage, viral hepatitis, or rapid progression of acute lymphocytic leukemia (ALL) in a child.

Alkaline Phosphatase

4.14   What is alkaline phosphatase?

Alkaline phosphatase (ALP) is an enzyme produced mainly in the liver, and is also produced by bones, kidneys, intestines, and placenta.

4.15   Why is the alkaline phosphatase test ordered?

The alkaline phosphatase test screens for liver disease, medication damage to the liver, rickets, osteomalacia, Paget's disease, and bone tumor.

4.16   How should the patient prepare for the alkaline phosphatase test?

There is no special preparation required for this test.

4.17   What should you assess in the patient prior to the Alkaline phosphatase test?

Assess if the patient is:
• Taking antibiotics
• Taking birth control pills
• Taking oral diabetes medication
• On aspirin therapy
• Pregnant, and the gestation age of the fetus. The placenta produces ALP in the third trimester
• Postmenopausal. The patient will have a high level of ALP.
• A child, since rapid bone growth increases ALP levels
• Using alcohol, since this affects the test results

4.18   What might a very high level of alkaline phosphatase indicate?

A very high level of alkaline phosphatase might indicate gallstones, hepatitis, obstructive jaundice, cancer metastasized to the liver, or liver disease.

4.19   Why might a pregnant woman have increased ALP?

It is normal for a pregnant woman in the third trimester to have increased ALP because the placenta makes ALP.

4.20   Why might a child have increased ALP?

It is normal for a child who is experiencing rapid bone growth to have an increased ALP.

Ammonia

4.21   How is ammonia formed in the body?

Ammonia is formed when bacteria in the intestines break down protein.

4.22   Why would ammonia levels increase in blood?

Ammonia is converted into urea by the liver, which is excreted by the kidney in urine. If the liver is unable to convert ammonia to urea, ammonia levels in blood increase, indicating that there may be a liver function problem.

4.23   Why is the ammonia test ordered?

An ammonia test is ordered to screen for liver function, Reye's syndrome, hyperalimentation, cirrhosis, and acute liver failure. The ammonia test is also a tool to assess for treatment of liver disease.

4.24   What signs indicate high ammonia levels in blood?

Signs of high ammonia levels in blood are confusion, sleepiness, hand tremors, or coma.

4.25 What should you assess in the patient before administering the ammonia test?

Assess if the patient:
- Has eaten and drunk anything other than water 8 hours before the test
- Smoked 8 hours before the test
- Performed strenuous exercise before the test
- Is constipated
- Has eaten a high or low protein diet
- Is taking furosemide, heparin, valproic acid, acetazolamide, neomycin, tetracycline, lactulose, Marplan, Nardil, diphenhydramine, or Parnate. The patient will be asked to refrain from taking these medications several days before the test.

4.26 What might a high ammonia level indicate?

A high ammonia level might indicate cirrhosis, hepatitis, Reye's syndrome, heart failure, bleeding from intestines or stomach, hemolytic disease of the newborn (incompatible blood types of mother and fetus), or kidney failure.

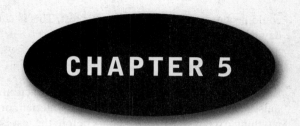

CHAPTER 5

Cardiac Enzymes and Markers Tests

5.1   Definition

When a patient is suspected of having a myocardial infarction, the healthcare provider will order cardiac enzymes and cardiac marker tests to determine if cardiac muscle enzymes appear in the patient's blood. Cardiac muscle contains enzymes. In a myocardial infarction, cardiac muscle is damaged, causing the release of cardiac enzymes into the bloodstream. It can take between 2 and 24 hours for cardiac muscle enzymes to reach a detectable level in blood. Healthcare providers typically use an EKG to diagnose the acute phase of a myocardial infarction. The cardiac enzyme and cardiac marker tests are used to confirm a previous acute myocardial infarction.

5.2   Brain Natriuretic Peptide (BNP) Test

The heart produces the hormone brain natriuretic peptide (BNP). A low level of BNP is normally found in blood. BNP level increases when the heart works harder for long periods, such as in heart failure. The brain natriuretic peptide test measures the level of BNP in the blood. The healthcare provider may order the N-terminal probrain-natriuretic peptide (NT-proBNP) test that measures the NT-proBNP hormone, which provides similar diagnostic results as the BNP test.

Why the Test Is Performed

The test is performed to screen for heart failure and to assess the treatment for heart failure.

Before Administering the Test

Assess if the patient:

- Has eaten or drunk anything except water for 12 hours before the test is administered
- Is taking diuretics or cardiac glycosides, which affect the test results
- Has had a heart attack, kidney dialysis and kidney disease, COPD
- Is taking Echinacea, valerian, or other herbs, since this can affect the test result. The patient may be required to stop taking these for several days before the test is administered.

How the Test Is Performed

A sample of blood is taken from the patient's vein. The patient will experience a tight feeling when the tourniquet is tightened, a pinch or nothing at all when the needle is inserted into the vein, and pressure when a gauze pad is pressed against the insertion site to stop bleeding. It can take up to 10 minutes for bleeding to stop if the patient is taking anticoagulants (aspirin, coumadin). A small bruise might appear at the insertion site, which could become swollen following this test. This is called phlebitis. Applying a warm compress several times a day will reduce the swelling.

Teach the Patient

Explain why the blood sample is taken, the function of BNP, and the meaning of abnormal values. The patient must refrain from ingesting Echinacea, valerian, or other herbs, and should refrain from eating or drinking anything except water for 12 hours before the test is administered.

Understanding the Test Results

Test results are available quickly. The laboratory determines normal values based on calibration of testing equipment with a control test. Test results are reported as high, normal, or low based on the laboratory's control test.

- Generally the normal range is: 0 to 99 pg/mL or 0 to 99 ng/L

A slightly high level may indicate minimum heart failure: 100 to 300 pg/mL or 100 to 300 ng/L.

A moderately high level may indicate mild heart failure: 300 pg/mL or 300 ng/L.
A high level may indicate moderate heart failure: 600 pg/mL or 600 ng/L.
A very high level may indicate severe heart failure: 900 pg/mL or 900 ng/L.

An abnormal level of BNP indicates there is increased pressure inside the heart, and may indicate heart failure if the patient is on kidney dialysis.

5.3 Cardiac Enzyme Studies

The cells of heart muscles and other tissues contain the enzyme creatinine phosphokinase (CK, CPK) and the protein troponin (TnT, TnI). Creatinine phosphokinase and troponin enter the blood when heart muscle and other tissues are damaged. If levels of creatinine phosphokinase and troponin are abnormal, the healthcare provider orders an electrocardiogram to differentiate between heart muscle damage and other tissue damage. Troponin and CPK-MB are mostly found in cardiac muscle. Blood samples are taken every 12 hours for 2 days following a suspected heart attack. It takes 6 hours for troponin levels to rise after a heart attack. The healthcare provider may order a myoglobin test along with the cardiac enzymes test to help diagnose a heart attack.

Why the Test Is Performed

The test is performed to screen for a heart attack, heart muscle injury following bypass surgery, and unstable angina. The test also assesses the results of percutaneous coronary intervention (PCI) or thrombolytic medication to restore blood flow through the coronary artery.

Before Administering the Test

Assess if the patient:

- Has Reye's syndrome, muscular dystrophy, myocarditis, autoimmune diseases, or cardiac disease
- Has undergone cardioversion or defibrillation
- Has recently received an intramuscular injection
- Has had recent surgery
- Has undergone strenuous exercise before the test is administered
- Is taking statins
- Abuses alcohol
- Has kidney failure

How the Test Is Performed

A sample of blood is taken from the patient's vein. The patient will experience a tight feeling when the tourniquet is tightened, a pinch or nothing at all when the needle is inserted into the vein, and pressure when a gauze pad is pressed against the insertion site to stop bleeding. It can take up to 10 minutes for bleeding to stop if the patient is taking anticoagulants (aspirin, coumadin). A small bruise might appear at the insertion site, which could become swollen following this test. This is called phlebitis. Applying a warm compress several times a day will reduce the swelling.

Teach the Patient

Explain why the blood sample is taken, that the patient should not exercise before the test is administered, that the patient should not receive an intramuscular injection before the test is administered, and that the healthcare provider may request that the patient stops taking statins for two weeks prior to the test.

Understanding the Test Results

Test results are available in 1 hour. The laboratory determines normal values based on calibration of testing equipment with a control test. Test results are reported as high, normal, or low based on the laboratory's control test.

- Normal troponin range is:
  - TnI: less than 0.3 mcg/L
  - TnT: less than 0.1 mcg/L
- Normal total creatine phosphokinase range is:
  - Men: 55 to 170 IU/L
  - Women: 30 to 135 IU/L
- Normal creatine phosphokinase-MB range is: less than 3.0 ng/mL

High troponin values may indicate cardiac muscle injury. The troponin level increases 4 hours after the cardiac muscle injury, and reaches the highest level 24 hours after the cardiac muscle injury. The troponin level returns to normal levels in 10 days following the cardiac muscle injury.

High total creatine phosphokinase values may indicate cardiac muscle injury or tissue injury. Total creatine phosphokinase increases 4 hours after the cardiac muscle injury, and reaches the highest level 24 hours after the cardiac muscle injury. The total creatine phosphokinase level returns to normal levels in 3 days following the cardiac muscle injury.

High creatine phosphokinase-MB values may indicate cardiac muscle injury. Creatine phosphokinase-MB increases 2 hours after the cardiac muscle injury, and reaches the highest level 24 hours after the cardiac muscle injury. The creatine phosphokinase-MB level returns to normal levels in 3 days following the cardiac muscle injury. If levels are high after 3 days, additional cardiac muscle is being damaged and the heart attack is continuing.

5.4 Homocysteine

Homocysteine is an amino acid found in blood. Increased homocysteine levels, along with increased levels of cholesterol, can lead to a risk of stroke, deep venous thrombosis, heart attack, and pulmonary embolism. The homocysteine test measures the level of homocysteine in blood. The healthcare provider may order the homocysteine test for a patient who has a family history of heart disease but who has not exhibited other risk factors. The healthcare provider may order a urine homocysteine test.

Why the Test Is Performed

The test is performed to assess risk for stroke and heart attack.

Before Administering the Test

The patient must avoid eating and drinking anything except water for 12 hours before the test is administered.
   Assess if the patient:

- Has eaten or drunk anything except water 12 hours before the test
- Is currently hypertensive
- Smokes

- Has psoriasis, leukemia, kidney disease, or homocystinuria
- Is experiencing menopause
- Is deficient in vitamin B_{12}, vitamin B_6, and folic acid
- Drinks three or more cups of coffee daily
- Is taking birth control pills, theophylline, tamoxifen, antibiotics, or anticonvulsants
- Has a family history of elevated homocysteine
- Is a diabetic

How the Test Is Performed

A sample of blood is taken from the patient's vein. The patient will experience a tight feeling when the tourniquet is tightened, a pinch or nothing at all when the needle is inserted into the vein, and pressure when a gauze pad is pressed against the insertion site to stop bleeding. It can take up to 10 minutes for bleeding to stop if the patient is taking anticoagulants (aspirin, coumadin). A small bruise might appear at the insertion site, which could become swollen following this test. This is called phlebitis. Applying a warm compress several times a day will reduce the swelling.

Teach the Patient

Explain why the sample is taken and that the patient cannot eat or drink anything except water 12 hours before the test. The healthcare provider may ask the patient to refrain from taking birth control pills, theophylline, tamoxifen, antibiotics, or anticonvulsants two weeks prior to the test.

Understanding the Test Results

The homocysteine test results are available in 24 hours. The laboratory determines normal values based on calibration of testing equipment with a control test. Test results are reported as high, normal, or low based on the laboratory's control test.

- Normal homocysteine test results: 4 to 14 µmol/L

A high homocysteine level may indicate homocystinuria, hypothyroidism, kidney disease, Alzheimer's disease, inflammatory bowel disease, or a diet deficient in vitamin B_{12}, vitamin B_6, or folic acid.

A low homocysteine level may indicate diabetes.
The homocysteine level naturally increases with age.

5.5   Renin Assay

Blood pressure is regulated by the renin-angiotensin system (RAS). Low blood pressure causes the secretion of the renin enzyme by the kidneys. The renin enzyme increases angiotensin production, which constricts blood vessels, resulting in increased blood pressure. Angiotensin causes the adrenal cortex to replace aldosterone, which causes the kidneys to retain water and sodium. This results in an increase in fluid volume and in blood pressure. The renin assay test measures the level of renin in blood. The healthcare provider may also order the aldosterone test. The renin stimulation test may be ordered if the renin level is low.

Why the Test Is Performed

The test is performed to assess the underlying cause of hypertension.

Before Administering the Test

Assess if the patient:

- Has eaten natural black licorice two weeks before the test
- Has ingested caffeine 24 hours before the test

- Has eaten or drunk 8 hours before the test
- Maintained a low sodium diet three days before the test
- Has taken beta-blockers, corticosteroids, ACE inhibitors, estrogen, aspirin, or diuretics four weeks before the test
- Has relaxed two hours before the first blood sample is taken
- Has ambulated for two hours after the first blood sample is taken and before the second blood sample is taken
- Is pregnant
- Was upright when the sample is taken

How the Test Is Performed

Avoid:

- Eating natural black licorice for 2 weeks before the test.
- Ingesting caffeine 24 hours before the test.
- Eating or drinking 8 hours before the test.

The patient must:

- Maintain a low sodium diet for 3 days before the test.
- Relax for 2 hours before the first blood sample is taken.
- Ambulate for 2 hours after the first blood sample is taken and before the second blood sample is taken.
- The patient should be upright when the sample is taken.

A sample of blood is taken from the patient's vein. The patient will experience a tight feeling when the tourniquet is tightened, a pinch or nothing at all when the needle is inserted into the vein, and pressure when a gauze pad is pressed against the insertion site to stop bleeding. It can take up to 10 minutes for bleeding to stop if the patient is taking anticoagulants (aspirin, coumadin). A small bruise might appear at the insertion site, which could become swollen following this test. This is called phlebitis. Applying a warm compress several times a day will reduce the swelling.

Teach the Patient

Explain why the sample is taken and that two samples are taken—one after resting for two hours and another after ambulating for two hours. The healthcare provider may ask the patient to refrain from taking Beta-blockers, corticosteroids, ACE inhibitors, estrogen, aspirin, or diuretics four weeks prior to the test. The patient should avoid eating natural black licorice for 2 weeks before the test, and ingesting caffeine 24 hours before the test. The patient should maintain a low sodium diet for 3 days before the test and avoid eating or drinking 8 hours before the test.

Understanding the Test Results

The renin assay test results are available quickly. The laboratory determines normal values based on calibration of testing equipment with a control test. Test results are reported as high, normal, or low based on the laboratory's control test.

- Normal renin assay test results (patient in upright position):
  - Age 20 years to 39 years (normal sodium diet): 0.1 to 4.3 ng/mL/hr
  - Age 20 years to 39 years (low sodium diet): 2.9 to 24 ng/mL/hr
  - Age 40 years and older (normal sodium diet): 0.1 to 3.0 ng/mL/hr
  - Age 40 years and older (low sodium diet): 2.9 to 10.8 ng/mL/hr

High renin assay test results may indicate malignant high blood pressure, kidney disease, blocked artery, cirrhosis, Addison's disease, and hemorrhage.

Low renin assay test results may indicate Conn's syndrome.

Solved Problems

Brain Natriuretic Peptide (BNP)

5.1   What is BNP?

The heart produces the hormone brain natriuretic peptide (BNP).

5.2   What happens to BNP in heart failure?

A low level of BNP is normally found in blood. The BNP level increases when the heart works harder for long periods, such as in heart failure

5.3   Why is the BNP test ordered?

The BNP test is ordered to screen for heart failure and assess the treatment for heart failure.

5.4   What should you determine before administering the BNP test?

Assess if the patient:
- Has eaten or drunk anything except water for 12 hours before the test is administered
- Is taking diuretics or cardiac glycosides, which affect the test results
- Has had a heart attack, kidney dialysis and kidney disease, and COPD
- Is taking Echinacea, valerian, or other herbs, since this can affect the test result. The patient may be required to stop taking these for several days before the test is administered.

5.5   What would you do if immediately prior to administering the BNP test the patient tells you that he had breakfast?

Do not administer the test. Reschedule the test and tell the patient to refrain from eating or drinking anything except water 12 hours before the test is administered.

5.6   What does an abnormal level of BNP indicate?

An abnormal level of BNP indicates there is increased pressure inside the heart and may indicate heart failure if the patient is on kidney dialysis.

Cardiac Enzyme Studies

5.7   What are creatinine phosphokinase and troponin?

The cells of heart muscles and other tissues contain the enzyme creatinine phosphokinase (CK, CPK) and the protein troponin (TnT, TnI).

5.8   Why are creatinine phosphokinase and the protein troponin measured?

Creatinine phosphokinase and troponin enter the blood when heart muscle and other tissues are damaged, and are used to determine if there is heart damage.

5.9   What happens if there is an abnormal level of creatinine phosphokinase and troponin in the blood?

If levels of creatinine phosphokinase and troponin are abnormal, the healthcare provider orders an electrocardiogram to differentiate between heart muscle damage and other tissue damage.

5.10   How long does it take for troponin levels to rise after a heart attack?

6 hours.

5.11   Following a suspected heart attack, when are blood samples taken from the patient?

Blood samples are taken every 12 hours for 2 days following a suspected heart attack.

5.12   Before administering the creatinine phosphokinase and troponin test, what would you assess in the patient?

Assess if the patient:
- Has Reye's syndrome, muscular dystrophy, myocarditis, autoimmune diseases, or cardiac disease
- Has undergone cardioversion or defibrillation

- Has recently received an intramuscular injection
- Has had recent surgery
- Has undergone strenuous exercise before the test is administered
- Is taking statins
- Abuses alcohol
- Has kidney failure

5.13 Why should the patient refrain from exercise before the test creatinine phosphokinase and troponin is administered?

Exercising might cause tissue damage, resulting in the release of creatinine phosphokinase and troponin into the blood. This can cause a false reading.

5.14 How long does it take for the troponin level to return to normal?

The troponin level returns to normal levels in 10 days following the cardiac muscle injury.

5.15 When is the highest level of creatinine phosphokinase and troponin reached following injury to the heart?

24 hours after the cardiac muscle injury.

5.16 What would you do if after the patient reported to the healthcare provider that she might have had heart damage 2 weeks ago, and the healthcare provider ordered a creatinine phosphokinase and troponin test?

Question the order, since levels of creatinine phosphokinase and troponin would have returned to normal levels even if the patient's statement is true.

Renin Assay

5.17 How does the renin-angiotensin system (RAS) work?

Low blood pressure causes the secretion of the renin enzyme by the kidneys, which increases angiotensin production. The increased angiotensin production constricts blood vessels and results in increased blood pressure. Angiotensin causes the adrenal cortex to replace aldosterone, which causes the kidneys to retain water and sodium. This results in an increase in fluid volume and in blood pressure.

5.18 Why is the renin test administered?

A high level of the renin enzyme indicates the cause of hypertension.

5.19 What happens to the patient if there is a low level of renin?

The patient may experience hypotension.

5.20 What would the healthcare provider order if the patient's renin level is low?

The renin stimulation test may be ordered in order to assess if the renin-angiotensin system is properly working.

5.21 What should be assessed in the patient before administering the renin test?

Assess if the patient:
- Has eaten natural black licorice two weeks before the test
- Has ingested caffeine 24 hours before the test
- Has eaten or drunk 8 hours before the test
- Maintained a low sodium diet three days before the test
- Has taken beta-blockers, corticosteroids, ACE inhibitors, estrogen, aspirin, or diuretics four weeks before the test
- Has relaxed two hours before the first blood sample is taken
- Has ambulated for two hours after the first blood sample is taken and before the second blood sample is taken
- Is pregnant

5.22   What position should the patient be placed in during the renin test?

Upright.

5.23   What should the patient avoid before the renin test?

The patient should avoid eating natural black licorice for two weeks before the test, ingesting caffeine 24 hours before the test, and eating or drinking 8 hours before the test.

5.24   What should the patient do before and during the renin test?

The patient should relax for two hours before the first blood sample is taken, ambulate for two hours after the first blood sample is taken and before the second blood sample is taken, and be upright when the sample is taken.

5.25   What would a high result of the renin test indicate?

A high result of the renin test indicates malignant high blood pressure, kidney disease, blocked artery, cirrhosis, Addison's disease, or hemorrhage.

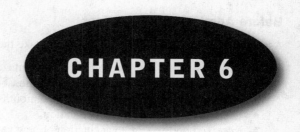

CHAPTER 6

Serologic Tests

6.1   Definition

Serology tests examine the patient's blood serum for antibodies. The presence of foreign protein in the body from a microorganism or from mismatched donated blood causes a reaction of the body's immune system. This reaction produces antibodies that destroy the foreign protein by metabolizing it into components that can be excreted safely by the body. Serology tests are used to diagnose an infection, if the patient has developed immunity to specific antigens, a patient's blood type, and if the patient has an autoimmune disorder. An autoimmune disorder occurs when the patient's immune system identifies the patient's own protein as a foreign protein, resulting in the patient's immune system creating antibodies to that protein

6.2   Immunoglobulins

Immunoglobulins are antibodies made by the immune system in response to a microorganism that enters the body, an allergen, and abnormal cells such as cancer cells. An antibody is specific to an antigen. The immunoglobulin test measures the level of an immunoglobulin in the patient's blood. A low level of a specific immunoglobulin increases the risk of repeated infections from an antigen. There are five major types of immunoglobulins:

1. **IgA**: This is found in tears and saliva and protects the ears, eyes, breathing passages, digestive tract, and vagina exposed to outside antigens (10% of immunoglobulins).
2. **IgG**: This is found in all body fluids and defends the body against viruses and bacteria. This immunoglobulin crosses the placenta (80% of immunoglobulins).
3. **IgM**: This is found in blood and lymph fluid and is the first response to infection (5% of immunoglobulins). Forms when an infection occurs for the first time.
4. **IgE**: This is found on mucous membranes, lungs, and skin and defends against allergens. A high level of IgE immunoglobulins is common in patients who are hyperallergenic, a condition known as *atopy* (less than 5% of immunoglobulins).
5. **IgD**: This is found in abdominal and chest tissues (less than 5% of immunoglobulins).

The immunoglobulins test is commonly administered as a follow up to an abnormal result from the *Total Blood Protein test* or from the *Blood Protein Electrophoresis test*.

Why the Test Is Performed

The test assesses levels of immunoglobulins to determine the strength of the patient's immune system, the patient's immunizations, and the effectiveness of treatment for infection and bone marrow cancer. The test also screens for allergies, autoimmune diseases, and multiple myeloma and macroglobulinemia cancers.

Before Administering the Test

Assess if there is reason for the patient not to take the test. Has the patient:

- Taken hydralazine (Apresoline), phenylbutazone, birth control pills, anticonvulsants (phenytoin), methotrexate, aminophenazone, asparaginase, and corticosteroids
- Received a blood transfusion within 6 months before the test
- Used alcohol or an illegal medication
- Received boosters of a vaccination or new vaccinations within 6 months before the test
- Received a radioactive scan within three days before the test
- Undergone radiation and chemotherapy treatment

How the Test Is Performed

Blood is drawn from an artery before it enters body tissues so that use of oxygen by tissues does not interfere with the measurement. The artery can be the **radial artery** (inside of the wrist) (typical), **femoral artery** (groin), or **brachial artery** (above crease in the elbow). A site that is infected, inflamed, or used for dialysis should not be used. An arterial catheter (thin tube) is placed in the artery if blood samples are collected at regular intervals. This increases patient comfort.

1. Seat the patient with the arm extended and the wrist resting on a small pillow.
2. Administer a local anesthetic if prescribed. Collecting blood from an artery is more painful than collecting blood from a vein.
3. Perform the Allen test to ensure there is normal blood flow.
   a. Stop the blood flow to both arteries to the hand until the hand becomes pale.
   b. Release and allow blood to flow through the arteries.
   c. The hand should regain normal color quickly, indicating injury to an artery. The immunoglobulin test will not block blood flow to the hand.
   d. If normal color is slow to return, then perform the Allen test on the other wrist. If color to this hand is also slow to return, then use an alternative site for the immunoglobulin.
4. Clean the puncture site with alcohol.
5. Instruct the patient to breathe normally.
6. Insert the needle into the artery.
7. Attach a test tube to the needle. Allow the blood to fill the test tube.
8. Place a gauze pad over the site while withdrawing the needle.
9. Apply firm pressure to the site for 10 minutes or longer until bleeding has stopped.

Explain to the patient that arteries are narrower and deeper than veins and are protected by nerves, making them sensitive to pain. Therefore there is more pain experienced collecting blood from an artery than collecting blood from a vein. Ask the patient if he/she wishes to have a local anesthetic. The patient may feel a brief pinch as the needle enters the skin. There are risks of nerve damage and a blockage of the artery as a result of the test, although incidents are rare. After the test, the patient may see a small bruise at the site. The patient may feel dizzy, lightheaded, and nauseated during the test. The patient should not lift or carry objects or exercise for 24 hours following the test.

Teach the Patient

No special preparation is needed for the test. Explain why the test is ordered. The immunoglobulin test can help the healthcare provider diagnose the infection.

Understanding the Test Results

Results are available in 2 days. The laboratory determines normal values based on calibration of testing equipment with a control test. Test results are reported as high, normal, or low based on the laboratory's control test.

- Generally, normal ranges are:
  ◦ IgA = 85 to 385 mg/dL
  ◦ IgG = 565 to 1,765 mg/dL
  ◦ IgM = 55 to 375 mg/dL

- ○ IgD = less than 8 mg/dL or 5 to 30 µg/L
- ○ IgE = 10 to 1,421 µg/L

Abnormal high values are not used to diagnose a condition. However, they can be a sign of:

- IgA: Systemic lupus erythematosus (SLE), rheumatoid arthritis, multiple myeloma, cirrhosis, or chronic hepatitis
- IgG: Chronic infection, multiple sclerosis (MS), multiple myeloma, chronic hepatitis
- IgM: Nephrotic syndrome, rheumatoid arthritis, macroglobulinemia, mononucleosis, viral hepatitis, parasite infection, or infection that started in the newborn before delivery
- IgD: multiple myeloma
- IgE: asthma, allergic reaction, parasite infection, atopic dermatitis, multiple myeloma

Abnormal low values are not used to diagnose a condition. However, they can be a sign of:

- IgA: Enteropathy, leukemia, nephrotic syndrome, ataxia-telangiectasia
- IgG: Leukemia, nephrotic syndrome, macroglobulinemia
- IgM: multiple myeloma, leukemia
- IgD: not significant
- IgE: ataxia-telangiectasia

6.3 Antinuclear Antibodies (ANA)

The antinuclear antibody (ANA) test measures the pattern and amount of these antibodies.

- In autoimmune diseases, the body produces antibodies that attach to and destroys the body's own cells.

Why the Test Is Performed

The test screens for rheumatoid arthritis, systemic lupus erythematosus (SLE), polymyositis, and scleroderma.

Before Administering the Test

No special patient preparation is necessary for the test. Ask the patient for a list of prescription and nonprescription medication that the patient has taken. Consult the laboratory to determine if these medications might affect the test results. Medication for high blood pressure, heart disease, and tuberculosis (TB) can cause the results to be high.

How the Test Is Performed

A sample of blood is taken from the patient's vein. The patient will experience a tight feeling when the tourniquet is tightened, a pinch or nothing at all when the needle is inserted into the vein, and pressure when a gauze pad is pressed against the insertion site to stop bleeding. It can take up to 10 minutes for bleeding to stop if the patient is taking anticoagulants (aspirin, coumadin). A small bruise might appear at the insertion site, which could become swollen following this test. This is called phlebitis. Applying a warm compress several times a day will reduce the swelling.

Teach the Patient

No special preparation is needed for the test. Explain why the test is ordered and that the test result is a sign and not a definitive diagnosis. Additional assessment must be made before a diagnosis is reached. Explain the conditions that can cause an elevated test result other than disease.

Understanding the Test Results

Results are available in 1 week. The laboratory determines normal values based on calibration of testing equipment with a control test. Test results are reported as high, normal, or low based on the laboratory's control test. Results are reported as a titer. A titer specifies how much of the sample of blood is diluted with saline before antibodies are no longer detected. The titer is reported as a ratio of parts of the blood sample and saline. The higher the second number of the ratio, the greater the number of antibodies in the blood sample.

- Generally normal range is:
  - 1:40 or less than 40

Abnormal high values are not used to diagnose a condition. However, it can be a sign of rheumatoid arthritis, systemic lupus erythematosus (SLE), scleroderma, polymyositis, Raynaud's syndrome, Addison's disease, Hashimoto's thyroiditis, hemolytic anemia, vitamin B_{12} deficiency, hepatitis, or idiopathic thrombocytopenia.

An elevated result can be caused by medication for high blood pressure, heart disease, tuberculosis, and a viral infection. Older adults also show an elevated result due to aging. A patient who has a family history of autoimmune disease may have an elevated result.

6.4   Human Immunodeficiency Virus (HIV) Tests

The human immunodeficiency virus (HIV) determines if a patient has HIV antibodies or the HIV's RNA in the patient's blood. The human immunodeficiency virus (HIV) infects the CD4+ white blood cells that are the body's defense against infection. There are two types of HIV:

1. **HIV–1** is common in nearly all acquired immunodeficiency syndrome (AIDS) cases.
2. **HIV–2** is associated with West Africa. HIV causes AIDS, which is incurable.

There is a period when the HIV infection is not detectable in a patient. This is called the *seroconversion period*, also known as the window period. The patient can spread HIV during this period. The seroconversion period can be as short as 2 weeks and as long as 6 months. After the seroconversion period, the human immunodeficiency virus test is able to detect HIV antibodies or the HIV's RNA in the patient's blood. Detecting HIV in a newborn is difficult because the newborn's blood still has HIV antibodies from either HIV positive parent for 18 months. Testing is performed when the patient exhibits symptoms of HIV, has HIV risk factors, is donating blood or organs, or is pregnant. An infected mother can be treated to decrease the likelihood that HIV will be passed to the fetus. There are several HIV tests:

- **Enzyme-linked immunosorbent assay (ELISA)**: The first test administered to screen a patient. This looks for HIV antibodies in the blood. If the test result is negative, then other tests are not performed. If the test result is positive, another ELISA test is performed. Other tests are performed if there are two positive ELISA tests because the ELISA test can produce a false positive.
- **Western blot**: This tests for HIV antibodies and is more difficult to perform than the ELISA test.
- **Polymerase chain reaction (PCR)**: This looks for HIV's RNA in the blood. PCR is used to identify a very recent infection and is administered to screen blood and organs before donations and when HIV antibody tests are inconclusive. The PCR test is not performed often, due to expense.
- **Indirect fluorescent antibody (IFA)**: This tests for HIV antibodies and is performed secondary to two positive ELISA tests.
- **Saliva test**: Tests the presence of HIV in saliva. Results must be confirmed by the Western blot test.
- **Rapid test kits**: Test results are available within a half an hour. Results must be confirmed by the Western blot test.
- **The P24 antigen assay**: Early after the infection, the presence of the P24 protein in blood is detectable earlier than the HIV antibody. The P24 antigen assay tests for the presence of the P24 protein in blood.
- **Home blood test kits**: Available without prescription. Samples are sent through the mail to the laboratory. Results are provided over the phone using an anonymous code.

Why the Test Is Performed

The test is performed to assess if the patient has been infected with HIV.

Before Administering the Test

If the patient is diagnosed with HIV, then the healthcare provider will order regular CD4+ count and Viral Load Measurement tests. The CD4+ count determines the impact HIV has on the immune system. The viral load measurement test determines the amount of HIV in the blood. Refer to the healthcare institution's policy on reporting positive test results.

Assess if the patient:

- Used corticosteroids, since this can affect the test results
- Has an autoimmune disease, syphilis, or leukemia. These can affect the test results.
- Consumed alcohol. This can affect the test results.
- Arranged for counselors to be available to assist the patient with the emotional, financial, and social repercussions of being HIV positive, should there be positive test results

How the Test Is Performed

The patient must consent to HIV testing. Tests are performed at 6 weeks, 3 months, and 6 months after the patient is exposed to HIV. The PCR test is performed days or a few weeks following exposure to HIV. There are no special preparations for this test.

A sample of blood is taken from the patient's vein. The patient will experience a tight feeling when the tourniquet is tightened, a pinch or nothing at all when the needle is inserted into the vein, and pressure when a gauze pad is pressed against the insertion site to stop bleeding. It can take up to 10 minutes for bleeding to stop if the patient is taking anticoagulants (aspirin, coumadin). A small bruise might appear at the insertion site, which could become swollen following this test. This is called phlebitis. Applying a warm compress several times a day will reduce the swelling.

Teach the Patient

Explain that HIV testing cannot be performed without the patient's consent and why the blood sample is taken. HIV testing is part of routine blood screening. HIV testing does not determine if the person has AIDS. A negative test result will require retesting at 6 weeks, 3 months, and 6 months after the patient is exposed to HIV because of the seroconversion period. It is difficult to detect HIV in a newborn for 18 months because the newborn has antibodies from the mother. A positive ELISA test result does not mean that the patient is HIV positive. Additional testing is necessary to confirm this result. Counselors will be available to assist the patient with the emotional, financial, and social repercussions of being HIV positive. Explain the benefits of early detection and treatment. Treatment can be given to an infected mother to decrease the likelihood that HIV will be passed to the fetus.

Understanding the Test Results

ELISA test results are available in 2 to 4 days. Results of other tests are available within 2 weeks.

- Normal (negative) is:
  - No HIV antibodies detected.
  - The test is repeated for 6 months if the test is negative. The immune system can take up to 6 months to produce detectable HIV antibodies.
- Uncertain (indeterminate) is:
  - Results are not clear if the patient is infected with HIV because another factor is possibly interfering with the results.
  - The PCR test is typically ordered.
  - After 6 months, the patient is said to be stable indeterminate and not infected with HIV.
- Abnormal (positive) is:
  - HIV antibodies are found in the patient's blood.
  - If the ELISA test is positive, the same blood sample is tested again. If the second ELISA test is positive, then the Western blot or IFA test is performed.
  - A patient is considered HIV positive if the Western blot, IFA, or PCR tests are positive confirming two positive ELISA test results.

6.5 CD4+ Count

The CD4+ count test measures the level of leukocytes to assess the patient's immune system. Three types of leukocytes (WBC) important to fighting infection are T-lymphocytes, T-cells, and T-helper cells. Patients who have a low CD4+ count are at risk for opportunistic infections. The CD4+ count test is used to assess the immune system of patients who have human immunodeficiency virus (HIV). The result of the CD4+ count test and the viral load test determines when antiretroviral treatment for HIV is started. The healthcare provider may also order the CD4+ percentage test that determines the percentage of CD4+ cells in the total number of lymphocytes and the CD8 count test, which determines the level of T suppressor cells.

Why the Test Is Performed

The test is performed to assess the patient's immune system, the progress of HIV, and the treatment for HIV. It also assists in the diagnosis of AIDS. Develop a baseline of CD4+ count. The healthcare provider compares CD4+ values over time to identify changes in levels.

Before Administering the Test

Note the time when the CD4+ blood sample is taken, since CD4+ cells are normally lower in the morning. Be sure that the blood sample is refrigerated.
Assess if the patient has:

- Influenza, pneumonia, or herpes simplex since these can affect the test results
- Taken corticosteroids or is undergoing chemotherapy

How the Test Is Performed

A sample of blood is taken from the patient's vein. The patient will experience a tight feeling when the tourniquet is tightened, a pinch or nothing at all when the needle is inserted into the vein, and pressure when a gauze pad is pressed against the insertion site to stop bleeding. It can take up to 10 minutes for bleeding to stop if the patient is taking anticoagulants (aspirin, coumadin). A small bruise might appear at the insertion site, which could become swollen following this test. This is called phlebitis. Applying a warm compress several times a day will reduce the swelling.

Teach the Patient

Explain why the blood sample is taken and that the healthcare provider may request that the patient stop taking corticosteroids for 2 weeks prior to the test.

Understanding the Test Results

Test results are available in 3 days.

- Normal CD4+ cell count range is:
  - Not infected with HIV: 600 to 1,200 cells/μL
  - Low risk for opportunistic infection: greater than 350 cells/μL

Low CD4+ cell count may indicate:

- 200 to 350 cells/μL: weak immune system, risk for opportunistic infection, start antiretroviral treatment, start prophylactic drugs for prevent of opportunistic infections (especially PCP)
- Under 200 cells/μL: high risk for opportunistic infection, acquired immunodeficiency syndrome (AIDS), start antiretroviral treatment, start prophylactic drugs for prevent of opportunistic infections (especially PCP)

6.6 Viral Load Measurement

The viral load measurement test determines the amount of HIV RNA in the patient's blood. The human immunodeficiency virus (HIV) in a patient's blood is determined by the presence of HIV RNA. The amount of HIV RNA indicates if the infection is decreasing, stabilized, or increasing. A viral load measurement test is administered when the patient is diagnosed with HIV and becomes the baseline. Results of subsequent viral load measurement tests are compared to the baseline to determine the infection's progress. There are three types of viral load measurement tests:

1. Branched DNA (bDNA) test
2. Nucleic acid sequence-based amplification (NASBA) test
3. Reverse-transcriptase polymerase chain reaction (RT-PCR) test

The healthcare provider may order the CD4+ count test along with the viral load measurement test, although the viral load measurement test is more accurate than the CD4+ count test to assess the progress of the HIV infection. The viral load measurement test is not used to diagnose HIV. A patient diagnosed with HIV who has a negative viral load measurement test result can infect another person.

Why the Test Is Performed

The test assesses treatment of HIV infection and progress of HIV infection.

Before Administering the Test

Assess if the patient has another infection or recently received immunizations.

How the Test Is Performed

- Baseline, then every 4 months if the patient is not receiving highly active antiretroviral therapy (HAART)
- Baseline, then 8 weeks after the start of HAART, and then every 4 months if the patient is receiving HAART

A sample of blood is taken from the patient's vein. The patient will experience a tight feeling when the tourniquet is tightened, a pinch or nothing at all when the needle is inserted into the vein, and pressure when a gauze pad is pressed against the insertion site to stop bleeding. It can take up to 10 minutes for bleeding to stop if the patient is taking anticoagulants (aspirin, coumadin). A small bruise might appear at the insertion site, which could become swollen following this test. This is called phlebitis. Applying a warm compress several times a day will reduce the swelling.

Teach the Patient

Explain why the sample is taken and that a negative test result does not mean that the patient is cured. The patient can still spread the infection.

Understanding the Test Results

The viral load measurement test results take 2 weeks. Normal viral load measurement test result is (negative): No HIV RNA is found in blood.

- An abnormal viral load measurement test result is: HIV RNA is found and is reported as copies/mL where a copy is an HIV RNA.

The viral load measurement test result is compared to the baseline test result and to previous test results to determine the trend of the infection.

6.7 Rheumatoid Factor (RF)

The rheumatoid factor test measures the amount of the rheumatoid factor in the blood sample. The *rheumatoid factor* (RF) is an autoantibody that destroys the patient's own tissues resulting in stiffness, joint pain, and inflammation. The rheumatoid factor test is used to differentiate rheumatoid arthritis from other forms of arthritis. There are two types of rheumatoid factor tests: (1) the agglutination test and (2) the nephelometry test. The rheumatoid factor is one of the other signs and symptoms 1used to diagnose rheumatoid arthritis. A patient may have a high level of rheumatoid factor but no symptoms of rheumatoid arthritis. However, the patient is likely to develop rheumatoid arthritis in the future. A patient may have a normal level of rheumatoid factor and symptoms of rheumatoid arthritis will likely require a second rheumatoid factor test.

Why the Test Is Performed

The test screens for rheumatoid arthritis.

Before Administering the Test

Assess the patient's age. Patients older than 65 years of age normally have a higher rheumatoid factor level.

How the Test Is Performed

A sample of blood is taken from the patient's vein. The patient will experience a tight feeling when the tourniquet is tightened, a pinch or nothing at all when the needle is inserted into the vein, and pressure when a gauze pad is pressed against the insertion site to stop bleeding. It can take up to 10 minutes for bleeding to stop if the patient is taking anticoagulants (aspirin, coumadin). A small bruise might appear at the insertion site, which could become swollen following this test. This is called phlebitis. Applying a warm compress several times a day will reduce the swelling.

Teach the Patient

Explain why the sample is taken and that the healthcare provider may ask for a second rheumatoid factor test if the first test is normal and the patient shows signs of rheumatoid arthritis.

Understanding the Test Results

The rheumatoid factor test results are available quickly. Results are reported as a titer. A titer specifies how much of the sample of blood is diluted with saline before antibodies are no longer detected. The titer is reported as a ratio of parts of the blood sample and saline. The higher the second number of the ratio, the greater number of antibodies in the blood sample.

- Normal test results: 1:20 to 1:40 or less

Higher levels may indicate: Rheumatoid arthritis, systemic lupus erythematosus (SLE), vasculitis, scleroderma, cirrhosis, hepatitis, leukemia, endocarditis, mononucleosis, malaria, tuberculosis, and syphilis.

Solved Problems

Immunoglobulins

6.1   What are immunoglobulins?

Immunoglobulins are antibodies made by the immune system in response to a microorganism that enter the body, an allergen, and abnormal cells such as cancer cells.

6.2   What are the five major types of immunoglobulins?

IgA, IgG, IgM, IgE, and IgD.

6.3   What is IgE?

IgE is found on mucous membranes, lungs, and skin and defends against allergens. A high level of IgE immunoglobulins is common in patients who are hyperallergenic. This type makes up less than 5% of immunoglobulins.

6.4   What is IgA?

IgA is found in tears and saliva and protects the ears, eyes, breathing passages, digestive tract, and vagina exposed to outside antigens. This type makes up 10% of immunoglobulins.

6.5 What is IgM?

IgM is found in blood and lymph fluid and is the first response to infection. This type makes up 5% of immunoglobulins and forms when an infection occurs for the first time.

6.6 Why is the Immunoglobulin test ordered?

The Immunoglobulin test assesses the levels of immunoglobulins to determine the strengths of the patient's immune system, the patient's immunization, and the effectiveness of treatment for infection and bone marrow cancer. The test screens for allergies, autoimmune diseases, multiple myeloma, and macroglobulinemia cancers.

6.7 What might cause a high value of IgA?

A high value of IgA can be caused by systemic lupus erythematosus (SLE), rheumatoid arthritis, multiple myeloma, cirrhosis, and chronic hepatitis.

6.8 What might a high value of IgE indicate?

A high value of IgE might indicate asthma, allergic reaction, parasite infection, atopic dermatitis, or multiple myeloma.

6.9 What might a lower value of IgG indicate?

A lower value of IgG might indicate leukemia, nephrotic syndrome, and macroglobulinemia.

Antinuclear Antibody

6.10 Why is the antinuclear antibody test ordered?

The test screens for rheumatoid arthritis, systemic lupus erythematosus (SLE), polymyositis, and scleroderma.

6.11 How could medication for high blood pressure affect the antinuclear antibody test?

Medication for high blood pressure, heart disease, and tuberculosis (TB) can cause the results to be high.

6.12 What is diagnosed by the results of the antinuclear antibody test?

The test result is a sign and not a definitive diagnosis. Additional assessment must be made before a diagnosis is reached.

6.13 How is the result of the antinuclear antibody test reported?

Results are reported as a titer.

6.14 What is a titer?

A titer specifies how much of the sample of blood is diluted with saline before antibodies are no longer detected. The titer is reported as a ratio of parts of the blood sample and saline. The higher the second number of the ratio, the greater the number of antibodies in the blood sample.

6.15 What might a high result of the antinuclear antibody test indicate?

A high result of the antinuclear antibody test might indicate rheumatoid arthritis, systemic lupus erythematosus (SLE), scleroderma, polymyositis, Raynaud's syndrome, Addison's disease, Hashimoto's thyroiditis, hemolytic anemia, vitamin B_{12} deficiency, hepatitis, or idiopathic thrombocytopenia.

6.16 Other than medication, what might cause a false elevated result of the antinuclear antibody test?

Older adults also show an elevated result due to aging. A patient who has a family history of autoimmune disease may have an elevated result.

Human Immunodeficiency Virus (HIV) Tests

6.17 Name two HIV tests.

HIV-1 is common in nearly all acquired immunodeficiency syndrome (AIDS) cases.

HIV-2 is associated with West Africa. HIV causes AIDS, which is incurable.

6.18   What does HIV infect?

The human immunodeficiency virus (HIV) infects the CD4+ white blood cells that are the body's defense against infection.

6.19   What is the seroconversion period?

There is a period when the HIV infection is not detectable in a patient. This is called the seroconversion period, also known as the window period. The patient can spread HIV during this period.

6.20   How long is the seroconversion period?

The seroconversion period can be as short as 2 weeks and as long as 6 months.

6.21   When should the HIV test be administered?

After the seroconversion period, the human immunodeficiency virus test is able to detect HIV antibodies or the HIV's RNA in the patient's blood. Testing is performed when the patient exhibits symptoms of HIV, has HIV risk factors, is donating blood or organs, or is pregnant. An infected mother can be treated, decreasing the likelihood that HIV will be passed to the fetus.

6.22   What are the HIV tests?

The HIV tests are enzyme-linked immunosorbent assay (ELISA), Western blot, polymerase chain reaction (PCR), indirect fluorescent antibody (IFA), saliva test, rapid test kits, and home blood test kits.

6.23   What is the enzyme-linked immunosorbent assay test?

The first test administered to screen a patient. This looks for HIV antibodies in the blood.

6.24   What would you expect if the enzyme-linked immunosorbent assay test is positive?

If the test result is positive, another ELISA test is performed. Other tests are performed if there are two positive ELISA tests, because the ELISA test can produce a false positive.

6.25   Why is the polymerase chain reaction administered?

This looks for HIV's RNA in the blood. PCR is used to identify a very recent infection and is administered to screen blood and organs before donations and when HIV antibody tests are inconclusive. The PCR test is not performed often, due to expense.

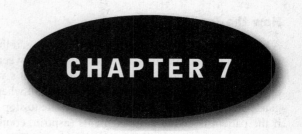

CHAPTER 7

Endocrine Tests

7.1 Definition

Endocrine tests are administered to assess if the patient is experiencing an endocrine disease. The *endocrine system* sends hormones via blood vessels to regulate bodily functions, including metabolism, growth, mood, and tissue function. Hormones are created, stored, and released by glands, and act as messengers signaling other glands and organs to react in a specific manner. Hormones are released based on existing hormone levels in the blood in order to keep hormonal levels in balance. For example, an excess amount of a hormone may cause the release of a different hormone that in turn causes the gland to stop or reduce excretion of the hormone, thereby bringing hormones in balance. Diseases can deregulate the release of hormones, resulting in underproduction or overproduction of one or more hormones.

7.2 Adrenocorticotropic Hormone (ACTH) and Cortisol

The adrenocorticotropic hormone test measures the level of ACTH in the blood. The hypothalamus releases corticotropin-releasing hormone (CRH), which causes the pituitary gland to release the adrenocorticotropic hormone (ACTH). ACTH causes the adrenal gland to release cortisol. Cortisol increases blood pressure and glucose and reduces immune responses. ACTH levels fall when cortisol levels rise, and ACTH levels rise when cortisol levels fall. The healthcare provider may request that an inferior petrosal sinus sample be taken from the inferior petrosal sinus near the pituitary gland to determine if the pituitary gland is producing ACTH, or if ACTH is made elsewhere in the patient's body. The patient may experience bruising if either the ACTH or cortisol levels are elevated.

Why the Test Is Performed

The test assesses pituitary gland function and the function of the adrenal glands.

Before Administering the Test

Assess the patient for conditions that might affect the test results:

- Intoxication
- Pregnancy
- Menstruation
- Emotional or physical stress or severe injury
- Whether the patient underwent a radioactive tracer medical test the week before the ACTH test
- Whether the patient is taking corticosteroids, which act like cortisol
- Whether the patient is taking amphetamines, insulin, or lithium carbonate, which causes the release of cortisol
- Has eaten or drunk 12 hours before the test
- Has exercised within the previous 12 hours

How the Test Is Performed

A blood specimen is taken, either in the morning, if the healthcare provider wants a peak level, or in the evening if a trough level is required. ACTH is highest between 6 a.m. and 8 a.m. and lowest between 6 p.m. and 11 p.m.

A sample of blood is taken from the patient's vein. The patient will experience a tight feeling when the tourniquet is tightened, a pinch or nothing at all when the needle is inserted into the vein, and pressure when a gauze pad is pressed against the insertion site to stop bleeding. It can take up to 10 minutes for bleeding to stop if the patient is taking anticoagulants (aspirin, coumadin). A small bruise might appear at the insertion site, which could become swollen following this test. This is called phlebitis. Applying a warm compress several times a day will reduce the swelling.

Teach the Patient

Do not exercise 12 hours before the test. Avoid stressful situations 12 hours before the test. Explain that there might be bruising if the ACTH and cortisol levels are high. The test cannot be taken if the patient is pregnant, menstruating, intoxicated, or if the patient has taken corticosteroids, amphetamines, insulin, and lithium carbonate. If the patient is taking these medications, then the patient must stop taking them for 2 days prior to the test. Explain when and why blood samples are taken, and that the healthcare provider may ask the patient not to eat or drink 12 hours before the test. The patient may be permitted to eat low-carbohydrate foods for 2 days before the test.

Understanding the Test Results

The result is available in 6 days. The laboratory determines normal values based on calibration of testing equipment with a control test. Test results are reported as high, normal, or low based on the laboratory's control test. Levels of ACTH vary by the minute, making test results difficult to interpret.

- Generally normal ranges for ACTH levels are:
  - 6 a.m. to 8 a.m.: less than 80 pg/mL or less than 18 pmol/L
  - 6 p.m. to 11 p.m.: less than 50 pg/mL or less than 11 pmol/L
- Generally normal ranges for cortisol levels are:
  - 6 a.m. to 8 a.m.: 5 to 23 μg/dL or 138 to 635 nmol/L
  - 6 p.m. to 11 p.m.: 3 to 13 μg/dL or 83 to 359 nmol/L

High levels may indicate physical or emotional stress, Addison's disease, Cushing's disease, adrenal gland tumor, or pituitary gland tumor.

Low levels may indicate head injury, stroke, pituitary gland damaged from radiation or surgery, pituitary gland tumor, or Adrenal gland tumor-Cushing's syndrome (increased release of cortisol).

Comparing levels of ACTH and cortisol can give an indication of the following diseases/conditions:

- High ACTH high cortisol = ACTH made outside the pituitary gland; Cushing's disease
- Low ACTH high cortisol = Adrenal tumor (Cushing's syndrome)
- High ACTH low cortisol = Addison's disease
- Low ACTH low cortisol = hypopituitarism

7.3   Overnight Dexamethasone Suppression Test

The overnight dexamethasone suppression test examines the patient's cortisol level after dexamethasone is administered. The pituitary gland releases ACTH whenever there is a low level of cortisol in the blood. ACTH signals the adrenal glands to release cortisol. An adrenal gland tumor causes the release of cortisol in the absence of ACTH. Dexamethasone is a medication similar to cortisol, in that dexamethasone signals the pituitary gland that there is a high level of cortisol in the blood, causing the pituitary gland to suppress the release of ACTH. The cortisol level should be lower because there is no ACTH in the blood to signal the adrenal glands to release cortisol. If cortisol levels remain high, this is a sign of Cushing's syndrome developing as a result of an adrenal gland tumor producing cortisol.

Why the Test Is Performed

The test assesses the function of the adrenal glands and screens for Cushing's syndrome.

Before Administering the Test

Assess the patient for conditions that might affect the test results by preventing a decrease in cortisol levels:

- Severe obesity
- Pregnancy
- Dehydration
- Uncontrolled diabetes
- Severe weight loss
- Acute alcohol withdrawal
- Severe injury
- Stress
- Taking birth control pills, phenytoin (Dilantin), MAOIs, lithium, morphine, aspirin, barbiturates, methadone, diuretics or Aldactone
- Assess the patient's metabolism
  - Some patients metabolize dexamethasone quickly, resulting in a lower than expected blood level when the blood specimen is taken.
  - In this case, the healthcare provider will increase the dose of dexamethasone.
  - The patient may be given up to eight doses of dexamethasone over two days.
- The patient should refrain from taking birth control pills, phenytoin (Dilantin), MAOIs, lithium, morphine, aspirin, barbiturates, methadone, diuretics, or Aldactone 48 hours before the blood specimen is drawn.
- A patient with high ACTH and cortisol levels may experience bruising

How the Test Is Performed

- Dexamethasone is administered at 11 p.m. the night before the test.
- Administer dexamethasone with antacid or milk to reduce the risk of heartburn or stomach upset.
- The patient is not permitted to eat or drink anything 12 hours before the specimen is drawn.
- A blood specimen is taken at 8 a.m.

A sample of blood is taken from the patient's vein. The patient will experience a tight feeling when the tourniquet is tightened, a pinch or nothing at all when the needle is inserted into the vein, and pressure when a gauze pad is pressed against the insertion site to stop bleeding. It can take up to 10 minutes for bleeding to stop if the patient is taking anticoagulants (aspirin, coumadin). A small bruise might appear at the insertion site, which could become swollen following this test. This is called phlebitis. Applying a warm compress several times a day will reduce the swelling.

Teach the Patient

Do not exercise 12 hours before the test. Avoid stressful situations 12 hours before the test. Do not eat or drink 12 hours before the test

Explain when and why the blood sample is taken, and that there might be bruising if the ACTH and cortisol levels are high. Inform the patient that the test cannot be taken if the patient has taken birth control pills, phenytoin (Dilantin), MAOIs, lithium, morphine, aspirin, barbiturates, methadone, diuretics, or Aldactone. If the patient is taking these medications, the patient must stop taking them for 2 days before the test.

Understanding the Test Results

The result is available in 3 days. The laboratory determines normal values based on calibration of testing equipment with a control test. Test results are reported as high, normal, or low based on the laboratory's control test. Further testing is indicated if there is a high cortisol level. Also, a normal result does not rule out Cushing's syndrome. The healthcare provider may prefer conducting a 24-hour urine free cortisol test, since this is not influenced by the timing of the blood specimen.

- Generally, normal ranges for cortisol levels are:
  - less than 5 μg/dL or less than 150 nmol/L

High levels may indicate Cushing's syndrome, hyperthyroidism, uncontrolled diabetes, heart failure, heart attack, poor diet, fever, alcoholism, depression, anorexia nervosa, or lung cancer.

7.4　Aldosterone Test

The aldosterone test determines the level of aldosterone in the blood. Kidneys release renin. Renin is a hormone that signals the adrenal glands to release aldosterone to control blood pressure and fluids and electrolytes balance by retaining fluid and sodium. This test is typically performed with the renin activity test. A patient who has muscle cramps, muscle weakness, tingling in the hands, or high blood pressure may have a high level of aldosterone.

Why the Test Is Performed

The test assesses for an adrenal gland tumor, the cause of high blood pressure, the cause of low potassium level in the blood, and an overactive adrenal gland.

Before Administering the Test

The aldosterone test is given as part of routine blood screening. There is no special preparation required for this test. If the test result is abnormal, the healthcare provider may order subsequent aldosterone tests. For subsequent aldosterone tests, the patient should:

- Refrain from eating natural black licorice two weeks prior to the test.
- Eat 3 grams per day of sodium for 2 weeks prior to the test.
- Avoid a low salt diet, since this increases aldosterone levels.
- Avoid a high salt diet, since this decreases aldosterone levels.
- Do not eat olives, soy sauce, pretzels, potato chips, canned soups, bacon, and vegetables.
- Know that he or she might be asked to stand, sit, and lie down when the test is administered, since the patient's position may affect the test results. Standing or sitting for 2 hours before the test increases the aldosterone level.

Assess:

- Prescription and nonprescription medication that the patient takes. Diuretics, estrogen, corticosteroids, progesterone, opiates, NSAIDs, heparin, and Aldactone medication affect the test and should be stopped two weeks before the test.
- If the patient is in the third trimester of pregnancy, since the aldosterone level can be high at this stage of pregnancy.
- If the patient is under emotional stress or experienced strenuous exercise prior to the test. This can affect the test results.
- The patient's age, since aldosterone levels decrease with age.

How the Test Is Performed

A sample of blood is taken from the patient's vein. The patient will experience a tight feeling when the tourniquet is tightened, a pinch or nothing at all when the needle is inserted into the vein, and pressure when a gauze pad is pressed against the insertion site to stop bleeding. It can take up to 10 minutes for bleeding to stop if the patient is taking anticoagulants (aspirin, coumadin). A small bruise might appear at the insertion site, which could become swollen following this test. This is called phlebitis. Applying a warm compress several times a day will reduce the swelling.

　　The healthcare provider may choose to use a 24-hour urine test in place of measuring aldosterone levels in the blood if the patient is unable to change positions.

Teach the Patient

Explain why the blood sample is taken, the function of aldosterone, and the meaning of abnormal values. The patient may be asked to stand, sit, and lie down during the test. The healthcare provider may ask the patient to stop taking diuretics, estrogen, corticosteroids, progesterone, opiates, NSAIDs, heparin, and Aldactone medication for

2 weeks prior to the test, since they can affect the test. Ask the patient to refrain from eating natural black licorice two weeks prior to the test, and to avoid a low or high salt diet.

Understanding the Test Results

Test results are available in 2 to 5 days. The laboratory determines normal values based on calibration of testing equipment with a control test. Test results are reported as high, normal, or low based on the laboratory's control test. The healthcare provider will likely order subsequent aldosterone tests if there is an abnormal result. The healthcare provider may order a potassium blood test if there is abnormal adrenal growth or overactive adrenal glands are suspected as the cause of an abnormal aldosterone test result.

- Generally, the normal range is:
  - Lying down: 3 to 10 ng/dL or 0.08 to 0.3 nmol/L
  - Standing or sitting: 5 to 30 ng/dL or 0.14 to 0.8 nmol/L
  - Child 1 year and older: 5 to 80 ng/dL or 0.14 to 2.13 nmol/L
  - Child under 1 year: 1 to 160 ng/dL or 0.03 to 2.26 nmol/L

High levels may indicate primary hyperaldosteronism, which directly affects the adrenal glands and the renin activity test is low. This may be an indication of adrenal hyperplasia or Conn's syndrome-adrenal gland tumor.

Secondary hyperaldosteronism does not directly affect the adrenal glands, and the renin activity test is high. This may indicate cirrhosis, heart failure, kidney disease, or preeclampsia.

Low levels may indicate Addison's disease.

7.5   Cortisol Test

The cortisol test determines the level of cortisol in blood. Cortisol, produced by the adrenal glands, is a hormone that causes an increase in blood pressure and glucose, while decreasing the immune response. Cortisol levels are the highest at 7 a.m. and the lowest 3 hours after sleep, based on the diurnal rhythm. However, the diurnal rhythm reverses if the patient works at night and sleeps during the day. The pituitary gland releases ACTH whenever there is a low level of cortisol in the blood. ACTH signals the adrenal glands to release cortisol. The healthcare provider may also order the dexamethasone suppression test, the adreno-corticotropic hormone test, or a 24-hour urine test.

Why the Test Is Performed

The test assesses the function of the pituitary gland and adrenal glands.

Before Administering the Test

- Ask the patient to lie down for 30 minutes to reduce stress levels.
- Assess if the patient:
  - Has had strenuous physical activity 24 hours before the test is administered
  - Is pregnant, since this can increase cortisol levels
  - Is hypoglycemic
  - Has had a radioactive scan a week before the test
  - Has taken amphetamines, estrogen, birth control pills, or corticosteroids, since these affect the test results
  - Has eaten or drunk before the test, since this can affect the test results

How the Test Is Performed

A blood sample is taken in the morning to measure peak level.

A sample of blood is taken from the patient's vein. The patient will experience a tight feeling when the tourniquet is tightened, a pinch or nothing at all when the needle is inserted into the vein, and pressure when a gauze pad is pressed against the insertion site to stop bleeding. It can take up to 10 minutes for bleeding to stop if the patient is taking anticoagulants (aspirin, coumadin). A small bruise might appear at the insertion site, which could become swollen following this test. This is called phlebitis. Applying a warm compress several times a day will reduce the swelling.

Teach the Patient

Explain why the blood sample is taken, that the healthcare provider may ask the patient not to eat or drink 12 hours before the test, and that the healthcare provider may ask the patient to stop taking amphetamines, estrogen, birth control pills, or corticosteroids for 2 weeks prior to the test, since these affect the test results.

Understanding the Test Results

Test results are available quickly. The laboratory determines normal values based on calibration of testing equipment with a control test. Test results are reported as high, normal, or low based on the laboratory's control test.

- Normal range is:
  - Adult – morning: 5 to 23 µg/dL or 138 to 635 nmol/L
  - Adult – afternoon: 3 to 13 µg/dL or 83 to 359 nmol/L
  - Children – morning: 3 to 21 µg/dL or 83 to 580 nmol/L
  - Children – afternoon: 3 to 10 µg/dL or 83 to 276 nmol/L
  - Newborn: 1 to 24 µg/dL or 27 to 663 nmol/L

High level values may indicate an adrenal gland tumor, overactive adrenal gland, Cushing's syndrome, Cushing disease, adenoma, depression, severe liver disease, obesity, hyperthyroidism, severe kidney disease, surgery, and sepsis.

Low level values may indicate Addison's disease, shock, Sheehan's syndrome, and autoimmune disease.

7.6 Estrogens

The estrogen test determines the level of estrogen in blood. *Estrogen* is a hormone produced in the ovaries, placenta, muscle tissue, adipose tissue, adrenal glands, and in the testicles in men. There are three types of estrogen hormones:

1. **Estradiol**: Estradiol is estrogen found in nonpregnant women. It varies with the menstrual cycle.
2. **Estriol**: Estriol is estrogen that is produced by the placenta and is measured in pregnant women who are at least in the ninth week of pregnancy.
3. **Estrone**: Estrone is estrogen measured in women who have finished menopause, and in both men and women suspected of having testicular cancer, ovarian cancer, or an adrenal gland tumor.

Estrogen levels can also be measured in urine. The healthcare provider may order a triple test or quad marker screen to assess for fetal birth defects. The maternal serum triple test measures levels of estrogen, alphafetoprotein (AFP) and human chorionic gonadotropin (hCG). The quad marker screen measures the same as the triple test, but also tests inhibit A hormone.

Why the Test Is Performed

The test assesses the affects of fertility therapy, abnormal sexual characteristics in men, estrogen-producing tumors, and fetal birth defects.

Before Administering the Test

Assess:

- The stage of the patient's menstrual cycle
- If the patient is pregnant
- If the patient has completed menopause
- If the patient is undergoing hormone replacement therapy

- The type of birth control that is used by the patient (if used)
- If the patient has undergone a radioactive scan in the week prior to administering the test
- If the patient has taken prednisone, Clomid, or Serophene, since these might affect the test result.

How the Test Is Performed

A sample of blood is taken from the patient's vein. The patient will experience a tight feeling when the tourniquet is tightened, a pinch or nothing at all when the needle is inserted into the vein, and pressure when a gauze pad is pressed against the insertion site to stop bleeding. It can take up to 10 minutes for bleeding to stop if the patient is taking anticoagulants (aspirin, coumadin). A small bruise might appear at the insertion site, which could become swollen following this test. This is called phlebitis. Applying a warm compress several times a day will reduce the swelling.

Teach the Patient

Explain why the blood sample is taken and that the healthcare provider may ask the patient to stop taking prednisone, Clomid, or Serophene for two weeks prior to the test.

Understanding the Test Results

Estrogen test results are available in 1 day. The laboratory determines normal values based on calibration of testing equipment with a control test. Test results are reported as high, normal, or low based on the laboratory's control test.

- Normal Estradiol range is:
  - Before menopause: 30 to 400 pg/mL
  - After menopause: 0 to 30 pg/mL
  - Men: 10 to 50 pg/mL
  - Children: 0 to 15 pg/mL
- Normal Estriol range in pregnant women is:
  - First trimester: less than 38 ng/mL
  - Second trimester: 38 to 140 ng/mL
  - Third trimester: 31 to 460 ng/mL

High estrogen values may indicate cirrhosis, multiple fetuses, early puberty, infertility treatment is working, ovarian cancer, testicular cancer, or adrenal gland tumor.

Low estrogen values may indicate Turner's syndrome, anorexia nervosa, dysfunctional pituitary gland, dysfunctional placenta, or fetal disorder.

7.7 Growth Hormone

The growth hormone test measures the level of growth hormone in blood. The human growth hormone (GH), secreted by the pituitary gland, stimulates cell growth and reproduction and growth factor 1 (IGF–1). The healthcare provider may order the growth factor 1 (IGF–1) test, the growth hormone suppression test (glucose loading test), and the growth hormone stimulation test (insulin tolerance test) along with the growth hormone test.

Why the Test Is Performed

The test assesses for abnormal growth, treatment for abnormal growth, and a pituitary gland tumor.

Before Administering the Test

Assess if the patient:

- Has eaten or drunk 10 hours before the test
- Has exercised 10 hours before the test
- Has rested for 30 minutes before the test

- Is taking St. John's Wort, insulin, estrogen, amphetamines, birth control pills or corticosteroids, since these can affect the test result
- Is hypoglycemic
- Is obese

How the Test Is Performed

- Avoid eating and drinking for 10 hours before the test.
- Avoid exercising 10 hours before the test.
- Rest for 30 minutes before the test.

A sample of blood is taken from the patient's vein. The patient will experience a tight feeling when the tourniquet is tightened, a pinch or nothing at all when the needle is inserted into the vein, and pressure when a gauze pad is pressed against the insertion site to stop bleeding. It can take up to 10 minutes for bleeding to stop if the patient is taking anticoagulants (aspirin, coumadin). A small bruise might appear at the insertion site, which could become swollen following this test. This is called phlebitis. Applying a warm compress several times a day will reduce the swelling.

Teach the Patient

Explain why the sample is taken, that the patient must avoid eating and drinking for 10 hours before the test, that the patient must avoid exercising 10 hours before the test, and that the patient must rest for 30 minutes before the test. The healthcare provider may want the patient to refrain from taking St. John's wort, insulin, estrogen, amphetamines, birth control pills, or corticosteroids 2 weeks before the test.

Understanding the Test Results

Normal growth hormone test results are available quickly. The laboratory determines normal values based on calibration of testing equipment with a control test. Test results are reported as high, normal, or low based on the laboratory's control test.

- Normal range of levels of growth hormone is:
  - Men: less than 5 ng/mL
  - Women: less than 10 ng/mL
  - Children: 0 to 10 ng/mL
  - Newborn: 10 to 40 ng/mL

High growth hormone levels may indicate acromegaly, gigantism, a pituitary gland tumor, starvation, diabetes, or kidney disease.

Low growth hormone levels may indicate dwarfism, hypopituitarism, or sarcoidosis.

7.8 Luteinizing Hormone (LH)

The luteinizing hormone (LH) test measures the level of luteinizing hormone in blood. *Luteinizing hormone* (LH) is produced by the pituitary gland. It stimulates production of testosterone, stimulates ovulation, and regulates the menstrual cycle. Home ovulation testing kits detect luteinizing hormone levels in urine.

Why the Test Is Performed

The test assesses for the underlying cause of infertility, infertility treatment, for the underlying cause of irregular menstrual period or amenorrhea, for menopause, for precocious puberty and delayed puberty, and for erectile dysfunction.

Before Administering the Test

Assess if/when the patient:

- Experienced the first day of the last menstrual period
- Experienced light or heavy bleeding on the first day of the menstrual period

- Has hyperthyroidism.
- Has undergone a radioactive tracer test one week prior to the test.
- Is taking phenothiazine, cimetidine, clomiphene, spironolactone, digitalis, naloxone, anticonvulsants, levodopa, and birth control pills a month before the test is administered.
- Has liver disease.

How the Test Is Performed

The healthcare provider may order several samples taken on one day or over several days.

A sample of blood is taken from the patient's vein. The patient will experience a tight feeling when the tourniquet is tightened, a pinch or nothing at all when the needle is inserted into the vein, and pressure when a gauze pad is pressed against the insertion site to stop bleeding. It can take up to 10 minutes for bleeding to stop if the patient is taking anticoagulants (aspirin, coumadin). A small bruise might appear at the insertion site, which could become swollen following this test. This is called phlebitis. Applying a warm compress several times a day will reduce the swelling.

Teach the Patient

Explain why the sample is taken, that the healthcare provider may order several samples taken on one day or over several days, and that the healthcare provider may ask the patient to refrain from taking phenothiazine, cimetidine, clomiphene, spironolactone, digitalis, naloxone, anticonvulsants, levodopa, and birth control pills a month before the test is administered.

Understanding the Test Results

The luteinizing hormone test results are available quickly. The laboratory determines normal values based on calibration of testing equipment with a control test. Test results are reported as high, normal, or low based on the laboratory's control test. Age, menstrual cycle, and stage of sexual development affect the test results.

- Normal luteinizing hormone test results:
  - Menstruating:
    - Follicular phase: 1 to 18 IU/L
    - Mid-cycle phase: 8.7 to 80 IU/L
    - Luteal phase: 0.5 to 18 IU/L
    - Post-menopause: 12 to 55 IU/L
  - Men: 1 to 9 IU/L
  - Before puberty: 0 to 1 IU/L
  - Male puberty: 0.4 to 7 IU/L
  - Female puberty: 0.4 to 12 IU/L

A high luteinizing hormone level may indicate (in women) polycystic ovary syndrome, early puberty, or no ovaries, and (in men) Klinefelter syndrome, no testicles, or malfunctioning testicles.

A low luteinizing level may indicate a malfunctioning pituitary gland, malfunctioning hypothalamus, anorexia nervosa, the patient being underweight, or that the patient is stressed.

7.9 Parathyroid Hormone (PTH)

The parathyroid hormone (PTH) test measures the level of parathyroid hormone in blood. The parathyroid glands release *parathyroid hormone* (PTH) when the calcium level in the blood is low, causing the kidneys to retain calcium, and bone to release calcium into the blood. PTH converts vitamin D to an active form, resulting in increased absorption of calcium by the intestine. Calcium and phosphorus have an inverse relationship. When the calcium level in the blood is high, phosphorus level in the blood is low. Therefore, PTH also controls the phosphorus level in blood. The parathyroid hormone test measures the level of PTH in blood. The healthcare provider may also order tests for calcium and phosphorus levels in the blood, and creatinine tests to assess kidney function.

Why the Test Is Performed

The test assesses for hyperparathyroidism and the underlying cause of an abnormal level of calcium in blood.

Before Administering the Test

Assess if the patient:

- Works days or nights to determine the patient's sleep habits
- Has high cholesterol levels
- Has high triglyceride levels
- Is pregnant
- Is breast-feeding
- Has eaten or drunk anything except water 10 hours before the test
- Has taken calcium supplements or is on a high calcium diet
- Has taken phosphorus supplements or is on a high phosphorus diet
- Has undergone a radioactive tracer test in the week prior to the test
- Has taken Tagamet, Betachron ER, or Inderal, since these medications lower test results
- Has taken diuretics, lithium, rifampin, furosemide, thiazide, or anticonvulsant medication, since these medications raise measured levels

How the Test Is Performed

- Avoid eating or drinking anything except water 10 hours before the test.
- Take the blood sample shortly after the patient awakens.

A sample of blood is taken from the patient's vein. The patient will experience a tight feeling when the tourniquet is tightened, a pinch or nothing at all when the needle is inserted into the vein, and pressure when a gauze pad is pressed against the insertion site to stop bleeding. It can take up to 10 minutes for bleeding to stop if the patient is taking anticoagulants (aspirin, coumadin). A small bruise might appear at the insertion site, which could become swollen following this test. This is called phlebitis. Applying a warm compress several times a day will reduce the swelling.

Teach the Patient

Explain why the sample is taken, that the patient needs to avoid eating or drinking anything except water 10 hours before the test, and that the sample will be taken shortly after the patient awakens. The healthcare provider may ask the patient to refrain from taking Tagamet, Betachron ER, Inderal, diuretics, lithium, rifampin, furosemide, thiazide, or anticonvulsant medication 2 weeks prior to the test.

Understanding the Test Results

The parathyroid hormone test results are available in 2 days. The laboratory determines normal values based on calibration of testing equipment with a control test. Test results are reported as high, normal, or low based on the laboratory's control test. Normal parathyroid hormone test results are 10 to 65 pg/mL.

High parathyroid hormone test results may indicate hyperplasia, a parathyroid tumor, a low level of calcium in blood, kidney disease, pancreatic cancer, lung cancer, ovarian cancer, absorption disorder of the intestines, or vitamin D deficiency.

Low parathyroid hormone test results may indicate Lymphoma, a low magnesium level in blood, excess calcium intake, malfunctioning parathyroid gland, multiple myeloma, or sarcoidosis.

7.10   Thyroid Hormone Tests

The thyroid hormone test measures the level of thyroid hormones in blood. The hypothalamus gland releases *thyrotropin-releasing hormone* (TRH), which stimulates the anterior pituitary gland to release *thyroid-stimulating hormone* (TSH). TSH causes the thyroid gland to release *thyroxine* (T4) and *triiodothyronine* (T3), both of which regulate metabolism. T4 and T3 are produced only if there is sufficient iodine in the thyroid gland.

T4 and T3 are transported in blood either freely or bound to globulin. Free T4 and T3 affect metabolism. The thyroid gland also releases calcitonin when the patient has hypercalcemia. Calcitonin regulates calcium levels in blood by moving calcium from the blood to bone. The thyroid hormone tests measure the level of T4 and T3 in the blood. There are four thyroid hormone tests:

1. **Total thyroxine (T4) test**: This test measures the amount of T4 hormone that is bound to globulin and the amount of unbound T4 hormone called free thyroxine in the blood.
2. **Free thyroxine (FT4) test**: This test measures the amount of unbound T4 hormone.
3. **Free thyroxine index (FTI) test**: This test compares the amount of bound thyroxine to total thyroxine, and thereby indirectly measures unbound thyroxine.
4. **Triiodothyronine (T3) test**: This test measures T3 hormone that is bound to globulin and the amount of unbound T3 hormone called free triiodothyronine.

Why the Test Is Performed

The test assesses for the underlying cause for an abnormal thyroid-stimulating hormone (TSH) test, hyperthyroidism, treatment of hyperthyroidism, hypothyroidism, and treatment of hypothyroidism.

Before Administering the Test

Assess if the patient:

- Is taking Dilantin, Tegretol, coumadin, aspirin, heparin, propranolol, lithium, amiodarone, estrogen, birth control pills, corticosteroids, or progesterone
- Is pregnant
- Has had an iodine dye X-ray four weeks before the test

How the Test Is Performed

A blood sample is taken either from a heel stick or from a vein.

Heel Stick: Several drops of blood are collected from the heel of a newborn or baby. The heel is cleaned using alcohol. A sterile lancet is used to puncture the heel. Several drops of blood are collected in a small test tube. A gauze pad is pressed over the site until bleeding stops. A small bandage is applied.

Vein: A sample of blood is taken from the patient's vein. The patient will experience a tight feeling when the tourniquet is tightened, a pinch or nothing at all when the needle is inserted into the vein, and pressure when a gauze pad is pressed against the insertion site to stop bleeding. It can take up to 10 minutes for bleeding to stop if the patient is taking anticoagulants (aspirin, coumadin). A small bruise might appear at the insertion site, which could become swollen following this test. This is called phlebitis. Applying a warm compress several times a day will reduce the swelling.

Teach the Patient

Explain why the sample is taken and that the healthcare provider may ask the patient to refrain from taking Dilantin, Tegretol, coumadin, aspirin, heparin, propranolol, lithium, amiodarone, estrogen, birth control pills, corticosteroids, or progesterone before the test.

Understanding the Test Results

The thyroid hormone test results are available in 3 days. The laboratory determines normal values based on calibration of testing equipment with a control test. Test results are reported as high, normal, or low based on the laboratory's control test.

- Normal test results:
  - Total thyroxine:
    - Adults: 5 to 14 mcg/dL
    - Children: 5.6 to 16.6 mcg/dL
    - Newborns: 9.8 to 22.6 mcg/dL

- ○ Total triiodothyronine:
  - ▪ Adults: 80 to 230 ng/dL
  - ▪ Children: 83 to 280 ng/dL
  - ▪ Newborns: 32 to 250 ng/dL
- ○ Free thyroxine: 0.8 to 2.4 ng/dL
- ○ Free thyroxine index:
  - ▪ Adults: 4.2 to 13
  - ▪ Children: 5 to 12.8
  - ▪ Newborns: 7.5 to 17.5
  - ▪ Free triiodothyronine: 0.2 to 0.6 ng/dL

High levels may indicate hyperthyroidism, Graves' disease, goiter, thyroiditis, or overdose of T4 replacement therapy.

Low levels may indicate hypothyroidism, thyroid radiation treatment, thyroid surgery, pituitary gland disorder, or thyroiditis.

7.11   Thyroid-Stimulating Hormone (TSH)

The thyroid stimulating hormone test measures the level of thyroid stimulating hormones in blood. The hypothalamus gland releases thyrotropin-releasing hormone (TRH), which stimulates the anterior pituitary gland to release thyroid-stimulating hormone (TSH). TSH causes the thyroid gland to release thyroxine (T4) and triiodothyronine (T3) both of which regulate metabolism. The thyroid-stimulating hormone test measures the level of thyroid-stimulating hormone in blood. The healthcare provider is likely to order the thyroid hormone tests along with the thyroid-stimulating hormone test.

Why the Test Is Performed

The test assesses for hyperpituitarism, treatment of hyperpituitarism, hypopituitarism, treatment of hypopituitarism, hypothalamus disorder, the underlying cause of hyperthyroidism, and the underlying cause of hypothyroidism.

Before Administering the Test

Assess if the patient:

- Is taking dopamine, Tegretol, coumadin, aspirin, heparin, corticosteroids, lithium, levodopa, propylthiouracil or Tapazole
- Is pregnant
- Is stressed
- Has had an iodine dye X-ray four weeks before the test

How the Test Is Performed

A sample of blood is taken from the patient's vein. The patient will experience a tight feeling when the tourniquet is tightened, a pinch or nothing at all when the needle is inserted into the vein, and pressure when a gauze pad is pressed against the insertion site to stop bleeding. It can take up to 10 minutes for bleeding to stop if the patient is taking anticoagulants (aspirin, coumadin). A small bruise might appear at the insertion site, which could become swollen following this test. This is called phlebitis. Applying a warm compress several times a day will reduce the swelling.

Teach the Patient

Explain why the sample is taken and that the healthcare provider may ask the patient to refrain from taking dopamine, Tegretol, coumadin, aspirin, heparin, corticosteroids, lithium, levodopa, propylthiouracil or Tapazole before the test.

Understanding the Test Results

The thyroid hormone test results are available in 3 days. The laboratory determines normal values based on calibration of testing equipment with a control test. Test results are reported as high, normal, or low based on the laboratory's control test.

- Normal test results:
  - Adults: 0.4 to 4.5 mIU/L
  - Newborns: 3 to 18 mIU/L

High levels may indicate hypothyroidism, pituitary gland tumor, or Hashimoto's thyroiditis.

Low levels may indicate hyperthyroidism, goiter, toxic nodule tumor, Graves' disease, or pituitary gland damage.

7.12 Testosterone

The testosterone test measures the level of testosterone in blood. The pituitary gland releases luteinizing hormone (LH) that stimulates the release of testosterone by the adrenal glands, testes, and ovaries. Testosterone is unbound in blood, called free, or bound to the sex hormone binding globulin (SHBG) protein in blood.

Why the Test Is Performed

The test assesses for the underlying cause of infertility, erectile dysfunction, osteoporosis in men, precocious puberty (boys), hirsutism in women, irregular menstruation, and the treatment for prostate cancer.

Before Administering the Test

Assess if the patient:

- Is taking birth control pills, digoxin, Aldactone, corticosteroids, testosterone, estrogen, barbiturates or seizure medication
- Has hyperthyroidism or hypothyroidism
- Is obese

How the Test Is Performed

A sample of blood is taken from the patient's vein. The patient will experience a tight feeling when the tourniquet is tightened, a pinch or nothing at all when the needle is inserted into the vein, and pressure when a gauze pad is pressed against the insertion site to stop bleeding. It can take up to 10 minutes for bleeding to stop if the patient is taking anti-coagulants (aspirin, coumadin). A small bruise might appear at the insertion site, which could become swollen following this test. This is called phlebitis. Applying a warm compress several times a day will reduce the swelling.

Teach the Patient

Explain why the sample is taken and that the healthcare provider may ask the patient to refrain from taking birth control pills, digoxin, Aldactone, corticosteroids, testosterone, estrogen, barbiturates, or seizure medication before the test.

Understanding the Test Results

The testosterone hormone test results are available in 2 days. The laboratory determines normal values based on calibration of testing equipment with a control test. Test results are reported as high, normal, or low based on the laboratory's control test.

- Normal test results:
  - Bound testosterone:
    - Men:
      - Older than 19 years: 280 to 1080 ng/dL

- 16 to 19 years: 250 to 910 ng/dL
- 14 to 15 years: 170 to 540 ng/dL
- 10 to 13 years: less than 300 ng/dL
- 7 months to 9 years: less than 30 ng/dL
  - Women:
    - Older than 16 years: less than 70 ng/dL
    - 14 to 15 years: less than 60 ng/dL
    - 10 to 13 years: less than 40 ng/dL
    - 7 months to 9 years: less than 30 ng/dL
  - Unbound testosterone: 0.3 to 2 pg/mL

High levels may indicate testicular cancer, adrenal gland cancer, ovarian cancer, polycystic ovary syndrome (PCOS), or precocious puberty (boys).

Low levels may indicate Klinefelter syndrome, cirrhosis, alcohol abuse, testicular disorder, or pituitary gland damage.

Solved Problems

Adrenocorticotropic Hormone (ACTH) and Cortisol

7.1 What causes the release of cortisol?

The hypothalamus releases corticotrophin-releasing hormone (CRH), which causes the pituitary gland to release the adrenocorticotropic hormone (ACTH). ACTH causes the adrenal gland to release cortisol. Cortisol increases blood pressure and glucose, and reduces the immune responses.

7.2 What is the relationship between ACTH and cortisol?

ACTH levels fall when cortisol levels rise, and ACTH levels rise when cortisol levels fall.

7.3 What does the adrenocorticotropic hormone test measure?

The adrenocorticotropic hormone test measures the level of ACTH in the blood.

7.4 Why is the adrenocorticotropic hormone test ordered?

To assess the function of the pituitary gland and the adrenal glands.

7.5 What should you assess before administering the adrenocorticotropic hormone test?

Assess the patient for conditions that might affect the test results: intoxication; pregnancy; menstruation; emotional or physical stress or severe injury; whether the patient underwent a radioactive tracer medical test the week before the ACTH test; whether the patient is taking corticosteroids (acts like cortisol), amphetamines, insulin, lithium carbonate (which causes the release of cortisol); has eaten or drunk 12 hours before the test; or has exercised within the previous 12 hours.

7.6 What should you teach the patient about the adrenocorticotropic hormone test?

Do not exercise 12 hours before the test. Avoid stressful situations 12 hours before the test. Explain when and why the blood samples are taken, that there might be bruising if the ACTH and cortisol levels are high, and that the test cannot be taken if the patient is pregnant, menstruating, intoxicated, or if the patient has taken corticosteroids, amphetamines, insulin, and lithium carbonate. If the patient is taking these medications, then the patient must stop taking them for 2 days before the test. The healthcare provider may ask the patient not to eat or drink anything 12 hours before the test. The patient may be permitted to eat low-carbohydrate foods for two days before the test.

Overnight Dexamethasone Suppression Test

7.7 What does the overnight dexamethasone suppression test measure?

The overnight dexamethasone suppression test examines the patient's cortisol level after dexamethasone is administered.

7.8 What is dexamethasone?

Dexamethasone is medication similar to cortisol, in that dexamethasone signals the pituitary gland that there is a high level of cortisol in the blood, causing the pituitary gland to suppress the release of ACTH.

7.9 After dexamethasone is administered to the patient, what should happen to the cortisol level?

The cortisol level should be lower because there is no ACTH in the blood to signal the adrenal glands to release cortisol. If cortisol levels remain high, then this is a sign of Cushing's syndrome, as a result of an adrenal gland tumor producing cortisol.

7.10 Why is the overnight dexamethasone suppression test ordered?

The overnight dexamethasone suppression test is ordered to assess the function of the adrenal glands and for Cushing's syndrome.

7.11 What must be considered before administering the Overnight Dexamethasone Suppression Test?

Assess the patient for conditions that might affect the test results by preventing a decrease in cortisol levels:
- Severe obesity, pregnancy, dehydration, uncontrolled diabetes, severe weight loss, acute alcohol withdrawal, severe injury, stress
- Taking birth control pills, phenytoin (Dilantin), MAOIs, lithium, morphine, aspirin, barbiturates, methadone, diuretics, or Aldactone

Assess the patient's metabolism:
- Some patients metabolize dexamethasone quickly, resulting in a lower than expected blood level when the blood specimen is taken.
- In this case, the healthcare provider will increase the dose of dexamethasone.
- The patient may be given up to eight doses of dexamethasone over two days.

The patient should refrain from taking birth control pills, phenytoin (Dilantin), MAOIs, lithium, morphine, aspirin, barbiturates, methadone, diuretics, or Aldactone 48 hours before the blood specimen is drawn.

7.12 What is an outward sign of a high ACTH and cortisol level?

A patient with a high ACTH and cortisol level may experience bruising.

7.13 What should you explain to the patient before administering the overnight dexamethasone suppression test?

Do not exercise 12 hours before the test. Avoid stressful situations 12 hours before the test. Explain when and why the blood sample is taken, that there might be bruising if the ACTH and cortisol levels are high, and that the test cannot be taken if the patient has taken birth control pills, phenytoin (Dilantin), MAOIs, lithium, morphine, aspirin, barbiturates, methadone, diuretics, or Aldactone. If the patient is taking these medications, the patient must stop taking them for 2 days before the test. Do not eat or drink 12 hours before the test

7.14 What might a high overnight dexamethasone suppression test result infer?

A high overnight dexamethasone suppression test result might infer Cushing's syndrome, hyperthyroidism, uncontrolled diabetes, heart failure, heart attack, poor diet, fever, alcoholism, depression, anorexia nervosa, or lung cancer.

Aldosterone Test

7.15 What is the relationship between renin and aldosterone?

Kidneys release renin. Renin is a hormone that signals the adrenal glands to release aldosterone to control blood pressure and fluids and the balance of electrolytes by retaining fluid and sodium.

7.16 What do you expect the healthcare provider to order when the aldosterone test is ordered?

The aldosterone test is typically performed with the renin activity test.

7.17 What might be an outward sign of high levels of aldosterone?

A patient who has muscle cramps, muscle weakness, tingling in the hands, or high blood pressure may have a high level of aldosterone.

7.18 Why is the aldosterone test ordered?

The aldosterone test is ordered to assess for an adrenal gland tumor, the cause of high blood pressure, the cause of a low potassium level in the blood, and for an overactive adrenal gland.

7.19 What special preparation is required before administering the aldosterone test?

There is no special preparation required for this test.

7.20 What would you expect the healthcare provider to do if the aldosterone test is abnormal?

If the test result is abnormal, the healthcare provider may order subsequent aldosterone tests. For subsequent aldosterone tests, the patient should:
• Refrain from eating natural black licorice two weeks prior to the test.
• Eat 3 grams per day of sodium for 2 weeks prior to the test.
• Avoid a low salt diet, since this increases aldosterone levels.
• Avoid a high salt diet, since this decreases aldosterone levels. Do not eat olives, soy sauce, pretzels, potato chips, canned soups, bacon, and vegetables.
• Know that he or she might be asked to stand, sit, and lie when the test is administered, since the patient's position may affect the test results. Standing or sitting for 2 hours before the test increases the aldosterone level.

7.21 What might a high level of aldosterone indicate?

Primary hyperaldosteronism directly affects the adrenal glands and the renin activity test is low (Adrenal hyperplasia, Conn's syndrome–adrenal gland tumor).

Secondary hyperaldosteronism does not directly affect the adrenal glands and the renin activity test is high (cirrhosis, heart failure, kidney disease, preeclampsia).

7.22 What might a low level of aldosterone indicate?

Addison's disease.

Cortisol Test

7.23 What does the cortisol test measure?

The cortisol test determines the level of cortisol in blood.

7.24 What might a high level of cortisol infer?

A high level of cortisol might infer an adrenal gland tumor, overactive adrenal gland, Cushing's syndrome, Cushing disease, adenoma, depression, severe liver disease, obesity, hyperthyroidism, severe kidney disease, surgery, or sepsis.

7.25 What might a low level of cortisol infer?

A low level of cortisol might infer Addison's disease, shock, Sheehan's syndrome, or autoimmune disease.

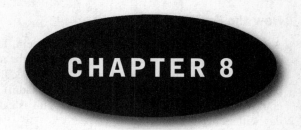

CHAPTER 8

Glucose Tests

8.1   Definition

Blood glucose must be maintained within a narrow range, which occurs naturally with the secretion of insulin and glucagon. There are two pancreatic endocrine hormones secreted by the islet cells in the pancreas: insulin and glucagon. Insulin and glucagon are secreted based on blood glucose levels. When blood glucose is elevated, the pancreas secretes insulin, which causes glucose to cross the cell membrane and allows it to be used for energy, resulting in a decrease in blood glucose. When blood glucose levels are low, the pancreas secretes glucagon, which signals the liver to release stored glucose into the blood, resulting in an increase in blood glucose. Other cells such as muscles also release glucose in response to glucagon. Failure of islet cells to properly function due to diseases such as diabetes can result in high levels of blood glucose (*hyperglycemia*) or low levels of blood glucose (*hypoglycemia*). Healthcare providers order glucose tests to monitor the blood glucose level. Based on the results of these tests, the healthcare provider may administer insulin or glucose to the patient.

8.2   C-Peptide

The C-peptide test measures the level of C-peptide in blood and is used to differentiate between type 1 and type 2 diabetes. Proinsulin is split into C-peptide and insulin. The level of C-peptide is considered equal to the amount of insulin, indicating the amount of insulin made by the pancreas. The healthcare provider will order a blood glucose test along with the C-peptide test. The healthcare provider may order a C-peptide stimulation test to differentiate between type 1 and type 2 diabetes. A patient with type 2 diabetes can develop a low C-peptide level over time.

Why the Test Is Performed

The test differentiates between type 1 and type 2 diabetes. It also assesses the result of removal of an insulinoma from the pancreas and the underlying cause of hypoglycemia.

Before Administering the Test

Assess if the patient:

- Ate or drank 8 hours before the test is administered
- Has taken insulin or oral type 2 diabetic medication, since this can affect the test result
- Has ingested alcohol, insulin, meglitinides or sulfonylureas, birth control pills, diuretics, or corticosteroids, since these can affect the test result
- Has kidney failure
- Is obese

How the Test Is Performed

A sample of blood is taken from the patient's vein. The patient will experience a tight feeling when the tourniquet is tightened, a pinch or nothing at all when the needle is inserted into the vein, and pressure when a gauze pad is pressed against the insertion site to stop bleeding. It can take up to 10 minutes for bleeding to stop if the patient is taking anticoagulants (aspirin, coumadin). A small bruise might appear at the insertion site, which could become swollen following this test. This is called phlebitis. Applying a warm compress several times a day will reduce the swelling.

Teach the Patient

Explain why the blood sample is taken, that the patient should not eat or drink 8 hours before the test is administered, and that the healthcare provider may ask the patient to stop taking alcohol, insulin, meglitinides or sulfonylureas, birth control pills, diuretics, or corticosteroids for 2 weeks prior to the test.

Understanding the Test Results

Test results are available quickly. The laboratory determines normal values based on calibration of testing equipment with a control test. Test results are reported as high, normal, or low based on the laboratory's control test. The blood glucose test is performed along with the C-peptide test and the results of both tests are compared to each other. Normal C-peptide range is: 0.78 to 1.89 ng/mL

High C-peptide and high blood glucose values may indicate type 2 diabetes, Cushing's syndrome, or insulin resistance.

High C-peptide and low blood glucose values may indicate an insulinoma–pancreatic insulin producing tumor, that the patient is taking sulfonylureas, that the patient is taking meglitinides, or metastasized insulinoma, if the insulinoma was removed.

Low C-peptide and low blood glucose values may indicate Addison's disease, liver disease, that the patient has taken insulin, or infection.

Low C-peptide and high blood glucose values may indicate type 1 diabetes or pancreatectomy.

8.3 D-xylose Absorption Test

The D-xylose absorption test measures the level of D-xylose in blood. *D-xylose* is a simple sugar that is absorbed by the intestine. D-xylose absorption can also be tested with a urine sample. A urine test is less accurate than the blood D-xylose absorption test for patients under 12 years of age. The healthcare provider may order an upper gastrointestinal series if the D-xylose test is positive.

Why the Test Is Performed

The test screens for malabsorption syndrome.

Before Administering the Test

- The patient should avoid fruits, jams, pastries, and jellies 1 day before the test is administered.
- Adult patients should avoid eating or drinking anything except water12 hours.
- Patients under 9 years of age should avoid eating or drinking anything except water 4 hours before the test.
- Patients are not permitted to eat or drink until the last blood sample is taken.
- The patient should rest quietly until the last blood sample is taken.
- Assess if the patient is:
  - Undergoing radiation treatment.
  - Taking aspirin, antibiotics, indomethacin, or cardiac medication, since these can affect the test result.

How the Test Is Performed

The patient drinks 8 ounces of water that contain 25 grams of D-xylose. A blood sample is taken two hours after drinking the water and again five hours after drinking the water.

A sample of blood is taken from the patient's vein. The patient will experience a tight feeling when the tourniquet is tightened, a pinch or nothing at all when the needle is inserted into the vein, and pressure when a gauze pad is pressed against the insertion site to stop bleeding. It can take up to 10 minutes for bleeding to stop if the patient is taking anticoagulants (aspirin, coumadin). A small bruise might appear at the insertion site, which could become swollen following this test. This is called phlebitis. Applying a warm compress several times a day will reduce the swelling.

Teach the Patient

Explain why the blood sample is taken and that the patient should avoid fruits, jams, pastries, and jellies 1 day before the test is administered. The patient should avoid eating or drinking anything except water for 12 hours before the test. Patients under 9 years of age should avoid eating or drinking anything except water for 4 hours before the test. The patient will not be permitted to eat or drink until after the last blood sample is taken, and will be asked to rest quietly until the last blood sample is taken.

Understanding the Test Results

Test results are available quickly. The laboratory determines normal values based on calibration of testing equipment with a control test. Test results are reported as high, normal, or low based on the laboratory's control test.

- Normal D-xylose range is:
  - Adult: 21 to 57 mg/dL
  - Under 13 years of age: greater than 20 mg/dL
  - Under 6 months of age: greater than 15 mg/dL

High D-xylose levels may indicate that the patient is undergoing radiation treatment, has Hodgkin's disease, or scleroderma.

Low D-xylose levels may indicate celiac disease, hookworms, malabsorption syndrome, inflammation of the intestine, Crohn's disease, giardiasis, or Whipple's disease.

8.4 Blood Glucose

The blood glucose tests measures the level of glucose in the blood. *Glucose* is the source of energy for cells and is transported into cells by insulin. As blood glucose levels rise following the ingestion of food, the pancreas releases insulin to move the glucose from blood into cells. Glucose levels can also be measured in urine. However, this is not used to diagnose or monitor glucose levels. The healthcare provider may order the glycohemoglobin (GHb) blood test, which is used to monitor blood glucose levels for the previous 120 days. The blood glucose test must be repeated on two different days for diagnosing diabetes.

- There are four blood glucose tests:
  1. **Oral glucose tolerance test (OGTT)**: This test measures the blood glucose levels at specific time intervals after the patient ingests a glucose drink. The oral glucose tolerance test is ordered to screen for gestational diabetes and to confirm positive results of other blood glucose tests.
  2. **Two hour postprandial blood sugar test**: This test measures blood glucose levels 2 hours after the patient ingests food.
  3. **Fasting blood sugar (FBS) test**: This test measures blood glucose levels after the patient has fasted for 8 hours. The FBS test is the initial test for diabetes.
  4. **Random blood sugar (RBS)**: This test measures blood glucose levels several times a day regardless of food intake.

Why the Test Is Performed

The test screens for diabetes and hypoglycemia. It also assesses the treatment for diabetes.

Before Administering the Test

Assess if the patient:

- Is ill. Illness can increase blood glucose levels and affect the test result.
- Smokes, since this can affect the test result.
- Uses caffeine, since this can affect the test result.
- Is experiencing stress, since this can affect the test result.
- Has eaten or fasted according to procedures for the blood glucose test.
- Has taken Dyrenium, dyazide, Dilantin, Lasix, niacin, Inderal, Esidrix, hydro par, oretic, prednisone, or birth control pills, since these may affect the test result.

How the Test Is Performed

- The fasting blood sugar (FBS) test requires the patient to fast for 8 hours before the test is administered.
- Insulin and other diabetic medications are withheld until the test is administered.
- Two-hour postprandial test requires the patient to eat a normal meal 2 hours before the test is administered.
- Oral glucose tolerance test requires the patient to fast 8 hours before the test.
- Ingesting water is permitted.
- A blood sample is taken to be used as a baseline.
- The patient ingests a glucose drink.
- A blood sample is taken in hourly intervals for 3 hours.

A sample of blood is taken from the patient's vein. The patient will experience a tight feeling when the tourniquet is tightened, a pinch or nothing at all when the needle is inserted into the vein, and pressure when a gauze pad is pressed against the insertion site to stop bleeding. It can take up to 10 minutes for bleeding to stop if the patient is taking anticoagulants (aspirin, coumadin). A small bruise might appear at the insertion site, which could become swollen following this test. This is called phlebitis. Applying a warm compress several times a day will reduce the swelling.

Teach the Patient

Explain why the blood sample is taken, the dietary restriction required by the test (if any), and that the healthcare provider may ask the patient to stop taking Dyrenium, dyazide, Dilantin, Lasix, niacin, Inderal, Esidrix, hydro par, oretic, prednisone, or birth control pills for two weeks prior to the test.

Understanding the Test Results

Blood glucose test results are available in 2 hours. The laboratory determines normal values based on calibration of testing equipment with a control test. Test results are reported as high, normal, or low based on the laboratory's control test.

- Normal blood glucose range is:
  - Fasting blood glucose test: 70 to 99 mg/dL
  - Two-hour postprandial blood sugar test: 70 to 145 mg/dL
  - Random blood sugar: 70 to 125 mg/dL

A high blood glucose level may indicate diabetes (fasting blood glucose test greater than 125 mg/dL), (2-hour postprandial blood sugar test greater than 199 mg/dL), (random blood sugar: greater than 199 mg/dL and the presence of symptoms of diabetes), prediabetes (fasting blood glucose test: 100 mg/dL and 125 mg/dL), acromegaly, Cushing's syndrome, stroke, heart attack, or that the patient has taken corticosteroid medication.

Low blood glucose may indicate hypoglycemia (FBS less than 40 mg/dL), insulinoma–insulin producing tumor, hypothyroidism, Addison's disease, kidney failure, malnutrition, cirrhosis, anorexia, or that the patient has taken insulin or other diabetes medication.

8.5 Glycohemoglobin (GHb)

The glycohemoglobin (GHb), commonly known as HgbAIC test, measures the level of glucose bound to hemoglobin. This differs from the blood glucose test, which measures the level of glucose in plasma. Glucose binds to hemoglobin in red blood cells, which has a life span of 120 days. The healthcare provider orders the glycohemoglobin test to assess if treatment is controlling diabetes, and if the patient has been adhering to the treatment over a 120-day period. The glycohemoglobin test can be administered at any time. However, the healthcare provider is likely to order the test four times a year. The glycohemoglobin test is not a replacement for the blood glucose test and cannot indicate hypoglycemia.

Why the Test Is Performed

The test assesses treatment for diabetes, and if the patient has been adhering to treatment for diabetes.

Before Administering the Test

Assess if the patient has:

- Had a blood transfusion in the past 120 days
- Hemolytic anemia, thalassemia, sickle cell anemia, polycystic ovary syndrome, pheochromocytoma, Cushing's syndrome, or kidney disease
- Had the spleen removed
- Taken corticosteroids

How the Test Is Performed

A sample of blood is taken from the patient's vein. The patient will experience a tight feeling when the tourniquet is tightened, a pinch or nothing at all when the needle is inserted into the vein, and pressure when a gauze pad is pressed against the insertion site to stop bleeding. It can take up to 10 minutes for bleeding to stop if the patient is taking anticoagulants (aspirin, coumadin). A small bruise might appear at the insertion site, which could become swollen following this test. This is called phlebitis. Applying a warm compress several times a day will reduce the swelling.

Teach the Patient

Explain why the sample is taken, why the test is administered several times during the year, and that the glycohemoglobin test is not an alternative to daily blood glucose tests.

Understanding the Test Results

Normal glycohemoglobin test results are available in 2 days. The laboratory determines normal values based on calibration of testing equipment with a control test. Test results are reported as high, normal, or low based on the laboratory's control test.

- Range of a normal glycohemoglobin level is:
  - Glycohemoglobin A1c: 4.5% to 5.7%
  - Total glycohemoglobin: 5.3% to 7.5%

High glycohemoglobin levels (8% or greater) may indicate poorly controlled diabetes, that the patient is undergoing corticosteroid treatment, Pheochromocytoma, polycystic ovary syndrome (PCOS), or Cushing's syndrome.

Solved Problems

C-Peptide

8.1   What does the C-peptide test measure?

The C-peptide test measures the level of C-peptide in blood and is used to differentiate between type 1 and type 2 diabetes.

8.2   How does the C-peptide test work?

Proinsulin is split into C-peptide and insulin. The level of C-peptide is considered equal to the amount of insulin, indicating the amount of insulin made by the pancreas.

8.3   Why is the C-peptide test ordered?

The C-peptide test is ordered to differentiate between type 1 and type 2 diabetes, and to assess the result of removal of an insulinoma from the pancreas and the underlying cause of hypoglycemia.

8.4   What should you assess before administering the C-peptide test?

Assess if the patient:
- Ate or drank 8 hours before the test is administered
- Has taken insulin or oral type 2 diabetic medication, since this can affect the test result
- Is ingesting or taking alcohol, insulin, meglitinides or sulfonylureas, birth control pills, diuretics, or corticosteroids, since these can affect the test result
- Has kidney failure
- Is obese

8.5   What might a high C-peptide level and high blood glucose level indicate?

A high C-peptide level and high blood glucose level might indicate type 2 diabetes, Cushing's syndrome, or insulin resistance.

8.6   What might a high C-peptide level and low blood glucose level indicate?

A high C-peptide level and low blood glucose level might indicate insulinoma–pancreatic insulin producing tumor, that the patient is taking sulfonylureas, that the patient is taking meglitinides, or metastasized insulinoma, if the insulinoma was removed.

8.7   What might a low C-peptide level and low blood glucose level indicate?

A low C-peptide level and low blood glucose level might indicate Addison's disease, liver disease, that the patient has taken insulin, or infection.

8.8   What might a low C-peptide level and high blood glucose level indicate?

A low C-peptide level and high blood glucose level might indicate type 1 diabetes and pancreatectomy.

D-xylose Absorption Test

8.9   What is D-xylose?

D-xylose is a simple sugar that is absorbed by the intestine.

8.10   Why is the D-xylose absorption test ordered?

The D-xylose absorption test is ordered to screen for malabsorption syndrome.

8.11   What must be considered before administering the D-xylose absorption test?

- The patient should avoid fruits, jams, pastries, and jellies 1 day before the test is administered.
- Adult patients should avoid eating or drinking anything except water 12 hours before the test.

- Patients under 9 years of age should avoid eating or drinking anything except water 4 hours before the test.
- Patients are not permitted to eat or drink until the last blood sample is taken.
- The patient should rest quietly until the last blood sample is taken.
- Assess if the patient is:
  - Undergoing radiation treatment.
  - Taking aspirin, antibiotics, indomethacin, or cardiac medication since these can affect the test result.

8.12   How is the D-xylose absorption test administered?

The patient drinks 8 ounces of water that contain 25 grams of D-xylose. A blood sample is taken two hours after drinking the water and again five hours after drinking the water.

8.13   What might a high D-xylose level indicate?

A high D-xylose level might indicate that the patient is undergoing radiation treatment, has Hodgkin's disease, or scleroderma.

8.14   What might a low D-xylose level indicate?

A low D-xylose level might indicate celiac disease, hookworms, malabsorption syndrome, inflammation of the intestine, Crohn's disease, giardiasis, or Whipple's disease.

Blood Glucose Test

8.15   What is glucose?

Glucose is the source of energy for cells, and is transported into cells by insulin.

8.16   What happens when food is ingested?

As blood glucose levels rise following the ingestion of food, the pancreas releases insulin to move the glucose from blood into cells.

8.17   Why is the glycohemoglobin (GHb) blood test ordered?

The glycohemoglobin (GHb) blood test is used to monitor blood glucose levels for the previous 120 days.

8.18   What does the fasting blood sugar (FBS) test measure?

This test measures blood glucose levels after the patient has fasted for 8 hours.

8.19   What does the oral glucose tolerance test (OGTT) measure?

This test measures the blood glucose levels at specific time intervals after the patient ingests a glucose drink. The oral glucose tolerance test is ordered to screen for gestational diabetes and to confirm positive results of other blood glucose tests.

8.20   What does the 2-hour postprandial blood sugar test measure?

This test measures blood glucose levels 2 hours after the patient ingests food.

8.21   What does the random blood sugar (RBS) test measure?

This test measures blood glucose levels several times a day, regardless of food intake.

8.22   What test is the initial test for diabetes?

The fasting blood sugar (FBS) test is the initial test for diabetes.

8.23   Why is blood glucose measured?

Blood glucose is measured to screen for diabetes and hypoglycemia, and to assess the treatment for diabetes.

8.24   What must be assessed before administering the blood glucose test?

Assess if the patient:
- Is ill. Illness can increase blood glucose levels and affect the test result.
- Smokes, since this can affect the test result.
- Uses caffeine, since this can affect the test result.
- Is experiencing stress, since this can affect the test result.
- Has eaten or fasted according to procedures for the blood glucose test.
- Has taken Dyrenium, dyazide, Dilantin, Lasix, niacin, Inderal, Esidrix, hydro par, oretic, prednisone, or birth control pills, since these may affect the test result.

8.25   Should the patient be administered insulin prior to the blood glucose test?

Insulin and other diabetic medications are withheld until the test is administered.

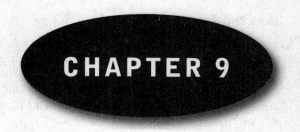

CHAPTER 9

Tumor Markers

9.1 Definition

A *tumor marker* is a substance, usually a protein, which is produced either by tumor cells or by other cells in response to the presence of a tumor. A *tumor* is uncontrollable growth of cells that may be malignant (cancerous) or benign (noncancerous). Blood tests are performed to detect the presence of tumor markers. The presence of a tumor marker does not mean that the patient has cancer. Conditions other than cancer can also generate the tumor marker. The absence of a tumor marker does not mean that the patient is cancer-free because many times early stages of cancer do not produce tumor markers. In addition to tumor markers, a patient's blood can also be tested for cancer genomics. *Cancer genomics* are mutations of specific genes, which are called *risk markers*. A risk marker indicates that a patient has a higher than normal risk for developing cancer. However, there is not a sign of cancer as yet. Conversely, the presence of the tumor marker indicates a possibility that a tumor is present.

9.2 Cancer Antigen 125 (CA–125)

The cancer antigen 125 test measures the level of the cancer antigen 125 in the blood. *Cancer antigen 125* (CA–125) is a protein attached to ovarian cancer cells and other cancer cells. The cancer antigen 125 test is not used to screen patients for ovarian cancer. The cancer antigen 125 test cannot differentiate between a benign or malignant ovarian tumor. The healthcare provider may order testing of peritoneal fluid to assess if cancer antigen 125 is present. A high level of cancer antigen 125 might be found months before other diagnostic tests indicate the return of previously treated ovarian cancer.

Why the Test Is Performed

Although the test isn't a reliable test for ovarian cancer, some healthcare provider may use the test as one of a number of ways to screen for ovarian cancer and other types of cancers. It also assesses the effectiveness of cancer treatment.

Before Administering the Test

Assess if the patient:

- Has undergone abdominal surgery in the previous 3 weeks
- Has undergone chemotherapy recently
- Has undergone a radioactive scan recently
- Is pregnant
- Is menstruating

How the Test Is Performed

A sample of blood is taken from the patient's vein. The patient will experience a tight feeling when the tourniquet is tightened, a pinch or nothing at all when the needle is inserted into the vein, and pressure when a gauze pad is pressed against the insertion site to stop bleeding. It can take up to 10 minutes for bleeding to stop if the patient is taking anticoagulants (aspirin, coumadin). A small bruise might appear at the insertion site, which could become swollen following this test. This is called phlebitis. Applying a warm compress several times a day will reduce the swelling.

Teach the Patient

Explain why the blood sample is taken, that this test is not used to screen for ovarian cancer, and that a positive result does not differentiate between a benign or malignant ovarian tumor.

Understanding the Test Results

Test results are available in 3 days. The laboratory determines normal values based on calibration of testing equipment with a control test. Test results are reported as high, normal, or low based on the laboratory's control test. Normal cancer antigen 125 range is less than 35 U/mL.

High cancer antigen 125 values may indicate ovarian cancer, cancer of the endometrium, cancer of the fallopian tubes, liver cancer, breast cancer, lung cancer, colon cancer, pancreatic cancer, esophagus cancer, stomach cancer, cancer of the peritoneum, lymphoma, pancreatitis, hepatitis, cirrhosis, lupus, endometriosis, pelvic inflammatory disease, uterine fibroids, menstruation, or pregnancy.

9.3   Carcinoembryonic Antigen (CEA)

The carcinoembryonic antigen test measures the level of carcinoembryonic antigen in blood. The *carcinoembryonic antigen* (CEA) is a protein present during fetal development. It terminates at birth. The carcinoembryonic antigen is produced in certain types of cancers. The carcinoembryonic antigen is not used to screen for early detection of a cancer and is not used to diagnose cancer. Most cancers do not cause high levels of the carcinoembryonic antigen. The healthcare provider may order test of peritoneal fluid and cerebrospinal fluid to determine if the cancer metastasized. Carcinoembryonic antigen may be normal, although the patient has cancer.

Why the Test Is Performed

The test screens for cancer and assesses the effectiveness of treatment for cancer and success of surgery to remove the cancer.

Before Administering the Test

Assess if the patient:

- Smokes, since it can affect the test result
- Has undergone chemotherapy recently
- Has undergone a radioactive scan recently
- Is pregnant
- Is menstruating

How the Test Is Performed

A sample of blood is taken from the patient's vein. The patient will experience a tight feeling when the tourniquet is tightened, a pinch or nothing at all when the needle is inserted into the vein, and pressure when a gauze pad is pressed against the insertion site to stop bleeding. It can take up to 10 minutes for bleeding to stop if the patient is taking anticoagulants (aspirin, coumadin). A small bruise might appear at the insertion site, which could become swollen following this test. This is called phlebitis. Applying a warm compress several times a day will reduce the swelling.

Teach the Patient

Explain why the blood sample is taken, that further testing is likely if there is a positive result, and that a negative result does not rule out cancer.

Understanding the Test Results

Test results are available in 3 days. The laboratory determines normal values based on calibration of testing equipment with a control test. Test results are reported as high, normal, or low based on the laboratory's control test.

- Normal carcinoembryonic antigen range is:
  - Nonsmoker: less than 3 ng/mL
  - Smoker: less than 5 ng/mL

High carcinoembryonic antigen values may indicate colon cancer, rectal cancer, lung cancer, breast cancer, pancreatic cancer, ovarian cancer, cancer has returned following treatment (successful treatment results in carcinoembryonic antigen levels returning to normal within six weeks of treatment), cancer has metastasized, pancreatitis, kidney failure, cirrhosis, peptic ulcer, COPD, inflammatory bowel disease, or Crohn's disease.

9.4 Prostate-Specific Antigen (PSA)

The prostate-specific antigen (PSA) test measures the level of prostate-specific antigen in blood. The prostate gland releases prostate-specific antigen (PSA) in low amounts. Increased amounts are released with an enlarged prostate gland, prostatitis, prostate cancer, and from injury resulting from a digital rectal exam, cystoscopy, or sexual activity. The prostate-specific antigen level can be normal in a patient who has prostate cancer. The prostate-specific antigen test is performed in conjunction with a digital rectal examination. The healthcare provider may also order the prostate-specific antigen density (PSAD) test to compare the PSA value to the prostate gland size; the prostate-specific antigen velocity test to determine if the PSA increases over time; the complex prostate-specific antigen (cPSA) to detect prostate cancer; and the transrectal ultrasound (TRUS) to measure the size of the prostate gland.

Why the Test Is Performed

The test screens for prostate cancer and assesses the treatment of prostate cancer.

Before Administering the Test

Assess if the patient:

- Has ejaculated 48 hours before the test
- Has a urinary tract infection
- Has been catheterized within the past eight weeks
- Has prostatitis
- Has undergone a prostate biopsy in the past eight weeks
- Is taking Avodart, proscar, finasteride, cytoxan, Neosar, methotrexate, or diethylstilbestrol

How the Test Is Performed

Do not ejaculate 48 hours before the test.

A sample of blood is taken from the patient's vein. The patient will experience a tight feeling when the tourniquet is tightened, a pinch or nothing at all when the needle is inserted into the vein, and pressure when a gauze pad is pressed against the insertion site to stop bleeding. It can take up to 10 minutes for bleeding to stop if the patient is taking anticoagulants (aspirin, coumadin). A small bruise might appear at the insertion site, which could become swollen following this test. This is called phlebitis. Applying a warm compress several times a day will reduce the swelling.

Teach the Patient

Explain why the sample is taken and that further testing is necessary if there is a high level of prostate-specific antigen in the blood. This does not mean that the patient has prostate cancer. A normal level of prostate-specific antigen does not mean that the patient is free from prostate cancer.

Understanding the Test Results

The prostate-specific antigen test results are available quickly.

- Normal test results (maximum level):
  - Less than 50 years of age: 2.5 ng/mL
  - 51 to 60 years of age: 3.5 ng/mL
  - 61 to 70 years of age: 4.5 ng/mL
  - Over 70 years of age: 6.5 ng/mL

Higher levels may indicate prostate cancer, benign prostatic hypertrophy (BPH), prostatitis, a recent catherization, or injury.

Solved Problems

Cancer Antigen 125

9.1   What is a tumor marker?

A tumor marker is a substance, usually a protein, which is produced either by tumor cells or by other cells in response to the presence of the tumor.

9.2   What is a tumor?

A tumor is uncontrollable growth of cells that may be malignant (cancerous) or benign (noncancerous).

9.3   Does the presence of a tumor indicate that the patient has cancer?

No. Conditions other than cancer can also generate the tumor marker.

9.4   Does the absence of a tumor marker indicate that the patient is cancer-free?

The absence of a tumor marker does not mean that the patient is cancer-free because many times early stages of cancer do not produce tumor markers.

9.5   What is CA–125?

Cancer antigen 125 (CA–125) is a protein attached to the ovarian cancer cells and other cancer cells.

9.6   What does the cancer antigen 125 test measure?

The cancer antigen 125 test measures the level of the cancer antigen 125 in the blood.

9.7   Can the cancer antigen 125 test differentiate between a benign or malignant tumor?

No.

9.8   What is the advantage of the cancer antigen 125 test in previously treated ovarian cancer?

A high level of cancer antigen 125 might be found months before other diagnostic tests indicate the return of previously treated ovarian cancer.

9.9   Why is the cancer antigen 125 test administered?

The test screens for ovarian cancer and other types of cancers. It also assesses the effectiveness of cancer treatment.

9.10   What should be assessed in the patient before the cancer antigen 125 test is administered?

Assess if the patient:
- Has undergone abdominal surgery in the previous three weeks
- Has undergone chemotherapy recently

- Has undergone a radioactive scan recently
- Is pregnant
- Is menstruating

9.11   What might a high level of cancer antigen 125 indicate?

A high level of cancer antigen 125 might indicate ovarian cancer, cancer of the endometrium, cancer of the fallopian tubes, liver cancer, breast cancer, lung cancer, colon cancer, pancreatic cancer, esophagus cancer, stomach cancer, cancer of the peritoneum, lymphoma, pancreatitis, hepatitis, cirrhosis, lupus, endometriosis, pelvic inflammatory disease, uterine fibroids, menstruation, or pregnancy.

Carcinoembryonic Antigen

9.12   What is CEA?

The carcinoembryonic antigen (CEA) is a protein present during fetal development that terminates at birth. The carcinoembryonic antigen is produced in certain types of cancers.

9.13   Do most cancers cause high levels of CEA?

No.

9.14   If CEA is high, what other test might the healthcare provider order?

The healthcare provider may order a test of peritoneal fluid and cerebrospinal fluid to determine if the cancer metastasized.

9.15   Why is the carcinoembryonic antigen test administered?

The carcinoembryonic antigen test is administered to screen for cancer. It also assesses the effectiveness of treatment for cancer and success of surgery to remove the cancer.

9.16   What should be assessed in the patient before the carcinoembryonic antigen test is administered?

Assess if the patient:
- Smokes, since it can affect the test result
- Has undergone chemotherapy recently
- Has undergone a radioactive scan recently
- Is pregnant
- Is menstruating

9.17   What is one of the most important facts to teach a patient about the carcinoembryonic antigen test?

A negative result does not rule out cancer.

9.18   What might a high carcinoembryonic antigen test result indicate?

A high carcinoembryonic antigen test might indicate colon cancer, rectal cancer, lung cancer, breast cancer, pancreatic cancer, ovarian cancer, that the cancer has returned following treatment (successful treatment results in carcinoembryonic antigen levels returning to normal within 6 weeks of treatment), that the cancer has metastasized, pancreatitis, kidney failure, cirrhosis, peptic ulcer, COPD, inflammatory bowel disease, or Crohn's disease.

Prostate-Specific Antigen (PSA)

9.19   What other test might a healthcare provider order in addition to the PSA test?

The healthcare provider may also order the prostate-specific antigen density (PSAD) test to compare the PSA value to the prostate gland size; the prostate-specific antigen velocity test to determine the if the PSA increases over time; the complex prostate-specific antigen (cPSA) to detect prostate cancer; and the transrectal ultrasound (TRUS) to measure the size of the prostate gland.

9.20   Why is the PSA test administered?

The PSA test is administered to screen for prostate cancer and assess the treatment of prostate cancer.

9.21   What should you assess before administering the PSA test?

Assess if the patient:
- Has ejaculated 48 hours before the test
- Has a urinary tract infection
- Has been catheterized within the past eight weeks
- Has prostatitis
- Has undergone a prostate biopsy in the past eight weeks
- Is taking Avodart, proscar, finasteride, cytoxan, Neosar, methotrexate, or diethylstilbestrol

9.22   Does a high PSA test result mean that the patient has prostate cancer?

No. Further testing is necessary if there is a high level of prostate-specific antigen in the blood. This does not mean that the patient has prostate cancer.

9.23   How would you respond if the patient appeared happy that he has a normal level of prostate-specific antigen?

Acknowledge the patient's feelings but also mention that a normal PSA level does not mean that the patient is free from prostate cancer.

9.24   What might a high PSA level indicate?

A high PSA level might indicate prostate cancer, benign prostatic hypertrophy (BPH), prostatitis, a recent catherization, or injury.

9.25   How would you interpret a PSA result of 4.5 ng/mL?

The result must be compared with the patient's age to assess whether or not the test results are normal.

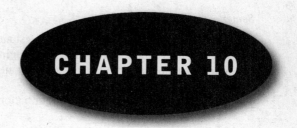

CHAPTER 10

Pregnancy and Genetic Tests

10.1   Definition

Pregnancy and genetic tests are ordered to determine the underlying cause of infertility and risk for genetic disorders that can affect the fetus or newborn. Pregnancy and genetic tests are ordered to screen patients for disorders when there are no telltale signs or symptoms. Pregnancy and genetic tests are also ordered when the healthcare provider is looking to confirm a sign or symptoms that something is outside of normal parameters. Pregnancy and genetic tests look for certain components in blood, such as the presence of antibodies or certain enzymes, or the levels of protein and hormones. Scientific research has determined that the absence or existence of these components in blood correlates to the presence or absence of a specific disorder.

10.2   Antisperm Antibody Test

The antisperm antibody test is administered to determine the cause of infertility. An immune system response can be caused by semen, resulting in antibodies attaching to and killing sperm, which causes immunologic infertility. These antibodies can be in blood, vaginal fluids, or semen. Antibodies can be made in a man if his sperm comes in contact with his immune system as a result of testicular injury, prostate gland infection, a vasectomy, or other surgeries that expose sperm to the immune system. Semen can cause an allergic reaction in a woman to her partner's sperm. Some healthcare providers question the usefulness of the test, since treatment is the same regardless of the test results.

Why the Test Is Performed

The test assesses if antisperm antibodies are in blood, vaginal fluid, or semen. Infertility may be caused by immunologic infertility.

Before Administering the Test

Patients may be embarrassed about collecting a sample. Confer with the healthcare provider if masturbation is against the patient's religious beliefs.

How the Test Is Performed

A sample of blood is taken from the patient's vein. The patient will experience a tight feeling when the tourniquet is tightened, a pinch or nothing at all when the needle is inserted into the vein, and pressure when a gauze pad is pressed against the insertion site to stop bleeding. It can take up to 10 minutes for bleeding to stop if the patient is taking anticoagulants (aspirin, coumadin). A small bruise might appear at the insertion site, which could become swollen following this test. This is called phlebitis. Applying a warm compress several times a day will reduce the swelling.

Semen sample from a male patient:

- Do not ejaculate for 2 days before the test and no longer than 5 days before the test.
- Collect semen samples after blood and vaginal fluid samples are taken.
- Samples cannot be taken by sexual intercourse and then withdrawn during ejaculation. Vaginal fluid may mix with the sperm.
- A semen sample is collected by masturbation.
  - Urinate
  - Wash and rinse your hands and penis
  - Collect the semen in a sterile cup
  - Do not use lubricants or condoms
  - Take sample to the lab within 30 minutes

Teach the Patient

Explain why the test is ordered and that the patient should not ejaculate for 2 days before the test and no longer than 5 days before the test. Explain how to collect the semen sample, to take the sample to the lab within 30 minutes, and not to use lubricants or condoms when collecting the sample. Ask the patient to consult his healthcare provider if masturbation is against the patient's religious beliefs.

Understanding the Test Results

- Negative test results: antisperm antibodies are not found.
- Positive test results: antisperm antibodies found.

10.3   Alpha-Fetoprotein (AFP) Test

The alpha-fetoprotein test is commonly administered as part of a maternal serum triple or quadruple screening test, which along with other factors, including the pregnant woman's age, is used to estimate the chances of birth defects. Alpha-fetoprotein (AFP) is produced by the fetal liver and is detectable in a pregnant woman's blood. The level of AFP rises gradually in the 14 weeks of gestation and continues rising until around week 34 of gestation, when the AFP level gradually decreases. A high level or low level of AFP is a sign that there may be a problem with the fetal development.

The maternal serum triple screening test examines levels of:

- Alpha-fetoprotein
- Beta human chorionic gonadotropin (beta-hCG)
- Unconjugated estriol or uE3 (estrogen)

The maternal serum quad screening test examines levels of the same substance as the maternal serum triple screening test and the hormone inhibin A. A healthcare provider may also administer the alpha-fetoprotein test in nonpregnant women and in children and men to assess for a number of other diseases that cause a high level of AFP in the blood. Half of patients diagnosed with certain cancers have normal alpha-fetoprotein test results. These include lymphoma, Hodgkin's disease, ovarian cancer, testicular cancer, renal cell cancer, and pancreatic cancer. The test is performed between 15 weeks and 20 weeks of gestation.

Why the Test Is Performed

The test assesses for fetal neural tube defects, spinal bifida, anencephaly, Edward syndrome (trisomy 18), Down syndrome (trisomy 21), omphalocele, hepatoma in patients who have chronic hepatitis B or cirrhosis, lymphoma, Hodgkin's disease, renal cell cancer, ovarian cancer, testicular cancer, pancreatic cancer, and effectiveness of cancer treatment.

Before Administering the Test

Address the patient's concerns. Inform the patient that the alpha-fetoprotein test results provide a sign of a disease or medical condition, but are not used to make a definitive diagnosis. AFP levels can be high and the fetus may be normal.

Assess:

- If the patient smokes. Smoking increases the AFP level in the blood.
- If the patient is an insulin-dependent diabetic.
- The patient's weight.
- The gestational age of the fetus.
- If the patient has undergone a test involving radioactive tracers in the previous two weeks, since this might affect the test results.
- If the patient is a diabetic who requires insulin injections to manage the diabetes.
- The patient is weighed before the blood sample is drawn. The results of the test are evaluated based on the patient's weight.
- The patient's race is noted. Normal values of AFP are higher in African-American women and lower for Asian women.

How the Test Is Performed

- The test is performed between 15 weeks and 20 weeks of gestation.
- The patient is weighed before the blood sample is drawn. The results of the test are evaluated based on the patient's weight.
- Estimate the gestation.
- Assess if the patient is a diabetic who requires insulin injections to manage the diabetes.
- The patient's race is noted. Normal values of AFP are higher in African-American women and lower for Asian women.

A sample of blood is taken from the patient's vein. The patient will experience a tight feeling when the tourniquet is tightened, a pinch or nothing at all when the needle is inserted into the vein, and pressure when a gauze pad is pressed against the insertion site to stop bleeding. It can take up to 10 minutes for bleeding to stop if the patient is taking anticoagulants (aspirin, coumadin). A small bruise might appear at the insertion site, which could become swollen following this test. This is called phlebitis. Applying a warm compress several times a day will reduce the swelling.

Teach the Patient

Explain why the blood sample is taken, that there is no special preparation required for the test, that weight, race, and gestational age are used to assess the test results, and that an abnormal test result does not mean there are developmental problems with the fetus. The test result is one of several signs that help the healthcare provider reach a diagnosis. A neural tube defect is not related to the mother's age. Neural tube defects occur without a family history of this problem.

Understanding the Test Results

The result is available quickly. The laboratory determines normal values based on calibration of testing equipment with a control test. Test results are reported as high, normal, or low based on the laboratory's control test. If high levels of AFP are detected, the healthcare provider will likely order an ultrasound and/or amniocentesis. An ultrasound confirms the gestational age. If the gestational age is different than the estimated gestational age, the AFP is adjusted using the multiple of median (MoM) factor. An AFP value that is 0.5 to 2.5 times the multiple of median factor is considered normal. A normal AFP level does not rule out a neural tube defect or Down syndrome. An abnormal AFP level is not an indication of a definitive diagnosis. Additional testing such as an ultrasound or amniocentesis will likely be ordered for abnormal results. The patient may have an abnormal AFP level in her blood and a normal AFP level in the amniocentesis, indicating low risk to the fetus.

- Generally, the normal range is:
  ○ Pregnant women 12 to 22 weeks gestation: 19 to 75 IU/mL or 7 to 124 µg/L or 7 to 124 ng/mL
  ○ Non-pregnant women and men: 0 to 6.4 IU/mL or 0 to 20 µg/L or 0 to 20 ng/mL

High levels may indicate neural tube defect, omphalocele (abdominal organs are outside of the abdomen wall; repaired by surgery), multiple fetus, deceased fetus, incorrect gestational age, alcohol abuse, cirrhosis, hepatitis B, lymphoma, Hodgkin's disease, ovarian cancer, testicular cancer, renal cell cancer, and pancreatic cancer.

Low levels may indicate Down syndrome (60% accuracy. Accuracy increases to 80% with the maternal serum triple screening test) or incorrect gestational age.

10.4 Follicle-Stimulating Hormone

The follicle-stimulating hormone test measures the level of the follicle-stimulating hormone in blood. The *follicle-stimulating hormone* (FSH) is produced by the pituitary gland and controls sperm production by the testes and egg production in the ovaries. Follicle-stimulating hormone level is constant in men and changes with the menstrual cycle in women, with the highest level occurring during ovulation. The healthcare provider may order the luteinizing hormone blood test, estrogen blood test, and the progesterone blood test in addition to the follicle-stimulating hormone test. The healthcare provider may order a sperm count or assessment of the patient's ovarian reserve.

Why the Test Is Performed

The test assesses for the underlying cause of infertility, abnormal menstrual periods, precocious puberty, the function of the pituitary gland, and abnormal development of sexual organs.

Before Administering the Test

Assess:

- The patient's age. Test results depend on the patient's age.
- If the patient uses herbal or natural substances.
- The first day of the patient's last menstrual period. Test results depend on the patient's menstrual cycle.
- Which day the patient experiences the heaviest bleeding during the menstrual period.
- If the patient has undergone a radioactive tracer in the previous 7 days before the test.
- If the patient has taken digitalis, cimetidine, levodopa, clomiphene, birth control pills, estrogen, and progesterone 4 weeks before the test, since these may affect the test result.

How the Test Is Performed

A blood sample may be taken each day for a period ordered by the healthcare provider if the patient experiences menstrual cycle problems or is unable to become pregnant.

A sample of blood is taken from the patient's vein. The patient will experience a tight feeling when the tourniquet is tightened, a pinch or nothing at all when the needle is inserted into the vein, and pressure when a gauze pad is pressed against the insertion site to stop bleeding. It can take up to 10 minutes for bleeding to stop if the patient is taking anticoagulants (aspirin, coumadin). A small bruise might appear at the insertion site, which could become swollen following this test. This is called phlebitis. Applying a warm compress several times a day will reduce the swelling.

Teach the Patient

Explain why the blood sample is taken, that several blood samples may be necessary, one each for a period ordered by the healthcare provider if the patient experiences menstrual cycle problems or is unable to become pregnant, and that the healthcare provider may ask the patient to stop taking digitalis, cimetidine, levodopa, clomiphene, birth control pills, estrogen, and progesterone for 4 weeks prior to the test.

Understanding the Test Results

Follicle-stimulating hormone test results are available in 1 day. The laboratory determines normal values based on calibration of testing equipment with a control test. Test results are reported as high, normal, or low based on the laboratory's control test.

- Normal follicle stimulating hormone range is:
  - Menstruating:
    - Follicular/luteal phase: 5 to 20 IU/L
    - Mid-cycle peak: 30 to 50 IU/L
  - Post menopause: greater than 49 IU/L
  - Men: 5 to 15 IU/L
  - Children before puberty: less than 7 IU/L

High follicle stimulating hormone may indicate: (for women) polycystic ovary syndrome (PCOS), ovarian failure before 40 years of age, or menopause; (for men) abnormal testicle functionality or Klinefelter syndrome; (for children) start of puberty.

Low follicle stimulating hormone may indicate: (for women) loss of ovulation; (for men) testicles not producing sperm; (for both genders) malnutrition, hypothalamus disorder, pituitary gland disorder, or stress.

10.5   Human Chorionic Gonadotropin (hCG)

The human chorionic gonadotropin test measures the level of human chorionic gonadotropin in blood. The hCG hormone test is typically ordered as part of a maternal serum screening test that is administered at 15 weeks of gestation. When a fertilized egg implants in the uterine wall, the placenta begins development. By the ninth day, the placenta produces human chorionic gonadotropin (hCG) hormone, which is detectable in the patient's blood. The level of the hCG hormone is used as a sign of pregnancy, which is confirmed by other tests. In a normal pregnancy, the level of the hCG hormone increases until 16 weeks of gestation and then gradually decreases until birth, when no hCG hormone is detectable. A lower level of hCG hormone might indicate an ectopic pregnancy and a higher level may indicate multiple fetuses.

The hCG hormone can also be produced by a molar pregnancy, choricocarcinoma (uterus cancer), ovarian cancer, or other tumors. Testicular cancer also produces the hCG hormone in men. A normal hCG hormone level does not rule out cancer. The level of the hCG hormone can be detected before the patient misses her menstrual period and as early as six days after attachment of the egg. The hCG hormone test is also available as a urine test (home pregnancy test), which determines if the hCG hormone is present, but does not measures the hormone's level. The hCG hormone level is high 4 weeks following an abortion.

Why the Test Is Performed

The test assesses for pregnancy, ectopic pregnancy, molar pregnancy, treatment for molar pregnancy, testicular cancer, and choricocarcinoma.

Before Administering the Test

Assess if the patient has:

- Received hCG hormone infertility treatment prior to administering the test
- Has taken Anergan, phenergan, Prorex, a diuretic, heparin, Ambien, Mellaril, Serentil, Stelazine, or compazine

How the Test Is Performed

A sample of blood is taken from the patient's vein. The patient will experience a tight feeling when the tourniquet is tightened, a pinch or nothing at all when the needle is inserted into the vein, and pressure when a gauze pad is pressed against the insertion site to stop bleeding. It can take up to 10 minutes for bleeding to stop if the patient is taking anticoagulants (aspirin, coumadin). A small bruise might appear at the insertion site, which could become swollen following this test. This is called phlebitis. Applying a warm compress several times a day will reduce the swelling.

Teach the Patient

Explain why the sample is taken, that the hCG hormone blood test confirms a home urine pregnancy test (however other tests are necessary to confirm the pregnancy), and that the healthcare provider may ask the patient not to take hCG hormone infertility treatment, Anergan, phenergan, Prorex, diuretic, heparin, Ambien, Mellaril, Serentil, Stelazine, or compazine for several weeks prior to the test.

Understanding the Test Results

The hCG hormone test results are available quickly. The laboratory determines normal values based on calibration of testing equipment with a control test. Test results are reported as high, normal, or low based on the laboratory's control test.

- Normal hCG hormone level is:
  - Men: Less than 5 IU/L
  - Non-pregnant women: Less than 5 IU/L
  - Pregnant women:
    - 24 to 28 days gestation: 5 to 100 IU/L
    - 4 to 5 weeks gestation: 50 to 500 IU/L
    - 5 to 6 weeks gestation: 100 to 10,000 IU/L
    - 14 to 16 weeks gestation: 12,000 to 270,000 IU/L
    - After 16 weeks gestation: Levels decrease

High hCG hormone levels may indicate: (in men) lung cancer, pancreatic cancer, colon cancer, liver cancer, or testicular cancer; (in nonpregnant women) lung cancer, pancreatic cancer, colon cancer, liver cancer, or ovarian cancer, choricocarcinoma; (in pregnant women) multiple fetuses, Down syndrome, molar pregnancy, or incorrect estimate of gestation.

Low hCG hormone levels may indicate: (in pregnant women) ectopic pregnancy, incorrect estimate of gestation, fetal death, or risk for spontaneous abortion.

10.6   Inhibin A Test

The hormone inhibin A test is a component of the quad screen tests that are administered at the twentieth week of gestation to determine if there is a risk of a birth defect in the fetus such as Down syndrome. *Inhibin A hormone* is secreted by the placenta and the level of the hormone is measured by the hormone inhibin A test. The quad screen test also includes the alpha-fetoprotein (AFP) test, beta human chorionic gonadotropin (beta-hCG) test, and the unconjugated estriol (uE3) test. The hormone inhibin A test is not used to diagnose the potential for birth defects. Further testing is required if the hormone inhibin A test is abnormal.

Why the Test Is Performed

The test assesses the risk for Down syndrome and other birth defects.

Before Administering the Test

Assess if the patient:

- Smokes
- Is obese
- Is a diabetic

How the Test Is Performed

A sample of blood is taken from the patient's vein. The patient will experience a tight feeling when the tourniquet is tightened, a pinch or nothing at all when the needle is inserted into the vein, and pressure when a gauze pad is pressed against the insertion site to stop bleeding. It can take up to 10 minutes for bleeding to stop if the patient is taking anticoagulants (aspirin, coumadin). A small bruise might appear at the insertion site, which could become swollen following this test. This is called phlebitis. Applying a warm compress several times a day will reduce the swelling.

Teach the Patient

Explain why the sample is taken and that an abnormal test result does not mean there is a birth defect. Further testing might be ordered by the healthcare provider.

Understanding the Test Results

- The inhibin A hormone test results are available quickly.
- High inhibin A hormone levels may indicate birth defects. Additional testing is required for positive diagnosis.

10.7   Prolactin

The prolactin test measures the level of prolactin in the blood. *Prolactin* is a hormone produced by the pituitary gland that increases during pregnancy causing an increase in milk product and enlargement of the mammary glands. A high level of progesterone that occurs during pregnancy prevents milk from ejecting. Progesterone levels fall after delivery. As the newborn sucks the nipple to cause ejection of milk from the breast, this action simulates release of prolactin, causing lactogenesis, resulting in increased production of milk. Prolactin levels return to normal after delivery if the mother is not breastfeeding.

Why the Test Is Performed

The test assesses for prolactinoma (pituitary gland tumor), underlying cause of amenorrhea, underlying cause of infertility, underlying cause of nipple discharge, and erectile dysfunction.

Before Administering the Test

Assess if the patient:

- Exercised 12 hours prior to the test
- Is under emotional stress
- Has difficulty sleeping
- Has undergone a radioactive tracer test one week prior to the test
- Is taking tricyclic antidepressants, birth control pills, phenothiazines, hypertensive medication, or cocaine
- Nipples have been stimulated within the previous day

How the Test Is Performed

- Avoid eating or drinking 12 hours before the test
- Take the blood sample 3 hours after the patient awakens
- Prolactin levels are normally higher in the morning
- Rest 30 minutes before taking the blood sample
- Avoid stimulating the nipples for 1 day prior to the test

A sample of blood is taken from the patient's vein. The patient will experience a tight feeling when the tourniquet is tightened, a pinch or nothing at all when the needle is inserted into the vein, and pressure when a gauze pad is pressed against the insertion site to stop bleeding. It can take up to 10 minutes for bleeding to stop if the patient is taking anticoagulants (aspirin, coumadin). A small bruise might appear at the insertion site, which could become swollen following this test. This is called phlebitis. Applying a warm compress several times a day will reduce the swelling.

Teach the Patient

Explain why the sample is taken, that the blood sample must be taken 3 hours after the patient awakens, that the patient must avoid simulating the nipples for 1 day prior to the test, that the patient will be asked to rest 30 minutes before the blood sample is taken, and that the healthcare provider may ask the patient to refrain from taking cocaine 12 hours prior to the test. Avoid eating or drinking 12 hours before the test.

Understanding the Test Results

The prolactin test results are available quickly. The laboratory determines normal values based on calibration of testing equipment with a control test. Test results are reported as high, normal, or low based on the laboratory's control test.

- Normal prolactin test results:
  - Pregnant: 20 to 400 ng/mL
  - Non-Pregnant: less than 25 ng/mL
  - Men: less than 20 ng/mL

High prolactin levels may indicate prolactinoma, idiopathic hyperprolactinemia, hypothyroidism, cirrhosis, or kidney disease.

10.8 Phenylketonuria (PKU) Test

The phenylketonuria (PKU) test measures the level of the phenylalanine hydroxylase enzyme in blood. *Phenylalanine* is an amino acid in breast milk, formula, dairy products, and meats. The body requires the phenylalanine hydroxylase enzyme to metabolize phenylalanine into tyrosine. *Phenylketonuria* (PKU) is a genetic disorder in which the patient is missing the phenylalanine hydroxylase enzyme and is therefore unable to metabolize phenylalanine, causing a buildup of phenylalanine level in the blood, which results in mental retardation and seizures. Newborns are administered the phenylketonuria (PKU) test between 12 hours and 28 hours after birth, and again a week after birth. Infants older than six weeks of age may be administered a phenylketonuria urine test if a phenylketonuria was not performed at birth. Newborns that are ill are retested three weeks after birth.

Why the Test Is Performed

The test assesses for phenylketonuria.

Before Administering the Test

Assess if the:

- Newborn ingested formula or breast milk for 48 hours prior to the test
- Newborn was born prematurely
- Patient has vomited prior to the test
- Patient is taking antibiotics

How the Test Is Performed

The newborn should ingest formula or breast milk for 48 hours prior to the test.

Heel Stick: Several drops of blood are collected from the heel of a newborn or baby. The heel is cleaned using alcohol. A sterile lancet is used to puncture the heel. Several drops of blood are collected in a small test tube. A gauze pad is pressed over the site until bleeding stops. A small bandage is applied.

The healthcare provider may order a blood sample taken from a vein to confirm a positive phenylketonuria test that used a sample from a heel stick.

Teach the Patient

Explain why the sample is taken and that the test may be repeated a week after birth. Inform the parents that the newborn must ingest formula or breast milk for 48 hours prior to the test.

Understanding the Test Results

The phenylketonuria test results are available quickly. Normal phenylketonuria test results are less than 3 mg/dL. High phenylketonuria test results may indicate phenylketonuria.

10.9 Tay-Sachs Test

The Tay-Sachs test measures the amount of hexosaminidase A in the blood. *Hexosaminidase A* is an enzyme that metabolizes *ganglioside*, which is a fatty acid. If the hexosaminidase A is not present, ganglioside accumulates in brain and nerve cells, resulting in neural damage. This is referred to as Tay-Sachs disease, which is an inherited disease. A positive result will be confirmed by genetic testing. The healthcare provider may order an amniocentesis or the chorionic villus sampling of the placenta to determine if the fetus has the hexosaminidase A enzyme.

Why the Test Is Performed

The test assesses for Tay-Sachs disease and if the patient is carrying the Tay-Sachs trait.

Before Administering the Test

Assess if the patient:

- Has had a blood transfusion 90 days prior to the test
- Is taking birth control pills
- Is pregnant

How the Test Is Performed

A sample of blood is taken from the patient's vein. The patient will experience a tight feeling when the tourniquet is tightened, a pinch or nothing at all when the needle is inserted into the vein, and pressure when a gauze pad is pressed against the insertion site to stop bleeding. It can take up to 10 minutes for bleeding to stop if the patient is taking anticoagulants (aspirin, coumadin). A small bruise might appear at the insertion site, which could become swollen following this test. This is called phlebitis. Applying a warm compress several times a day will reduce the swelling.

Teach the Patient

Explain why the sample is taken, that the test result may indicate that the patient carries the Tay-Sachs trait and recommend genetic counseling, and that the healthcare provider may ask the patient to refrain from taking birth control pills prior to the test.

Understanding the Test Results

The Tay-Sachs test results are available quickly. The laboratory determines normal values based on calibration of testing equipment with a control test. Test results are reported as high, normal, or low based on the laboratory's control test.

- Normal test results:
  - Total hexosaminidase: 10.4 to 23.8 U/L
  - Percentage of blood level: 56% to 80%

A half-normal level may indicate that the patient is a carrier of the Tay-Sachs trait.

No hexosaminidase A enzyme may indicate Tay-Sachs disease or Sandhoff's disease (missing hexosaminidase A and hexosaminidase B).

10.10   Sickle Cell Test

The sickle cell test determines if the patient has sickled blood cells, which is an abnormal form of hemoglobin. Normal red blood cells contain hemoglobin A. In sickle cell disease, red blood cells contain hemoglobin S, which causes the red blood cell to form a sickle shape and is therefore called a *sickled blood cell*. Sickle cell disease is an autosomal recessive disease where the sickle cell gene must be inherited from both parents. Patients with sickled blood cells can experience a sickle cell crisis when sickled blood cells block blood vessels, resulting in decreased blood flow. Sickled blood cells are destroyed faster than normal red blood cells, leading to sickle cell anemia. The patient should undergo genetic counseling if the patient has the sickle cell trait or sickle cell disease. The healthcare provider may order the HPLC test to examine the patient's DNA for the sickle cell gene. Sickle cell disease is more prevalent in African Americans. Healthcare providers commonly test newborns for the sickle cell trait although infants under 6 months old can have false-negative test results, since they have fetal hemoglobin in their blood, and therefore the sickle cell test is repeated after 6 months of age. The health-care provider may order the sickle cell test for a fetus using chorionic villus sampling (CVS) or amniocentesis.

Why the Test Is Performed

The test assesses for the sickle cell trait and sickle cell disease.

Before Administering the Test

- Assess if the patient has received a blood transfusion within three months before the test is administered.
- The patient should undergo genetic counseling if the test is positive for sickle cell trait or sickle cell disease.

How the Test Is Performed

A sample of blood is taken from the patient's vein. The patient will experience a tight feeling when the tourniquet is tightened, a pinch or nothing at all when the needle is inserted into the vein, and pressure when a gauze pad is pressed against the insertion site to stop bleeding. It can take up to 10 minutes for bleeding to stop if the patient is taking anticoagulants (aspirin, coumadin). A small bruise might appear at the insertion site, which could become swollen following this test. This is called phlebitis. Applying a warm compress several times a day will reduce the swelling.

Teach the Patient

Explain why the sample is taken and that the patient should receive genetic counseling if the sickle cell trait or sickle cell disease is present.

Understanding the Test Results

The sickle cell test result is available quickly. A normal sickle cell test result is normal hemoglobin presence. An abnormal sickle cell test result is some presence of Hemoglobin S.

- Sickle cell trait: 35%–45% of red blood cells have Hemoglobin S.
- Sickle cell disease: Nearly all red blood cells have Hemoglobin S.

10.11   Hemochromatosis Gene Test (HFE)

The hemochromatosis gene test (HFE) determines if the patient has the hemochromatosis gene. The hemochromatosis gene increases the absorption of iron (hemochromatosis), which causes a buildup of iron in the liver, heart, blood, joints, skin, and pancreas, resulting in joint pain, weight loss, and decreased energy. This can lead to arrhythmia, cirrhosis, diabetes, heart failure, arthritis, and change in skin color. Existence of the hemochromatosis gene means that the patient has an increased chance of having hemochromatosis, but does not mean that the patient has hemochromatosis. The hemochromatosis gene test may not rule out the existence of the hemochromatosis gene. The test detects the most common hemochromatosis gene mutation, but not all mutations. It is advised that the patient consult a genetic counselor before the test is administered to discuss the risks of developing hemochromatosis. The healthcare provider will order the test if close family members have hemochromatosis. The healthcare provider might order the ferritin level test and transferrin saturation test to measure the level of iron in the patient's blood.

Why the Test Is Performed

The test screens for the presence of the hemochromatosis gene. The test assesses the underlying cause of hemocromatosis. If positive, other tests for hemocromatosis are not necessary. The test also assesses the treatment for hemocromatosis.

Before Administering the Test

Assess if the patient has:

- Received a blood transfusion within a week before the test is administered
- Undergone genetic counseling prior to the test

How the Test Is Performed

A sample of blood is taken from the patient's vein. The patient will experience a tight feeling when the tourniquet is tightened, a pinch or nothing at all when the needle is inserted into the vein, and pressure when a gauze pad is pressed against the insertion site to stop bleeding. It can take up to 10 minutes for bleeding to stop if the patient is taking anticoagulants (aspirin, coumadin). A small bruise might appear at the insertion site, which could become swollen following this test. This is called phlebitis. Applying a warm compress several times a day will reduce the swelling.

Teach the Patient

Explain why the sample is taken, that the patient should receive genetic counseling prior to the test, and that a positive test result does not mean that the patient will develop hemochromatosis. It means that the patient is at risk for developing hemochromatosis.

Understanding the Test Results

The hemochromatosis gene test result is available in 2 weeks.

- A normal hemochromatosis gene test result is (negative): No mutation found.
- An abnormal hemochromatosis gene test result is (positive): Mutation found. The patient has a risk of developing hemochromatosis.

Solved Problems

Antisperm Antibody Test

10.1 Why is the antisperm antibody test administered?

The antisperm antibody test is administered to assess if antisperm antibodies are in blood, vaginal fluid, or semen, and to assess if infertility may be caused by immunologic infertility.

10.2 What should you be concerned about before administering the antisperm antibody test?

Patients may be embarrassed about collecting a sample. Confer with the healthcare provider if masturbation is against the patient's religious beliefs.

10.3 How is a semen sample collected?

A semen sample is collected by masturbation. Urinate. Wash and rinse your hands and penis. Collect the semen in a sterile cup. Do not use lubricants or condoms. Take the sample to the lab within 30 minutes.

10.4 What should you explain to the patient before administering the antisperm antibody test?

Explain why the test is ordered, that the patient should not ejaculate for 2 days before the test and no longer than 5 days before the test; how to collect the semen sample; that the patient should take the sample to the lab within 30 minutes; and that the patient should not use lubricants or condoms when collecting the sample. Ask the patient to consult his healthcare provider if masturbation is against the patient's religious beliefs.

10.5 What does a positive antisperm antibody test result mean?

Positive test results mean that antisperm antibodies are found.

Alpha-Fetoprotein (AFP) Test

10.6   What is alpha-fetoprotein?

Alpha-fetoprotein (AFP) is produced by the fetal liver and is detectable in a pregnant woman's blood.

10.7   What might a high level of AFP indicate?

A high level or low level of AFP is a sign that there may be a problem with fetal development.

10.8   When does a high level of AFP occur?

The level of AFP rises gradually in the first 14 weeks of gestation and continues rising until around week 34, when the AFP level gradually decreases.

10.9   What does the maternal serum triple screening test examine?

The maternal serum triple screening test examines levels of alpha-fetoprotein, beta human chorionic gonadotropin (beta-hCG), and unconjugated estriol or uE3 (estrogen).

10.10   What does the maternal serum quad screening test examine?

The maternal serum quad screening test examines the same substances as the maternal serum triple screening test, and the hormone inhibin A.

10.11   Why is the AFP test administered to men?

A healthcare provider may also administer the alpha-fetoprotein test in nonpregnant women, children, and men to assess for a number of other diseases that cause a high level of AFP in the blood. Half of patients diagnosed with certain cancers have normal alpha-fetoprotein test results. These include lymphoma, Hodgkin's disease, ovarian cancer, testicular cancer, renal cell cancer, and pancreatic cancer.

10.12   Why is the AFP test ordered?

The AFP test is ordered to assess for fetal neural tube defects, spinal bifida, anencephaly, Edward syndrome (trisomy 18), Down syndrome (trisomy 21), omphalocele, hepatoma in patients who have chronic hepatitis B or cirrhosis, lymphoma, Hodgkin's disease, renal cell cancer, ovarian cancer, testicular cancer, pancreatic cancer, and effectiveness of cancer treatment.

10.13   What must be assessed before administering the AFP test?

Assess:
- If the patient smokes. Smoking increases the AFP level in the blood.
- If the patient is an insulin dependent diabetic.
- The patient's weight.
- The gestational age of the fetus.
- The patient's race.
- If the patient has undergone a test involving radioactive tracers in the previous two weeks, since this might affect the test results.

10.14   When is the AFP test administered?

The test is performed between 15 weeks and 20 weeks of gestation.

10.15   Why is the patient weighed before administering the FPA test?

The patient is weighed before the blood sample is drawn. The results of the test are evaluated based on the patient's weight.

10.16   What factor does race play in the results of the FPA test?

The patient's race is noted. Normal values of AFP are higher in African-American women and lower in Asian women.

10.17   What should be explained to the patient before administering the FPA test?

Explain why the blood sample is taken, that weight, race, and gestational age are used to assess the test results, and that there is no special preparation required for the test. An abnormal test result does not mean there are developmental problems with the fetus. The test result is one of several signs that help the healthcare provider reach a diagnosis. A neural tube defect is not related to the mother's age. Neural tube defects occur without a family history of this problem.

10.18   What does a high level of AFP mean?

If high levels of AFP are detected, the healthcare provider is likely to order an ultrasound and/or amniocentesis. An ultrasound confirms the gestational age. If the gestational age is different than the estimated gestational age, the AFP is adjusted using the multiple of median (MoM) factor. An AFP value that is 0.5 to 2.5 times the multiple of median factor is considered normal.

10.19   Is an abnormal AFP value a definitive diagnosis?

An abnormal AFP level is not an indication of a definitive diagnosis. Additional testing such as an ultrasound or amniocentesis will likely be ordered for abnormal results.

Human Chorionic Gonadotropin (HCG)

10.20   Why is the hCG test administered?

The level of the hCG hormone is used as a sign of pregnancy, which is confirmed by other tests.

10.21   When is the hCG test administered?

The hCG hormone test is typically ordered as part of a maternal serum screening test that is administered at 15 weeks of gestation.

10.22   When does the hCG level decrease?

In a normal pregnancy, the level of the hCG hormone increases until 16 weeks of gestation and then gradually decreases until birth, when no hCG hormone is detectable.

10.23   What might a low level of hCG hormone indicate?

A lower level of hCG hormone might indicate an ectopic pregnancy.

10.24   What can also produce the hCG hormone?

The hCG hormone can also be produced by a molar pregnancy, choricocarcinoma (uterus cancer), ovarian cancer, or other tumors.

10.25   How early in a pregnancy can the hCG hormone level be detected?

The level of the hCG hormone can be detected before the patient misses her menstrual period, and as early as six days after attachment of the egg.

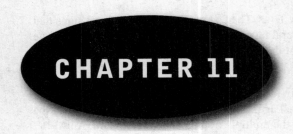

CHAPTER 11

Infection Tests

11.1 Definition

Inflammation can be the result of the immune system's response to an infection caused by a microorganism. A sample of blood, infected tissue, or body fluid such as urine and sputum are taken from the patient. Laboratory specialists place the sample in a culture dish. The culture dish contains nutrients that encourage the microorganism to replicate. The laboratory specialist then performs tests to identify the microorganism. Once identified, the laboratory specialist recommends the most sensitive medication and the minimum dose to effectively kill the microorganism. In this way, the proper dose of the right medication can be prescribed, reducing the risk that the microorganism will become resistant to the medication.

11.2 Antibody Tests

Antibody tests assess antibodies in the patient's blood. *Antibodies* are proteins made by the immune system that bind to bacteria, viruses, and other microorganisms to destroy the microorganism. Antibodies can also bind to red blood cells, destroying them also. Antibodies are created as a result of:

- **Blood transfusions reaction**: The transfused blood has different antigens on the surface of its red blood cells than the patient's red blood cells, causing the immune system to produce antibodies that attack the transfused red blood cells.
- **Rhesus factor sensitization**: The Rh antigen is in the fetus's blood (Rh positive), but not in the pregnant woman's blood (Rh negative). During delivery, the fetus blood mixes with the mother's blood, causing the mother's immune system to create antibodies against the baby's red blood cells. The mother becomes Rh sensitive. The antibodies can attack the fetus's red blood cells in future pregnancies if the fetus is Rh positive. Women with Rh-negative blood are given the Rh immune globulin (RhoGAM) that typically stops Rh sensitivity.
  - *Rh antibody titer*: The test performed in early pregnancy to determine the mother's blood type and to determine if the mother is Rh negative.
- **Autoimmune hemolytic anemia**: The patient's immune system creates antibodies against the patient's red blood cells.
  - *Direct Coombs Test*: Identifies antibodies attached to the patient's red blood cells. This test is performed:
    - On a newborn whose mother is Rh-negative to determine if the antibodies crossed the placenta into the newborn's blood.
    - On a patient who received a blood transfusion to determine if there is a transfusion reaction.
    - On a patient to determine if an autoimmune response is occurring.
  - *Indirect Coombs Test*: Identifies antibodies that have not but could attach to the patient's red blood cells if the patient's blood is mixed. This test is performed:
    - On the blood transfusion recipient or donor before the transfusion to identify if antibodies exists in the donor's blood.

Why the Test Is Performed

The test assesses blood transfusion reaction or potential reaction, Rh factor sensitization, and autoimmune hemolytic anemia.

Before Administering the Test

Assess if one or more of these reasons for the patient not to take the test exist:

- A history of blood transfusions
- Recently administering contrast material IV or dextran injections
- Pregnant in the previous three months
- Has taken cephalosporins, tetracyclines, tuberculosis medication, sulfa medication, or insulin

How the Test Is Performed

A sample of blood is taken from the patient's vein. The patient will experience a tight feeling when the tourniquet is tightened, a pinch or nothing at all when the needle is inserted into the vein, and pressure when a gauze pad is pressed against the insertion site to stop bleeding. It can take up to 10 minutes for bleeding to stop if the patient is taking anticoagulants (aspirin, coumadin). A small bruise might appear at the insertion site, which could become swollen following this test. This is called phlebitis. Applying a warm compress several times a day will reduce the swelling.

Teach the Patient

Explain that no special preparation is needed for the test, why the test is ordered, and Rh sensitivity and the administration of Rh immune globulin vaccine (RhoGAM), if the patient is Rh negative.

Understanding the Test Results

- Negative test results:
  - No antibodies were found in the patient's blood (direct Coombs test).
  - The patient's blood is compatible with the transfusion donor's blood (indirect Coombs test).
  - Rh negative mother is not Rh sensitized (indirect Coombs test). The mother is administered the Rh immune globulin vaccine (RhoGAM®).
- Positive test results:
  - The patient's blood contains antibodies for the patient's red blood cells (direct Coombs test).
  - The patient's blood is incompatible with the transfusion donor's blood (indirect Coombs test). The blood is not transfused.
  - Rh negative mother is Rh sensitized (indirect Coombs test). The healthcare provider monitors the pregnancy closely to prevent problems with the fetus if the fetus is Rh positive.

11.3   Blood Culture

A blood culture identifies the microorganism that has invaded the patient. Blood can be infected by bacteria or fungi. A blood culture identifies the bacteria or fungi by allowing the microorganism to grow in a controlled environment and then examining the microorganism under a microscope. The healthcare provider typically orders a sensitivity test along with the blood culture. The sensitivity test identifies medication that kills the microorganism.

Why the Test Is Performed

The test assesses the existence of bacteria or fungi in blood, endocarditis, the medication that will kill the microorganism, the cause of unexplained fever, and the effect of treatment of a microorganism infection.

Before Administering the Test

- Assess if the patient has recently been administered antibiotics, since this can affect the test results.

How the Test Is Performed

- A blood sample is taken from three different veins and at two different times to assure that bacteria on the skin does not contaminate the blood sample.
- Patients who have a catheter in their veins will have the blood sample taken from the catheter.

A sample of blood is taken from the patient's vein. The patient will experience a tight feeling when the tourniquet is tightened, a pinch or nothing at all when the needle is inserted into the vein, and pressure when a gauze pad is pressed against the insertion site to stop bleeding. It can take up to 10 minutes for bleeding to stop if the patient is taking anticoagulants (aspirin, coumadin). A small bruise might appear at the insertion site, which could become swollen following this test. This is called phlebitis. Applying a warm compress several times a day will reduce the swelling.

Teach the Patient

Explain why the blood sample is taken, that multiple samples may be taken from different sites and at different times, and that the results of the sensitivity test will direct the healthcare provider to prescribe the medication that will effectively kill the microorganism.

Understanding the Test Results

Test results for bacteria infection are normally available in 3 days but can take longer than 10 days. Test results for a fungal infection can take up to 30 days.

- Normal is negative: No bacteria or fungi found in the blood sample.
- Normal false-negative: Improper processing or improper sampling results in bacteria or fungi not found in the blood sample but patient's blood is infected.
- Abnormal is positive: Bacteria or fungi found in the blood sample.
- Abnormal false-positive: Contaminated sample or improper processing results in bacteria or fungi found in the blood sample but not in the patient's blood.

11.4 Mononucleosis Tests

The mononucleosis tests identify antibodies for the Epstein-Barr virus in the blood sample. The Epstein-Barr virus causes mononucleosis. There are two kinds of mononucleosis tests:

1. **Monospot Test**: This test identifies heterophil antibodies that form between two weeks and nine weeks after the patient becomes infected.
2. **EBV Antibody Test**: This test is ordered when the patient shows symptoms of mononucleosis and the monospot test is negative.

Why the Test Is Performed

The test assesses for infectious mononucleosis.

Before Administering the Test

- A false-negative result can occur if the test is administered within 2 weeks of the patient being infected.
- Assess if the patient has lymphoma, hepatitis, rubella, cytomegalovirus, or lupus.

How the Test Is Performed

A sample of blood is taken from the patient's vein. The patient will experience a tight feeling when the tourniquet is tightened, a pinch or nothing at all when the needle is inserted into the vein, and pressure when a gauze pad is pressed against the insertion site to stop bleeding. It can take up to 10 minutes for bleeding to stop if the patient is taking anticoagulants (aspirin, coumadin). A small bruise might appear at the insertion site, which could become swollen following this test. This is called phlebitis. Applying a warm compress several times a day will reduce the swelling.

Finger Stick: Several drops of blood are collected from the finger. The finger is cleaned using alcohol. A sterile lancer is used to puncture the finger. Several drops of blood are collected in a small test tube. A gauze pad is pressed over the site until bleeding stops. A small bandage is applied.

Teach the Patient

Explain why the blood sample is taken and that a false-negative result can occur if the test is administered within two weeks of the patient being infected.

Understanding the Test Results

The presence of the IgG antibody indicates that the patient was exposed to the Epstein-Barr virus in the past. Most adults have the IgG antibody.

- Monospot test results are available in 1 hour.
  - Normal (negative) heterophil antibody range is: 0.
  - High (positive) heterophil antibody levels greater than 0 may indicate mononucleosis, rheumatoid arthritis, leukemia, hepatitis, or lymphoma.

EBV Antibody Test results are available in 3 days. Results are reported as a titer. A titer specifies how much of the sample of blood is diluted with saline before antibodies are no longer detected. The titer is reported as a ratio of parts of the blood sample and saline. The higher the second number of the ratio, the greater number of antibodies in the blood sample. Normal (negative) EBV antibody titer range is below 1 to 40 (1:40). High (positive) EBV antibody titer may indicate mononucleosis.

11.5   Helicobacter Pylori Tests

Helicobacter pylori tests detect *Helicobacter pylori* (*H. pylori*) bacteria. *Helicobacter pylori* (*H. pylori*) is a bacterium that infects the stomach and duodenum that may result in a peptic ulcer. Many patients have *H. pylori* but few develop peptic ulcer disease. All tests may produce a false-negative result if the *H. pylori* count is low and undetectable. A stomach biopsy may produce a false-negative result if the sample was not infected. The blood test for *H. pylori* antibodies may give a false-positive result since antibodies are present years after the *H. pylori* infection is resolved. There are four tests used to detect *H. pylori*:

1. ***H. pylori* blood antibody test**: This test determines if the blood sample has *H. pylori* antibodies.
2. **Urea breath test**: This test determines the presence of *H. pylori* in the stomach.
3. ***H. pylori* stool antigen test**: This test determines the presence of *H. pylori* antigens in feces.
4. **Stomach biopsy**: This is the endoscopy removal of the lining of the stomach and small intestine, which is examined for the presence of *H. pylori*.

Why the Tests Are Performed

The tests assess for the presence of *H. pylori* and if the treatment for *H. pylori* is successful.

Before Administering the Tests

Assess if the patient:

- Is pregnant or breastfeeding. The Urea Breath test is not performed
- Has taken antibiotics. This can reduce the *H. pylori* count.
- Has taken Prilosec, Carafate, Pepcid, Aciphex, Zantac or Pepto-Bismol, since these can affect the test result

How the Test Is Performed

A sample of blood is taken from the patient's vein. The patient will experience a tight feeling when the tourniquet is tightened, a pinch or nothing at all when the needle is inserted into the vein, and pressure when a gauze pad is pressed against the insertion site to stop bleeding. It can take up to 10 minutes for bleeding to stop if the patient is taking anticoagulants (aspirin, coumadin). A small bruise might appear at the insertion site, which could become swollen following this test. This is called phlebitis. Applying a warm compress several times a day will reduce the swelling.

Teach the Patient

Explain why the sample is taken, how to take a stool collection at home (if necessary), that there is no long-term affect of swallowing a capsule or water containing radioactive material in the urea breath test, and that the healthcare provider may want the patient to refrain from taking Prilosec, Carafate, Pepcid, Aciphex, Zantac, or Pepto-Bismol 12 hours before the test.

Understanding the Test Results

- Blood test results are available in 1 day.
  - Normal result is: No *H. pylori* antibodies.
  - Abnormal blood test result is: Presences of *H. pylori* antibodies.
- Urea breath test results are available in 3 hours.
  - Normal result is: No tagged hydrocarbon.
  - Abnormal breath test result is: Tagged hydrocarbon present.
- Stool antigen test results are available in 3 hours.
  - Normal result is: No *H. pylori* antigens.
  - Abnormal stool antigen test result is: Presence of *H. pylori* antigens.
- Stomach biopsy test result is available between 2 and 10 days.
  - Normal result is: No *H. pylori*.
  - Abnormal stomach biopsy test result is: Presences of *H. pylori*.

11.6   Herpes Tests

Herpes tests determine the presence of the herpes simplex virus (HSV). Herpes simplex virus (HSV) causes painful blister-like sores on the skin and mucous membrane of the mouth, vagina, penis, urethra, rectum, nose, and throat. HSV–1 can infect the genitals. HSV–2 can infect the newborn if the mother has HSV–2. HSV–2 can infect the mouth. There is no cure for herpes simplex virus. However, the herpes simplex virus can go into remission. Fatigue, stress, or sunlight can cause herpes simplex virus sores to recur. *Varicella zoster* is a type of herpes virus that is better known as shingles and chickenpox. There are two types of herpes simplex virus:

1. **Herpes simplex virus type 1(HSV–1)**: Commonly called a fever blister or cold sore that appears on the lips, it is spread by direct contact or indirectly through sharing eating utensils.
2. **Herpes simplex virus type 2(HSV–2)**: Commonly called genital herpes, it appears on the penis or vagina and is spread by direct contact.

There are four common tests of herpes simplex virus:

1. **Herpes simplex virus antibody test**: This test identifies HSV antibodies in the blood but cannot differentiate between HSV–1 and HSV–2. It can produce a false negative result since the immune system takes several days to develop sufficient antibodies to be detected by the herpes simplex virus antibody test.
2. **Polymerase chain reaction (PCR) test**: This test differentiates between HSV–1 and HSV–2 in cell scraping.
3. **Herpes virus antigen detection test**: This test detects antigens on cells scraped from the herpes simplex virus sore using a microscope.
4. **Herpes viral culture**: This test cultures cells or fluid from a herpes simplex virus sore to determine if the sore is from HSV–2.

Why the Tests Are Performed

The tests assess for herpes simplex virus and identify the type of herpes simplex virus.

Before Administering the Test

Assess if the patient (or sample):

- Has had sexual contact before the test results are known
- Urinated 2 hours before the test if the sore is on the urethra
- Douched 24 hours before the test if the sore is on the cervix
- Has taken ganciclovir, acyclovir, valacyclovir, or famciclovir
- Is taken from a crusted sore

How the Test Is Performed

See How to Collect a Viral Culture, Viral Antigen, Polymerase Chain Reaction (PCR) tests

A sample of blood is taken from the patient's vein. The patient will experience a tight feeling when the tourniquet is tightened, a pinch or nothing at all when the needle is inserted into the vein, and pressure when a gauze pad is pressed against the insertion site to stop bleeding. It can take up to 10 minutes for bleeding to stop if the patient is taking anticoagulants (aspirin, coumadin). A small bruise might appear at the insertion site, which could become swollen following this test. This is called phlebitis. Applying a warm compress several times a day will reduce the swelling. The POC kit tests for HSV–2 antibodies in blood in 10 minutes.

Finger Stick: Several drops of blood are collected from the finger. The finger is cleaned using alcohol. A sterile lancer is used to puncture the finger. Several drops of blood are collected in a small test tube. A gauze pad is pressed over the site until bleeding stops. A small bandage is applied.

Teach the Patient

Explain why the sample is taken, that the patient should not douche 24 hours before the test if the sore is on the cervix, that the patient should not urinate 2 hours before the test if the sore is on the urethra, that the patient should not have sexual contact before the test results are known, and that the healthcare provider may request that the patient may avoid taking ganciclovir, acyclovir, valacyclovir, or famciclovir for 2 weeks prior to the test.

Understanding the Test Results

Rapid herpes simplex virus culture test results take 3 days. The herpes simplex virus culture test results take 14 days. The herpes simplex virus antigen test results take 1 day. The polymerase chain reaction (PCR) test takes 3 days. The antibody blood test takes 2 days.

- Normal herpes simplex virus test result is (negative): No HSV, no HSV antigen, no HSV DNA, no HSV antibodies.
- Abnormal herpes simplex virus test result is: HSV, HSV antigen, HSV DNA, HSV antibodies present.
- A negative test does not rule out a herpes simplex virus infection. Additional testing is necessary if symptoms appear.

11.7 Lyme Disease Test

The Lyme disease tests detect Borrelia burgdorferi bacteria antibodies in blood. The Borrelia burgdorferi bacteria is carried by ticks and transmitted by a tick bite. The healthcare provider orders the Lyme disease tests if the patient has symptoms of Lyme disease or is known to have been exposed to tick bites. The healthcare provider will order at least two of three Lyme disease tests:

1. Indirect fluorescent antibody (IFA)
2. Enzyme-linked immunosorbent assay (ELISA): Quickest and most sensitive test for Lyme disease
3. Western blot test: Confirms positive IFA and ELISA test results

Test results can produce a false positive because Borrelia burgdorferi bacteria antibodies remain in the patient's blood years after the Borrelia burgdorferi bacteria was killed. Lyme disease test results can produce a false negative if performed within 2 months of the tick bite, because the patient's immune system may take 2 months to produce a detectable amount of Borrelia burgdorferi bacteria antibodies.

Why the Test Is Performed

The tests assess for Lyme disease.

Before Administering the Test

Assess if the patient:

- Has a viral or bacterial infection
- Has a high lipid level
- Has ever been diagnosed with Lyme disease
- Has ever been exposed to ticks

How the Test Is Performed

A sample of blood is taken from the patient's vein. The patient will experience a tight feeling when the tourniquet is tightened, a pinch or nothing at all when the needle is inserted into the vein, and pressure when a gauze pad is pressed against the insertion site to stop bleeding. It can take up to 10 minutes for bleeding to stop if the patient is taking anticoagulants (aspirin, coumadin). A small bruise might appear at the insertion site, which could become swollen following this test. This is called phlebitis. Applying a warm compress several times a day will reduce the swelling.

Teach the Patient

Explain why the sample is taken, that a negative test result does not rule out Lyme disease since the immune system can take 2 months to develop detectable antibodies, that a positive test result must be confirmed by another Lyme disease test (which is usually the Western blot test), and that a positive test result does not mean that the patient has Lyme disease since detectable antibodies remain in the blood for years after a Borrelia burgdorferi bacteria infection. The patient may have been infected in the past but is not currently infected.

Understanding the Test Results

The Lyme disease test results are available in 2 weeks. The laboratory determines normal values based on calibration of testing equipment with a control test. Test results are reported as high, normal, or low based on the laboratory's control test. Results are reported as a titer. A titer specifies how much of the sample of blood is diluted with saline before antibodies are no longer detected. The titer is reported as a ratio of parts of the blood sample and saline. The higher the second number of the ratio, the greater the number of antibodies in the blood sample.

- Normal Lyme disease test results (Negative):
  - IFA: less than 1:256
  - ELISA: no Borrelia burgdorferi bacteria antibodies found
  - Western blot test: no Borrelia burgdorferi bacteria antibodies found
- Abnormal Lyme disease:
  - IFA: greater than 1:256
  - ELISA: Borrelia burgdorferi bacteria antibodies found
  - Western blot test: Borrelia burgdorferi bacteria antibodies found

11.8   Rubella Test

The rubella test determines if the patient has antibodies to the rubella virus. Rubella (German measles) is a virus that causes congenital rubella syndrome (CRS) if a pregnant woman is infected with the rubella virus and transmits the rubella virus to the fetus in the first trimester. Congenital rubella syndrome consists of birth defects and possibly a miscarriage or stillbirth. The rubella test detects rubella virus antibodies in the blood. There are two rubella virus antibodies that are detected:

1. **IgM antibody**: The patient currently has or recently had a rubella virus infection.
2. **IgG antibody**: The patient has immunity against the rubella virus. The rubella virus antibody developed from a previous rubella virus infection or from the rubella virus vaccination.

Why the Test Is Performed

The test assesses if the patient is immune to the rubella virus and if the patient currently or recently has had a rubella virus infection.

Before Administering the Test

- A woman who wants to become pregnant must receive the rubella test to assess if she is immune to the rubella virus.
- A woman who is not immune to the rubella virus can receive the rubella vaccination but must wait one month after receiving the vaccination before becoming pregnant.
- A pregnant woman who is not immune to the rubella virus cannot receive the rubella vaccination during the pregnancy and must avoid anyone who is at risk of being infected with the rubella virus.

How the Test Is Performed

A sample of blood is taken from the patient's vein. The patient will experience a tight feeling when the tourniquet is tightened, a pinch or nothing at all when the needle is inserted into the vein, and pressure when a gauze pad is pressed against the insertion site to stop bleeding. It can take up to 10 minutes for bleeding to stop if the patient is taking anticoagulants (aspirin, coumadin). A small bruise might appear at the insertion site, which could become swollen following this test. This is called phlebitis. Applying a warm compress several times a day will reduce the swelling.

Teach the Patient

Explain why the sample is taken, that if the patient is pregnant she should avoid others who might be at risk for a rubella virus infection unless she is immune to the rubella virus, and that the patient should have the rubella test before becoming pregnant. The healthcare provider is likely to order the rubella vaccination if she is not immune. She must wait 1 month after the vaccination before becoming pregnant.

Understanding the Test Results

The rubella test results are available quickly. Results are reported as a titer. A titer specifies how much of the sample of blood is diluted with saline before antibodies are no longer detected. The titer is reported as a ratio of parts of the blood sample and saline. The higher the second number of the ratio, the greater the number of antibodies in the blood sample.

- Normal test results (positive): 1:10 to 1:20
- Lower levels may indicate (negative): risk for rubella virus infection

11.9　Syphilis Tests

The syphilis tests identify Treponema pallidum antibodies in a blood sample. *Treponema pallidum* is the bacterium that causes syphilis. A positive venereal disease research laboratory (VDRL) test or rapid plasma reagin (RPR) test does not mean that the patient has syphilis. Other conditions can cause a positive test result. Fluorescent treponemal antibody absorption (FTA-ABS), Microhemagglutination assay (MHA-TP), and Treponema pallidum particle agglutination assay (TPPA) remain positive even after the patient is successfully treated for syphilis. VDRL and RPR tests are negative when treatment for syphilis is successful. A negative result does not rule out syphilis, since detectable antibodies can take 4 weeks to develop following the initial infection. Many syphilis tests can use either a blood sample or a sample of spinal fluid. Consult the healthcare facility's policy for reporting diagnosed cases of syphilis to the local health department. There are seven types of syphilis tests:

1. **Venereal disease research laboratory (VDRL)**: This test identifies anti-cardiolipin antibodies that are produced by a patient who has syphilis. Diseases including syphilis cause the production of anti-cardiolipin antibodies. Therefore this test is used for screening but not diagnosing syphilis.
2. **Rapid plasma reagin (RPR)**: This test is similar to VDRL, except antibodies can be detected without the aid of a microscope.
3. **Enzyme immunoassay (ELIA)**: This test identifies Treponema pallidum antibodies and is used for screening for syphilis. Additional testing is necessary to diagnose syphilis.
4. **Fluorescent treponemal antibody absorption (FTA-ABS)**: This test identifies Treponema pallidum antibodies after the fourth week after the initial infection and is used to confirm other positive test results.
5. **Treponema pallidum particle agglutination assay (TPPA)**: This test is similar to the FTA-ABS except it is not used to test spinal fluid.
6. **Darkfield microscopy**: This test identifies the Treponema pallidum bacterium under a darkfield microscope and is used to diagnose the early stage of syphilis.
7. **Microhemagglutination assay (MHA-TP)**: This test is similar to TPPA.

Why the Test Is Performed

The test assesses for syphilis infection and treatment for syphilis infection.

Before Administering the Test

Assess if the patient has:

- Had a blood transfusion recently
- Has liver disease, yaws, lupus, or HIV
- Has taken antibiotics

How the Test Is Performed

A sample of blood is taken from the patient's vein. The patient will experience a tight feeling when the tourniquet is tightened, a pinch or nothing at all when the needle is inserted into the vein, and pressure when a gauze pad is pressed against the insertion site to stop bleeding. It can take up to 10 minutes for bleeding to stop if the patient is taking anticoagulants (aspirin, coumadin). A small bruise might appear at the insertion site, which could become swollen following this test. This is called phlebitis. Applying a warm compress several times a day will reduce the swelling.

Teach the Patient

Explain why the sample is taken, that the sex partner must also be tested, that the patient should refrain from sexual intercourse until the test shows that that patient and the sex partner are no longer infected, that a diagnoses of syphilis may have to be reported to the health department, and that a negative test may not rule out syphilis since detectable antibodies can take four weeks to develop following the initial infection.

Understanding the Test Results

The syphilis test results are available in 10 days.

- Normal test results (nonreactive/negative): No antibodies found. No Treponema pallidum bacterium seen under the microscope.
- Abnormal test results (reactive/positive): Antibody regain found. Treponema pallidum bacterium seen under the microscope.
- Inconclusive test results (equivocal): Unclear if antibody regain found. Unclear if Treponema pallidum bacterium is seen under the microscope.

Solved Problems

Antibody Tests

11.1   What are antibodies?

Antibodies are proteins made by the immune system that bind to bacteria, viruses, and other microorganisms to destroy the microorganism.

11.2   How are antibodies created?
- Blood transfusions reaction: The transfused blood has different antigens on the surface of its red blood cells than the patient's red blood cells, which causes the immune system to produce antibodies that attack the transfused red blood cells.
- Rhesus factor sensitization: The Rh antigen is in the fetus's blood (Rh positive), but not in the pregnant woman's blood (Rh negative).
- Autoimmune hemolytic anemia: The patient's immune system creates antibodies against the patient's red blood cells

11.3   What is the purpose of the direct Coombs test?

The purpose of the direct Coombs test is to identify antibodies attached to the patient's red blood cells.

11.4   What is an Rh antibody titer?

An Rh antibody titer is the test performed in early pregnancy to determine the mother's blood type and to determine if the mother is Rh negative.

11.5   What is the indirect Coombs test?

The indirect Coombs test identifies antibodies that have not but could attach to the patient's red blood cells if the patient's blood is mixed with the fetal blood.

11.6   Why are antibody tests performed?

To assess blood transfusion reaction or potential reaction, Rh factor sensitization, and autoimmune hemolytic anemia.

11.7   What should be assessed before administering the antibody test?

Assess if there is reason for the patient not to take the test, such as a history of blood transfusions, recently administering contrast material IV or dextran injections, the patient was pregnant in the previous three months, or has taken cephalosporins, tetracyclines, tuberculosis medication, sulfa medication, or insulin.

11.8   What does a positive result of an antibody test mean?

Positive test results mean that the patient's blood contains antibodies for the patient's red blood cells (direct Coombs test), the patient's blood is incompatible with transfusion donor's blood (indirect Coombs test)—the blood is not transfused, or the Rh negative mother is Rh sensitized (indirect Coombs test). The healthcare provider monitors the pregnancy closely to prevent problems with the fetus if the fetus is Rh positive.

11.9   What does a negative result of an Rh sensitized test mean?

The Rh negative mother is not Rh sensitized (indirect Coombs test). The mother is administered the Rh immune globulin vaccine (RhoGAM).

Blood Culture

11.10   What is a blood culture?

A blood culture identifies the microorganism that has invaded the patient.

11.11   Why is the sensitivity test ordered?

The sensitivity test identifies the medication that kills the microorganism.

11.12   Why is a blood culture ordered?

A blood culture assesses the existence of bacteria or fungi in blood, for endocarditis, medication that will kill the microorganism, the cause of unexplained fever, and the effect of treatment of a microorganism infection.

11.13 What should be assessed before administering the blood culture?

Assess if the patient has recently been administered antibiotics, since this can affect the test results.

11.14 How long might a blood culture for a fungus infection take before results are known?

Test results for a fungus infection can take up to 30 days.

11.15 What is an abnormal false positive of a blood culture?

Abnormal false-positive: Contaminated sample or improper processing results in bacteria or fungi found in the blood sample but not in the patient's blood.

11.16 What is a false negative of a blood culture?

Improper processing or improper sampling results in bacteria or fungi not found in the blood sample, but the patient's blood is infected.

11.17 How is blood cultured in a laboratory?

A blood culture identifies the bacteria or fungi by allowing the microorganism to grow in a controlled environment and then examining the microorganism under a microscope.

Mononucleosis Tests

11.18 What is a monospot test?

The monospot test identifies heterophil antibodies that form between 2 weeks and 9 weeks after the patient becomes infected.

11.19 What is an EBV antibody test?

The EBV antibody test is ordered when the patient shows symptoms of mononucleosis and the monospot test is negative.

11.20 What causes mononucleosis?

The Epstein-Barr virus causes mononucleosis.

11.21 Why might a false-negative result occur in a mononucleosis test?

A false-negative result can occur if the test is administered within 2 weeks of the patient being infected.

11.22 What should be assessed before administering the mononucleosis test?

Assess if the patient has lymphoma, hepatitis, rubella, cytomegalovirus, or lupus.

11.23 What might be meant by a high monospot test?

High (positive) heterophil antibody levels greater than 0 may indicate mononucleosis, rheumatoid arthritis, leukemia, hepatitis, or lymphoma.

11.24 What might a high EBV Antibody Test result mean?

Mononucleosis.

11.25 What does the presence of the IgG antibody indicate?

The presence of the IgG antibody indicates that the patient was exposed to the Epstein-Barr virus in the past. Most adults have the IgG antibody.

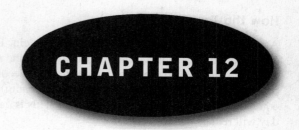

CHAPTER 12

Renal Function Tests

12.1 Definition

Renal function tests measure the capacity of the kidneys to filter waste from blood and excrete urine. Metabolic waste is carried by the blood to the kidneys. The *glomerulus* is the functional unit of the kidneys that acts as a filter to remove waste from the blood, which is collected in a tubule as urine. Metabolic waste such as sodium, potassium, and phosphorus can be reused by the body and are returned to the blood by the kidneys. The remaining waste is excreted as urine. Renal function is measured in percentages. A person with two healthy kidneys has 100% renal function. A person with one healthy kidney and one kidney in total renal failure is said to have 50% renal function. A person will experience health problems if the person has 25% or less renal function. Dialysis is typically ordered for a patient with less than 15% renal function. Renal failure occurs when the glomeruli no longer filter waste from the blood. This can occur suddenly (acute renal failure) in response to illness, medications, accidents, and poisons. It can also happen slowly (chronic kidney disease) from illnesses such as diabetes and high blood pressure. Chronic kidney disease can lead to end-stage renal disease where all or nearly all renal function is permanently destroyed.

12.2 Blood Urea Nitrogen

The blood urea nitrogen (BUN) test measures the level of nitrogen in the blood derived from urea. Ammonia is formed when bacteria in the intestines break down protein. Ammonia is then converted into urea by the liver, which is excreted by the kidney in urine. Urea contains nitrogen. The blood urea nitrogen (BUN) test measures the level of nitrogen in the blood derived from urea. The BUN test is typically performed with the creatinine test. The healthcare provider uses the BUN to creatinine ratio to evaluate the patient's condition.

Why the Test Is Performed

The test screens for kidney function and dehydration. The test assesses the treatment for kidney disease and kidney dialysis.

Before Administering the Test

Assess:

- If the patient has eaten meat or protein prior to the administration of the test
- If the patient has taken Fungizone, Garamycin, Nebcin, Chloromycetin, Nafcillin, Kantrex, tetracycline, or diuretics
- The patient's age, since BUN levels increase with age

How the Test Is Performed

A sample of blood is taken from the patient's vein. The patient will experience a tight feeling when the tourniquet is tightened, a pinch or nothing at all when the needle is inserted into the vein, and pressure when a gauze pad is pressed against the insertion site to stop bleeding. It can take up to 10 minutes for bleeding to stop if the patient is taking anticoagulants (aspirin, coumadin). A small bruise might appear at the insertion site, which could become swollen following this test. This is called phlebitis. Applying a warm compress several times a day will reduce the swelling.

Teach the Patient

Explain why the blood sample is taken, that the patient should avoid eating meat or protein for 24 hours before the test is administered, and that the healthcare provide may ask the patient to stop taking Fungizone, Garamycin, Nebcin, chloromycetin, nafcillin, Kantrex, tetracycline, or diuretics for 2 weeks prior to the test.

Understanding the Test Results

Test results are available in 1 day. The laboratory determines normal values based on calibration of testing equipment with a control test. Test results are reported as high, normal, or low based on the laboratory's control test.

- Normal BUN range is: 10 to 20 mg/dL
- Normal BUN to creatinine ratio: 10:1 to 20:1

High BUN values may indicate kidney disease, kidney stone, Addison's disease, kidney tumor, burns, heart failure, GI bleeding, dehydration, or a high protein diet.

A high BUN to creatinine ratio may indicate respiratory tract bleeding, GI tract bleeding, shock, kidney failure, urinary tract blockage, or dehydration.

Low BUN values may indicate malnutrition, liver damage, overhydration, or a low protein diet.

A low BUN to creatinine ratio may indicate rhabdomyolysis, cirrhosis, SIADH, or muscle injury. *Hint*: the BUN level is higher than the creatinine level in dehydration. Both BUN and creatinine levels are high when there is blockage of urine flow.

12.3   Creatinine and Creatinine Clearance

The Creatinine and creatinine clearance tests measure the levels of creatinine to determine kidney function. Creatine phosphate provides energy to skeletal muscles. After 7 seconds of intense effort, creatine phosphate converts to creatine. Creatine is metabolized into creatinine and is carried in blood to the kidneys for filtering and excreted in urine. If kidneys are malfunctioning, creatinine levels in the blood increase and creatinine levels in urine decrease. There are three types of creatinine tests:

1. **Blood creatinine level test**: This test measures the level of creatinine in blood.
2. **Creatinine clearance test**: This test measures creatinine in a 24-hour urine sample and measures the level of creatinine in blood.
3. **Blood urea nitrogen to creatinine ratio (BUN: creatinine)**: This test compares the results of the blood urea test with the blood creatinine level test to assess for dehydration.

A normal blood creatinine level does not rule out kidney disease. Urea is a byproduct of protein metabolism in the liver that is excreted in urine. Fetal kidney function is assessed by testing the level of creatinine in amniotic fluid. The healthcare provider may order the glomerular filtration rate test to determine kidney function.

Why the Test Is Performed

The test screens for kidney function and dehydration.

Before Administering the Test

Assess if the patient:

- Performed strenuous exercise during the two days prior to the test
- Has taken:
  - Blood creatinine level test: Diuretics, Proloprim, Trimpex, Aldomet, Tagamet, ascorbic acid, cephalosporin, or Mefoxin
  - Creatinine clearance test: Dilantin, cephalosporin, captopril, ascorbic acid, Garamycin, Tagamet, Proloprim, Trimpex, Cardioquin, Quinaglute, quinine, Quinidex, amphotericin B, or procainamide
  - BUN to creatinine ratio test: Tetracycline or Tagamet
- Ingested protein for one day prior to the test
- Drunk coffee or tea before the creatinine clearance test, since these increase urine production

How the Test Is Performed

A sample of blood is taken from the patient's vein. The patient will experience a tight feeling when the tourniquet is tightened, a pinch or nothing at all when the needle is inserted into the vein, and pressure when a gauze pad is pressed against the insertion site to stop bleeding. It can take up to 10 minutes for bleeding to stop if the patient is taking anticoagulants (aspirin, coumadin). A small bruise might appear at the insertion site, which could become swollen following this test. This is called phlebitis. Applying a warm compress several times a day will reduce the swelling.

See 24-Hour Urine Collection.

Teach the Patient

Explain why the sample is taken. The patient should avoid:

- Strenuous exercise for two days prior to the test
- Ingesting protein for one day prior to the test
- Drinking coffee and tea before the creatinine clearance test, since these increase urine production.

Explain that the healthcare provider may ask the patient to refrain from taking these medications prior to the test:

- *Blood creatinine level test*: Diuretics, Proloprim, Trimpex, Aldomet, Tagamet, ascorbic acid, cephalosporin or Mefoxin
- *Creatinine clearance test*: Dilantin, cephalosporin, captopril, ascorbic acid, Garamycin, Tagamet, Proloprim, Trimpex, Cardioquin, Quinaglute, quinine, Quinidex, amphotericin B or procainamide
- *BUN to creatinine ratio test*: Tetracycline or Tagamet

Understanding the Test Results

The creatinine blood level test and creatinine clearance test results are available quickly. The laboratory determines normal values based on calibration of testing equipment with a control test. Test results are reported as high, normal, or low based on the laboratory's control test.

- Normal test results:
  - Blood creatinine level:
    - Men: 0.6 to 1.2 mg/dL
    - Women: 0.5 to 1.1 mg/dL
    - 13 years old to 19 years old: 0.5 to 1.0 mg/dL
    - 6 months to 12 years old: 0.3 to 0.7 mg/dL
    - Newborns: 0.3 to 1.2 mg/dL
  - Creatinine clearance:
    - Men: 90 to 140 mL/min.
    - Women: 87 to 107 mL/min

- ○ BUN to creatinine ratio:
  - ▪ Over 11 months of age: 10:1 to 20:1
  - ▪ Under 12 months of age: 30:1 or less

Higher levels may indicate: (creatinine blood level) kidney disorder, shock, kidney stones, dehydration, rhabdomyolysis, acromegaly, gigantism, polymyositis, muscular dystrophy, urinary tract blockage, or cancer; (creatinine clearance) muscle injury, pregnancy, hypothyroidism, burns, strenuous exercise, or carbon monoxide poisoning; (BUN to creatinine ratio) dehydration, kidney stone, shock, or acute kidney failure.

Lower levels may indicate: (blood creatinine levels) protein deficient diet, decreased muscle mass, pregnancy, or liver disease; (creatinine clearance) cirrhosis, dehydration, infection, kidney disorder, urinary tract blockage, or reduced blood to the kidneys; (BUN to creatinine ratio) protein deficient diet, cirrhosis, rhabdomyolysis, SIADH, cancer, or pregnancy.

Solved Problems

Renal Function Tests

12.1   What metabolic waste can be reused by the body?

Metabolic waste such as sodium, potassium, and phosphorus can be reused by the body and are returned to the blood by the kidneys.

12.2   How is renal function measured?

Renal function is measured in percentages. A person with two healthy kidneys has 100% renal function. A person with one healthy kidney and one kidney in total renal failure is said to have 50% renal function.

12.3   At what level of renal function will a patient be placed on dialysis?

Dialysis is typically ordered for a patient with less than 15% renal function.

12.4   When does renal failure occur?

Renal failure occurs when the glomerulus no longer filters waste from the blood.

12.5   What type of renal failure occurs as a result of diabetes and high blood pressure?

Chronic kidney disease.

12.6   What causes acute renal failure?

This can occur suddenly in response to illness, medications, accidents, and poisons.

Blood Urea Nitrogen

12.7   What does the blood urea nitrogen test measure?

The blood urea nitrogen (BUN) test measures the level of nitrogen in the blood.

12.8   What is the source of the nitrogen in blood?

Urea.

12.9   What is the source of urea?

Ammonia is formed when bacteria in the intestines break down protein. Ammonia is then converted into urea by the liver.

12.10   Why is the blood urea nitrogen test ordered?

The test screens for kidney function and dehydration. The test assesses for the treatment for kidney disease and kidney dialysis.

12.11   What must be considered before administering the blood urea nitrogen test?

Assess:
- If the patient has eaten meat or protein prior to the administration of the test
- If the patient has taken Fungizone, Garamycin, Nebcin, chloromycetin, nafcillin, Kantrex, tetracycline, or diuretics
- The patient's age, since BUN levels increase with age.

12.12 What might a high blood urea nitrogen test value mean?

High BUN values may indicate kidney disease, kidney stones, Addison's disease, kidney tumor, burns, heart failure, GI bleeding, dehydration, or a high protein diet.

12.13 What might a high BUN to creatinine ratio value mean?

A high BUN to creatinine ratio may indicate respiratory tract bleeding, GI tract bleeding, shock, kidney failure, urinary tract blockage, or dehydration.

12.14 What might a low blood urea nitrogen test value mean?

Low BUN values may indicate malnutrition, liver damage, overhydration, or a low protein diet.

12.15 What might a low BUN to creatinine ratio value mean?

A low BUN to creatinine ratio may indicate rhabdomyolysis, cirrhosis, SIADH, or muscle injury.

12.16 What might a high level of BUN and creatinine level mean?

Both BUN and creatinine levels are high when there is blockage of urine flow.

Creatinine and Creatinine Clearance

12.17 What is creatine?

Creatine phosphate provides energy to skeletal muscles. After seven seconds of intense effort, creatine phosphate converts to creatine.

12.18 What is the difference between creatine and creatinine?

Creatine is metabolized into creatinine and is carried in blood to the kidneys for filtering and excreted in urine.

12.19 What happens if kidneys malfunction?

If kidneys are malfunctioning, creatinine levels in the blood increase and creatinine levels in urine decrease.

12.20 What does the creatinine clearance test measure?

The creatinine clearance test measures creatinine in a 24-hour urine sample and measures the level of creatinine in blood.

12.21 What does the BUN:creatinine test measure?

The BUN:creatinine test compares the results of the blood urea test with the blood creatinine level test to assess for dehydration.

12.22 How is the fetal kidney function assessed?

Fetal kidney function is assessed by testing the level of creatinine in amniotic fluid.

12.23 What must be assessed before the creatinine tests are administered?

Assess if the patient:
- Performed strenuous exercise two days prior to the test
- Has taken:
  - Blood creatinine Level Test: Diuretics, Proloprim, Trimpex, Aldomet, Tagamet, ascorbic acid, cephalosporin, or Mefoxin
  - Creatinine clearance test: Dilantin, cephalosporin, Captopril, ascorbic acid, Garamycin, Tagamet, Proloprim, Trimpex, Cardioquin, Quinaglute, quinine, Quinidex, amphotericin B or procainamide
  - BUN to creatinine ratio test: Tetracycline or Tagamet
- Ingested protein for one day prior to the test
- Drunk coffee or tea before the creatinine clearance test, since these increase urine production

12.24 What might a high level of creatinine indicate?

A high level of creatinine may indicate kidney disorder, kidney stones, dehydration, shock, rhabdomyolysis, acromegaly, gigantism, polymyositis, muscular dystrophy, a urinary tract blockage, or cancer.

12.25 What might a high level result of the creatinine clearance test indicate?

A high level result of the creatinine clearance test may indicate muscle injury, pregnancy, hypothyroidism, burns, strenuous exercise, or carbon monoxide poisoning.

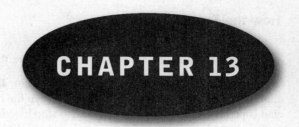

CHAPTER 13

Pancreas and Lipid Metabolism Tests

13.1 Definition

Healthcare providers order lipid metabolism tests to determine the level of lipids in the patient's blood stream and pancreatic tests to determine pancreatic function. The pancreas produces insulin and glucagon along with digestive enzymes that are used by the small intestine to break down carbohydrates, protein, and fat. *Lipids* are compounds used to store energy, develop cell membranes, and are elements of vitamins and hormones. Lipids combine with protein to form lipoprotein. Common lipoproteins in the body are cholesterol and triglycerides. Cholesterol is released into the bloodstream mostly by the liver and other organs, although some cholesterol is ingested in food. Two types of cholesterol are *high-density lipoprotein (HDL)* and *low-density lipoprotein (LDL)*. There is a balance between LDL and HDL. LDL is distributed to cells throughout the body by the bloodstream. Excess LDL is removed by HDL from the blood and transported to the liver, where LDL is metabolized into bile acids and excreted from the body. An imbalance occurs when too much LDL is in the blood, leading to accumulation of LDL on the artery walls. This causes a narrowing of the arteries and leads to a blockage. The healthcare provider is likely to order a lipase test along with the amylase test. *Lipase* is an enzyme that is produced only by the pancreas. The amylase test may also be performed with the creatinine test to help the healthcare provider diagnose pancreatitis.

13.2 Amylase

The amylase test measures the amount of amylase in blood. *Amylase* is an enzyme that breaks down starch into sugar. Amylase is produced by salivary glands and the pancreas. There is normally a low level of amylase in blood unless the salivary glands or pancreas is blocked or damaged.

Why the Test Is Performed

The test screens for pancreatic disease, pancreatitis, and inflammation of the salivary glands. It also assesses the treatments for pancreatic and salivary glands disease.

Before Administering the Test

Assess if the patient:

- Refrained from eating and drinking anything except water 2 hours before the test
- Drank alcohol 24 hours before the test
- Took codeine, morphine, diuretics, coumadin, indocin, aspirin, or birth control pills, since these can affect the test results
- Has chronic kidney disease, since this can cause high levels of amylase
- Has liver or pancreas damage, since this can affect the test result

How the Test Is Performed

- Refrain from eating or drinking anything except water for 2 hours before the test
- Avoid drinking alcohol for 24 hours before the test

A sample of blood is taken from the patient's vein. The patient will experience a tight feeling when the tourniquet is tightened, a pinch or nothing at all when the needle is inserted into the vein, and pressure when a gauze pad is pressed against the insertion site to stop bleeding. It can take up to 10 minutes for bleeding to stop if the patient is taking anticoagulants (aspirin, coumadin). A small bruise might appear at the insertion site, which could become swollen following this test. This is called phlebitis. Applying a warm compress several times a day will reduce the swelling.

Teach the Patient

Explain why the blood sample is taken, the function of amylase, and the meaning of abnormal values. Explain that the patient must refrain from eating or drinking anything except water for 2 hours before the test and avoid drinking alcohol for 24 hours before the test, and that the patient should tell the healthcare provider if he or she is taking codeine, morphine diuretics, coumadin, indocin, aspirin, or birth control pills, since these can affect the test results.

Understanding the Test Results

Test results are available within 3 days. The laboratory determines normal values based on calibration of testing equipment with a control test. Test results are reported as high, normal, or low based on the laboratory's control test. Generally the normal range is: 60 to 180 U/L. High values are normal for older adults and pregnant women. The patient may have chronic pancreatitis, even if there is a low amylase level. Children have very little amylase until they reach their first birthday, and then their amylase is at the normal adult level.

A high level may indicate pancreatitis, pancreatic cancer, mumps, bowel infarction, inflammation of the salivary glands, cystic fibrosis, diabetic ketoacidosis, gallstones, stomach ulcer, macroamylasemia, or ectopic pregnancy.

A low level may indicate preeclampsia, advanced cystic fibrosis, severe liver disease, or macroamylasemia.

13.3 Lipase

The lipase test measures the level of lipase in blood. *Lipase* is an enzyme in the pancreas. Levels of lipase in the blood increase when the pancreatic duct is blocked or there is damage to the pancreas. The lipase test does not diagnose pancreatic disorder. A high level of lipase in blood requires additional testing. The healthcare provider may order the amylase test at the same time as the lipase test.

Why the Test Is Performed

The test screens for pancreatic disease, pancreatitis, and cystic fibrosis. The test also assesses treatment for pancreatitis and cystic fibrosis.

Before Administering the Test

Assess if the patient has:

- Eaten or drunk anything except water 12 hours before the test is administered
- High cholesterol, varicose veins, kidney disease, diabetes, or high blood pressure
- Taken narcotics, anticoagulants, or cholinergics

How the Test Is Performed

- Avoid eating or drinking anything except water 12 hours before the test is administered.

A sample of blood is taken from the patient's vein. The patient will experience a tight feeling when the tourniquet is tightened, a pinch or nothing at all when the needle is inserted into the vein, and pressure when a gauze pad is pressed against the insertion site to stop bleeding. It can take up to 10 minutes for bleeding to stop if the patient is taking anticoagulants (aspirin, coumadin). A small bruise might appear at the insertion site, which could become swollen following this test. This is called phlebitis. Applying a warm compress several times a day will reduce the swelling.

Teach the Patient

Explain why the sample is taken, that the patient must not eat or drink anything except water 12 hours before the test is administered, and that the healthcare provider may ask the patient to refrain from taking narcotics, anticoagulants, or cholinergics 2 weeks before the test is administered.

Understanding the Test Results

The lipase test results are available in 12 hours. The laboratory determines normal values based on calibration of testing equipment with a control test. Test results are reported as high, normal, or low based on the laboratory's control test.

- Normal lipase test results: less than 200 U/L

A high lipase level may indicate pancreatic cancer, pancreatitis, pancreatic disease, cholecystitis, gallstones, bowel obstruction, infarction, chronic kidney disease, inflammation, infection, drug abuse, or peptic ulcer disease.

13.4 Cholesterol and Triglycerides Tests

The cholesterol and triglycerides tests profile the lipoprotein to measure components of cholesterol. Cholesterol is produced in the liver and used for cell growth and hormone production. Cholesterol attaches to a protein in the blood, forming a lipoprotein. Excess cholesterol in the blood forms plaque on the side of blood vessels that can lead to cardiovascular disorders. These components are:

- **Total cholesterol**: Total cholesterol is the total amount of LDL and HDL in the blood sample.
- **Low density lipoprotein (LDL)**: LDL transports lipids from the liver. High levels of LDL increase the risk of cardiovascular disorders.
- **Very low density lipoprotein (VLDL)**: VLDL distributes triglycerides that are produced in the liver. High levels of VLDL increase the risk of cardiovascular disorders.
- **High density lipoprotein (HDL)**: HDL binds with lipids in the blood returning lipids to the liver, where lipids are metabolized. High levels of HDL decrease the risk of cardiovascular disorders.
- **Triglycerides**: Triglycerides are stored lipids. High levels of triglycerides and high levels of LDL increase the risk of cardiovascular disorders.

Why the Test Is Performed

The test screens for lipid disorder and assesses the treatment of lipid disorder.

Before Administering the Test

Assess if the patient:

- Has eaten or drunk anything12 hours before the test is administered
- Has eaten a high fatty diet 24 hours before the test is administered
- Has exercised before the test is administered
- Has undergone a radioactive scan within a week before the test
- Has an infection, hyperthyroidism, hypothyroidism, cirrhosis, hepatitis, diabetes, kidney disease
- Is malnourished
- Abuses alcohol and medication
- Is undergoing alcohol or medication withdrawal

- Is pregnant
- Has taken androgens, birth control pills, corticosteroids, estrogen, niacin, antibiotics, tranquilizers, or diuretics

How the Test Is Performed

A sample of blood is taken from the patient's vein. The patient will experience a tight feeling when the tourniquet is tightened, a pinch or nothing at all when the needle is inserted into the vein, and pressure when a gauze pad is pressed against the insertion site to stop bleeding. It can take up to 10 minutes for bleeding to stop if the patient is taking anticoagulants (aspirin, coumadin). A small bruise might appear at the insertion site, which could become swollen following this test. This is called phlebitis. Applying a warm compress several times a day will reduce the swelling.

Teach the Patient

Explain why the blood sample is taken, not to eat or drink anything except water 12 hours before the test, not to eat a fatty diet 24 hours before the test, not to exercise before the test, and that the healthcare provider may request that the patient stop taking androgens, birth control pills, corticosteroids, estrogen, niacin, antibiotics, tranquilizers, or diuretics for 2 weeks prior to the test.

Understanding the Test Results

Test results are available in 1 day. The laboratory determines normal values based on calibration of testing equipment with a control test. Test results are reported as high, normal, or low based on the laboratory's control test.

- Normal total cholesterol range: less than 240 mg/dL
- Normal HDL range: greater than 40 mg/dL
- Normal total cholesterol: HDL ratio range is: less than 5:1
- Normal LDL range: less than 160 mg/dL
- Normal VLDL range: less than 160 mg/dL
- Normal triglycerides range: less than 200 mg/dL

Lower HDL and higher LDL, VLDL, and triglycerides increase the risk of cardiovascular disorders: coronary artery disease, acute coronary syndrome, and heart attack.

Solved Problems

Pancreas and Lipid Metabolism

13.1 What are lipids?

Lipids are compounds used to store energy, develop cell membranes, and are elements of vitamins and hormones.

13.2 What is produced by the pancreas?

The pancreas produces insulin and glucagon along with digestive enzymes that are used by the small intestine to break down carbohydrates, protein, and fat.

13.3 Name two lipoproteins.

Common lipoproteins in the body are cholesterol and triglycerides.

13.4 What releases cholesterol into the bloodstream?

Cholesterol is released into the bloodstream mostly by the liver and other organs, although some cholesterol is ingested in food.

13.5 What are two types of cholesterol?

Two types of cholesterol are high-density lipoprotein (HDL) and low-density lipoprotein (LDL).

13.6   How is excess LDL removed?

Excess LDL is removed by HDL from the blood and transported to the liver where LDL is metabolized into bile acids and excreted from the body.

13.7   What might happen when there is too much LDL in the bloodstream?

An imbalance occurs when too much LDL is in the blood, leading to the accumulation of LDL on the artery walls. This causes a narrowing of the arteries and leads to a blockage.

Amylase

13.8   Why is the amylase test performed with the creatininine test?

The amylase test may also be performed with the creatinine test to help the healthcare provider diagnose pancreatitis.

13.9   What is amylase?

Amylase is an enzyme that breaks down starch into sugar. Amylase is produced by salivary glands and the pancreas.

13.10   Is there normally low or high levels of amylase in blood?

There is normally a low level of amylase in blood unless the salivary glands or pancreas are blocked or damaged.

13.11   Why is the amylase test ordered?

The test screens for pancreatic disease, pancreatitis, and inflammation of the salivary glands. The test also assesses the treatment for pancreatic and salivary glands disease.

13.12   What must be assessed before administering the amylase test?

Assess if the patient:
- Refrained from eating and drinking anything except water 2 hours before the test
- Drank alcohol 24 hours before the test
- Has taken codeine, morphine, diuretics, coumadin, indocin, aspirin or birth control pills, since these can affect the test results
- Has chronic kidney disease, since this can cause high levels of amylase
- Has liver or pancreas damage, since this can affect the test result

13.13   What must the patient learn before the amylase test is administered?

Explain why the blood sample is taken, the function of amylase and the meaning of abnormal values, that the patient must refrain from eating or drinking anything except water for 2 hours before the test and avoid drinking alcohol for 24 hours before the test, and that the patient should tell the healthcare provider if he or she is taking codeine, morphine diuretics, coumadin, indocin, aspirin, or birth control pills, since these can affect the test results.

13.14   Are high levels of amylase normal?

High values are normal for older adults and pregnant women.

13.15   What might a healthcare provider order if there is a high amylase level?

High levels may indicate pancreatitis, pancreatic cancer, mumps, bowel infarction, inflammation of the salivary glands, cystic fibrosis, diabetic ketoacidosis, gallstones, stomach ulcer, macroamylasemia, or ectopic pregnancy.

13.16   What might a low level of amylase indicate?

A low level of amylase may indicate preeclampsia, advanced cystic fibrosis, severe liver disease, or macroamylasemia.

13.17   What level of amylase would you expect for a three-year-old child?

Children have very little amylase until they reach their first birthday and then their amylase is at the normal adult level.

Lipase

13.18 What is lipase?

Lipase is an enzyme in the pancreas.

13.19 What might cause a high level of lipase in the blood stream?

Levels of lipase in the blood increase when the pancreatic duct is blocked or there is damage to the pancreas.

13.20 Is a high lipase level used to diagnose pancreatic disorders?

The lipase test does not diagnose pancreatic disorder. A high level of lipase in blood requires additional testing.

13.21 Why is a patient administered the lipase test?

The test screens for pancreatic disease, pancreatitis, and cystic fibrosis. The test assesses treatment for pancreatitis and cystic fibrosis.

13.22 What should be assessed before administering the lipase test?

Assess if the patient has:
- Eaten or drunk anything except water 12 hours before the test is administered
- High cholesterol, varicose veins, kidney disease, diabetes, or high blood pressure
- Taken narcotics, anticoagulants, or cholinergics

13.23 What might a high level of lipase indicate?

A high lipase level may indicate pancreatic cancer, pancreatitis, pancreatic disease, cholecystitis, gallstones, bowel obstruction, infarction, chronic kidney disease, inflammation, infection, drug abuse, or peptic ulcer disease.

13.24 What is the function of cholesterol?

Cholesterol is produced in the liver and used for cell growth and hormone production.

13.25 What is the VLDL test?

Very low-density lipoprotein (VLDL) distributes triglyceride that is produced in the liver. High levels of VLDL increase the risk of cardiovascular disorders.

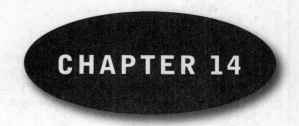

CHAPTER 14

Diagnostic Radiologic Tests

14.1 Definition

Radiologic tests provide a view inside the body. Radiologic tests use X-rays to view inside the body without opening the skin. An X-ray remains a cost-effective way to identify many common disorders, although primitive when compared with computed tomography (CT), computed axial tomography (CAT) scans, and magnetic resonance imaging (MRI). The X-ray is absorbed by dense objects and passes through less dense objects. Dense objects such as bone appear white on the X-ray file. Less dense objects, such as air, appear black, while fluid and fat appear as a lighter shade of gray.

14.2 How an X-ray Is Taken

The patient is positioned between the X-ray machine and photographic film. The X-ray machine focuses the X-ray beam at the area of the patient's body that is being examined. A portion of the X-ray beam passes through the patient's body, striking the photographic film and leaving a black area on the photographic film. Another portion of the X-ray beam is absorbed by bone and other dense tissue in the patient's body, which appear as shades of grey on the photographic film, depending on the density of the tissue. Areas that are not X-rayed are protected by a lead apron, when possible, to prevent X-rays from reaching those areas. An X-ray does not provide a good image of cartilage, ligaments, tendons, and other soft tissues. The healthcare provider is likely to order a CT scan or MRI to examine soft tissue.

Teach the Patient

Explain that an X-ray may not be taken if the patient is pregnant, the level of radiation will not have any long-term effects for the patient, and the healthcare provider may require specific preparation depending on the part of the body being X-rayed. Explain that any jewelry in the vicinity of the X-ray site must be removed, a radiologist is usually the healthcare professional who reads the X-ray, and that the patient may be required to remove clothing and wear a gown during the X-ray. Explain that the patient will be asked to lie still and hold his or her breath when the X-ray is taken, that the X-ray room is cool, and that the patient may feel uncomfortable while positioning for the X-ray. Assess if the patient has signed a consent form.

14.3 Abdominal X-ray

An abdominal X-ray shows the position, size, and shape of the:

- Stomach
- Diaphragm
- Liver
- Spleen

- Large intestines
- Small intestines

Ovaries are not protected with a lead apron during the X-ray because it is located at the site of the X-ray. An abdominal X-ray cannot detect ulcers or bleeding.

The healthcare provider may also order a CT scan, ultrasound, or IV pyelograph.

A KUB X-ray is an abdominal X-ray that examines the kidneys, uterus, and bladder.

Why the Test Is Performed

The test assesses the underlying cause of abdominal or flank pain, confirms the position of nasogastric tube, nephrostomy tube, V-P shunt, dialysis catheter, locates an ingested foreign body, assesses the underlying cause of vomiting and nausea, assesses for intestinal blockage, and assesses for perforation in the intestine or stomach.

Before Administering the Test

Assess if the patient:

- Is pregnant. An ultrasound is ordered instead of an X-ray if the patient is pregnant, to protect the fetus from radiation exposure.
- Has taken Pepto-Bismol (bismuth) or barium four days prior to the test. Bismuth and barium might obstruct the X-ray beam.
- Has an empty bladder

How the Test Is Performed

- The patient may be asked to stand between the X-ray machine and the photographic film or lie on his or her back or side on the X-ray table.
- The patient lies on his or her back:
  - A lead apron is placed over the lower pelvic area to protect the area from X-rays.
  - The X-ray machine is positioned over the abdomen.
  - The patient is asked to lie still and hold his or her breath when the X-ray is taken.
  - An X-ray is taken.
- The patient is asked to stand between the X-ray machine and the photographic film:
  - The patient is asked to stand still and hold his or her breath when the X-ray is taken.
  - An X-ray is taken.
- See How an X-ray Is Taken.

Teach the Patient

Explain why the X-ray is being taken, what the patient can expect in the X-ray room, that the patient should not take Pepto-Bismol (bismuth) or barium four days prior to the test, and that the patient will need to empty his or her bladder before the test.

Understanding the Test Results

The test takes 10 minutes. The results are ready within 15 minutes or two days, depending on the patient's condition.

- Normal:
  - Normal position, size, and shape of the stomach, diaphragm, liver, spleen, large and small intestines
  - No growths
  - Normal amounts of air, fluid, or stool
- Abnormal:
  - Abnormal position, size, and shape of the stomach, diaphragm, liver, spleen, large and small intestines
  - Blockage
  - Perforation in the intestine or stomach (Conn syndrome)

- ○ Abnormal amounts of air, fluid, or stool
- ○ Kidney stones
- ○ Gallstones
- ○ Foreign object located
- ○ Growths

14.4   Extremity X-ray

An extremity X-ray shows damage to:

- Hands
- Wrists
- Arms
- Feet
- Ankles
- Knees
- Hips
- Legs

The healthcare provider may not order an X-ray if the results of the X-ray would not alter treatment of the disorder.

The healthcare provider may order a bone scan, CT scan, or MRI if the X-ray does not reveal a disorder. The healthcare provider may order opposing extremities to be X-rayed to compare extremities.

Why the Test Is Performed

Assess for:

- Fractures
- Dislocation
- Tumors
- Deformities/degeneration
- Fluid around joints
- Growth
- The underlying cause of pain in the extremity
- Alignment following treatment
- Infection
- Foreign objects

Before Administering the Test

Assess if the patient:

- Is pregnant. An ultrasound is ordered instead of an X-ray if the patient is pregnant, to protect the fetus from radiation exposure.
- Can remain still during the X-ray

How the Test Is Performed

- The patient sits, stands, or lies down, depending on the extremity being examined.
- The extremity is positioned in front of the X-ray machine and held in place by an apparatus, if necessary.
- An X-ray is taken.
- See How an X-ray Is Taken.

Teach the Patient

Explain why the X-ray is being taken, what the patient can expect in the X-ray room, and that the patient will need to hold the extremity still when the X-ray is taken.

Understanding the Test Results

The test takes 10 minutes. The results are ready within 15 minutes or two days depending on the patient's condition.

- Normal:
  - No fracture
  - No dislocation
  - No tumors
  - No deformities
  - No fluid around joints
  - Normal growth
  - Extremity is aligned
  - No infection
  - No foreign objects
- Abnormal:
  - Signs of fracture
  - Signs of dislocation
  - Signs of tumors
  - Signs of deformities
  - Signs of fluid around joints
  - Abnormal growth
  - Extremity misaligned
  - Signs of infection
  - Signs of foreign objects

14.5   Spinal X-ray

The Spinal X-ray assesses the spine.

- The spine consists of 33 vertebrae, nearly all separated by a disc that absorbs shock related to movement.
- A *disc* is cartilage.
- Strained back muscles or ligaments are not visible on an X-ray.
- If the patient has a cervical collar, an X-ray will be taken and read to determine if the cervical collar can be removed without causing further injury.
- There are four types of spinal X-rays:
  1. **Cervical spine X-ray**: 7 vertebrae in the cervical area of the spine
  2. **Thoracic spine X-ray**: 12 vertebrae in the thoracic area of the spine
  3. **Lumbosacral spine X-ray**: 5 vertebrae in the lumbar area of the spine and 5 vertebrae in the sacrum area
  4. **Sacrum/coccyx X-ray**: 5 vertebrae in the sacrum area and 4 vertebrae in the coccyx area

Why the Test Is Performed

The test assesses for fracture, dislocation, tumors, deformities/degeneration, curvature of the spine, bone spurs, the underlying cause of weakness, pain, or numbness, and alignment following treatment.

Before Administering the Test

Assess if the patient:

- Is pregnant. An ultrasound is ordered instead of an X-ray if the patient is pregnant, to protect the fetus from radiation exposure.
- Is morbidly overweight, since this can blur details of the X-ray
- Has taken Pepto-Bismol (bismuth) or barium 4 days prior to the test. Bismuth and barium might obstruct the X-ray beam.
- Can remain still during the X-ray

How the Test Is Performed

- The patient lies on an X-ray table.
- The X-ray machine is positioned over the site.
- The patient is asked to lie still and hold his or her breath when the X-ray is taken.
- An X-ray is taken (up to five X-rays may be taken).
- See How an X-ray Is Taken.

Teach the Patient

Explain why the X-ray is being taken, what the patient can expect in the X-ray room, that the patient should not take Pepto-Bismol (bismuth) or barium 4 days prior to the test, and that the patient will need to lie still when the X-ray is taken.

Understanding the Test Results

The test takes 15 minutes. The results are ready within 15 minutes or 2 days, depending on the patient's condition.

- Normal:
  - No fracture
  - No dislocation
  - No tumors
  - No deformities/degeneration
  - Spine is aligned
  - No bone spurs
- Abnormal:
  - Signs of fracture
  - Signs of dislocation
  - Signs of tumors
  - Signs of deformities/degeneration
  - Spine is misaligned
  - Signs of bone spurs

14.6   Mammogram

A mammogram is an X-ray that detects palpable and non-palpable cysts or masses in the breast and is used to screen for signs of breast cancer. A breast ultrasound determines if a mass is a cyst or solid mass. Suspicious masses are biopsied to determine if the mass is cancerous. A mammogram is not normally performed if the patient is pregnant. If the mammogram must be performed, a lead apron is placed over the patient's abdomen. A mammogram is performed on a patient who has had breast implants. A mammogram is not performed if the patient is breast-feeding. A digital mammogram is considered to have the same accuracy as an X-ray mammogram. The healthcare provider may order the breast cancer (BRCA) gene test if there is a pattern of breast cancer in the patient's family. The healthcare provider must provide the patient with the original mammogram images if requested. A normal mammogram does not rule out breast cancer. Results may be difficult to interpret if the patient is obese.

Why the Test Is Performed

The test assesses if the patient has cysts, solid masses, or calcification in the breast. It also assesses the underlying cause of breast discomfort.

Before Administering the Test

Assess if the patient:

- Is pregnant
- Is breast-feeding
- Has breast implants

- Removed all powders, deodorant, ointments, or perfume from the breast, since these may appear on the X-ray image
- Scheduled the test within 2 weeks after the end of the patient's menstrual period to reduce tenderness of the patient's breasts
- Had any previous breast biopsies; identify their locations

How the Test Is Performed

- Remove all powders, deodorant, ointments, or perfume from the breast, since these may appear on the X-ray image.
- Schedule the mammogram within two weeks after the end of the patient's menstrual period to reduce tenderness of the patient's breasts.
- Remove the patient's clothes above the waist and provide the patient with a gown.
- The patient stands or sits.
- Each breast is placed on the X-ray plate.
- A second plate is placed on top of the breast.
- The breast is compressed.
- The patient is asked to hold her breath while the X-ray is taken.
- X-ray images are taken from the top and side of the breast.
- See How an X-ray Is Taken.

Teach the Patient

Explain why the mammogram is being taken, the procedure for taking the mammogram, that the breast is compressed to obtain the best possible view of the breast, that the test will be uncomfortable but not painful, that the patient should not use powders, deodorant, ointments or perfume on the breasts the day of the mammogram, and that the patient should schedule the mammogram 2 weeks after the end of the patient's menstrual period to reduce tenderness of the breasts.

Understanding the Test Results

The test takes 15 minutes. The results are ready within 15 minutes or ten days, depending on the patient's condition.

- Normal:
  - No cyst
  - No solid mass
  - Normal tissue
  - Clear ducts
- Abnormal:
  - Signs of cyst
  - Signs of solid mass
  - Signs of calcification

14.7   Chest X-ray

A chest X-ray shows the position, size, and shape of the collarbone, breastbone, heart, airway, lungs, thoracic spine, ribs, lymph nodes, and blood vessels. *Hint*: The healthcare provider may also order an echocardiography, ultrasound, MRI, or a CT.

Why the Test Is Performed

The test assesses for pulmonary disease or disorders, the underlying cause of chest pain or respiratory problems, the underlying cause of cardiac problems, a chest injury, and positioning of a medical device. The test also identifies foreign objects in the airway and esophagus.

Before Administering the Test

Assess if the patient:

- Is pregnant
- Is able to hold his/her breath
- Has removed all jewelry in the thoracic area, since these may appear on the X-ray image
- Is obese
- Has scars in the thoracic area that might appear on the X-ray

How the Test Is Performed

- Remove the patient's clothes above the waist and provide the patient with a gown.
- The patient stands or sits in front of or lies down on the X-ray plate.
- The patient is asked to hold his or her breath while the X-ray is taken.
- X-ray images are taken from the front and side.
- See How an X-ray Is Taken.

Teach the Patient

Explain why the X-ray is being taken, the procedure for taking the X-ray, and that the patient should remove all jewelry in the thoracic area.

Understanding the Test Results

The test takes approximately 15 minutes and the results are ready within 15 minutes or 2 days, depending on the patient's condition.

- Normal:
    - Normal size and shape of the collarbone, breastbone, heart, airway, lungs, thoracic spine, ribs, lymph nodes, and blood vessels
    - No abnormal fluid seen
    - Medical device is in the proper position
- Abnormal:
    - Abnormal position, size, and shape of the collarbone, breastbone, heart, airway, lungs, thoracic spine, ribs, lymph nodes, and blood vessels
    - Abnormal fluid seen
    - Medical device is not in the proper position

14.8   Dental X-ray

Dental X-rays are used to assess the condition of the patient's jaw, mouth, and teeth. There are four types of dental X-rays:

1. **Panoramic (orthopantogram)**: This assesses the temporomandibular joints, the jaw, sinuses, teeth, and nasal area for tumors, fractures, cysts, and impacted teeth, but not cavities.
2. **Occlusal**: This assesses the palate and lower portions of the mouth for fractures, cleft palate, abscesses, tumors, cysts, and immature teeth.
3. **Bitwing**: This is a single view of the upper and lower back teeth and used to assess the formation of teeth, bone loss, infection, and tooth decay.
4. **Periapical**: This is a view of a tooth and used to assess abscesses, tumors, cysts, and the overall status of the patient's teeth.

Why the Test Is Performed

The test assesses for cysts, tumors, abscesses, the underlying cause of mouth and sinus pain, the health and position of teeth, and for abnormal structures in the mouth and jaw.

Before Administering the Test

Assess if the patient:

- Is pregnant
- Is able to open his or her mouth enough to insert the X-ray film carrier into his or her mouth
- Has foreign objects in his or her mouth, such as body piercing, retainers, dentures, braces, or bridges

How the Test Is Performed

- The patient sits.
- The patient bites down on the X-ray film carrier that holds the X-ray film.
- X-ray image is taken.
- In a panoramic X-ray, the patient places his head in the arm of the X-ray machine and the arm rotates while taking the X-ray image.
- See How an X-ray Is Taken.

Teach the Patient

Explain why the X-ray is being taken and the procedure for taking the X-ray.

Understanding the Test Results

The test takes a few minutes. The results are ready within 15 minutes.

- Normal:
  ○ Normal position, size, and shape of the temporomandibular joints, the jaw, sinuses, teeth, mouth, and nasal area.
- Abnormal:
  ○ Tooth decay
  ○ Abnormal position, size, and shape of the temporomandibular joints, the jaw, sinuses, teeth, mouth, and nasal area.

14.9 Facial X-ray

A facial X-ray is used to assess facial bones, sinuses, and the orbital cavity. The healthcare provider may also order a CT scan.

Why the Test Is Performed

The test assesses for cysts, tumors, abscesses, the underlying cause of sinus pain, fractures, and foreign objects.

Before Administering the Test

Assess if the patient:

- Is pregnant
- Is able to sit still for the X-ray
- Has a prosthetic eye
- Has a neck injury
- Has body piercing in the area being X-rayed
- Has removed eyeglasses

How the Test Is Performed

- The patient sits.
- The patient must remove eyeglasses and body piercing in the area of the X-ray.
- The patient must hold his or her head still. A brace may be provided to stabilize the patient's head.

- X-ray image is taken.
- See How an X-ray Is Taken.

Teach the Patient

Explain why the X-ray is being taken and the procedure for taking the X-ray.

Understanding the Test Results

The test takes 30 minutes. The results are ready within 15 minutes.

- Normal:
  - Normal position, size, and shape of bones in the face and the orbital cavity
- Abnormal:
  - Inflammation
  - Infection
  - Abnormal position, size, and shape of bones in the face and the orbital cavity
  - Cysts, tumors, abscesses
  - Foreign object

14.10   Skull X-ray

A skull X-ray is used to assess the skull and sinuses. The healthcare provider may also order a CT scan.

Why the Test Is Performed

The test assesses for cysts, tumors, abscesses, the underlying cause of sinus pain, fractures, and foreign objects.

Before Administering the Test

Assess if the patient:

- Is pregnant
- Is able to sit still for the X-ray
- Has a prosthetic eye
- Has a neck injury
- Has body piercing in the area being X-rayed
- Has removed eyeglasses

How the Test Is Performed

- The patient sits.
- The patient must remove eyeglasses and body piercing in the area of the X-ray.
- The patient must hold his or her head still. A brace may be provided to stabilize the patient's head.
- X-ray image is taken. Several images are taken: front, back, top, and sides.
- See How an X-ray Is Taken.

Teach the Patient

Explain why the X-ray is being taken and the procedure for taking the X-ray.

Understanding the Test Results

The test takes 30 minutes. The results are ready within 15 minutes.

- Normal:
  - Normal position, size, and shape of bones in the skull and the orbital cavity

- Abnormal:
  - Inflammation
  - Infection
  - Abnormal position, size, and shape of bones in the skull
  - Cysts, tumors, abscesses
  - Foreign object

Solved Problems

Diagnostic Radiologic Test

14.1   How does an X-ray work?

The patient is positioned between the X-ray machine and photographic film. The X-ray machine focuses the X-ray beam at the area of the patient's body that is being examined. A portion of the X-ray beam passes through the patient's body, striking the photographic film and leaving a black area on the photographic film. Another portion of the X-ray beam is absorbed by bone and other dense tissue in the patient's body, which appears as shades of grey on the photographic film, depending on the density of the tissue.

Areas that are not X-rayed are protected by a lead apron, when possible, to prevent X-rays from reaching those areas. The X-ray is absorbed by dense objects and passes through less dense objects. Dense objects such as bone appear white on the X-ray file. Less dense objects such as air appear black, fluid and fat appear as a lighter shade of gray.

14.2   Why are X-ray tests still ordered by healthcare providers when more advanced methods such as CT, CAT scans, and MRIs are available?

An X-ray remains a cost-effective way to identify many common disorders, although primitive when compared with CT, CAT scans, and MRI.

14.3   Why would a healthcare provider not order an X-ray if it is suspected that the patient has an injured ligament?

An X-ray does not provide a good image of cartilage, ligaments, tendons, and other soft tissues.

14.4   What would you teach a patient before sending the patient for an X-ray?

Explain that an X-ray may not be taken if the patient is pregnant, the level of radiation will not have any long-term effects for the patient, the healthcare provider may require specific preparation, depending on the part of the body being X-rayed; any jewelry in the vicinity of the X-ray site must be removed, a radiologist is usually the healthcare professional who reads the X-ray, the patient may be required to remove clothing and wear a gown during the X-ray, the patient will be asked to lie still and hold his or her breath when the X-ray is taken, the X-ray room is cool, and the patient may feel uncomfortable while positioning for the X-ray.

Abdominal X-ray Test

14.5   Why is an abdominal X-ray ordered?

An abdominal X-ray shows the position, size, and shape of the stomach, diaphragm, liver, spleen, large intestines, and small intestines.

14.6   Are the ovaries protected with a lead apron during an abdominal X-ray?

Ovaries are not protected with a lead apron during the X-ray because the apron is located at the site of the X-ray.

14.7   How would you respond if the patient asks for an abdominal X-ray to determine if he has a stomach ulcer?

Abdominal X-rays cannot detect ulcers or bleeding.

14.8   What is a KUB X-ray?

A KUB X-ray is an abdominal X-ray that examines the kidneys, uterus, and bladder.

14.9 Why is an abdominal X-ray ordered?

An abdominal X-ray is ordered to assess the underlying cause of abdominal or flank pain, confirm position of nasogastric tube, nephrostomy tube, V-P shunt, or dialysis catheter, locate an ingested foreign body, assess the underlying cause of vomiting and nausea, assess for intestinal blockage, and assess for perforation in the intestine or stomach.

14.10 What do you assess before administering an abdominal X-ray?

Assess if the patient:
- Is pregnant. An ultrasound is ordered instead of an X-ray if the patient is pregnant, to protect the fetus from radiation exposure.
- Has taken Pepto-Bismol (bismuth) or barium four days prior to the test. Bismuth and barium might obstruct the X-ray beam.
- Has an empty bladder

14.11 What might be abnormal findings of an abdominal X-ray?

Some abnormal findings of an abdominal X-ray are abnormal position, size, and shape of the stomach, diaphragm, liver, spleen, large and small intestines; blockage; perforation in the intestine or stomach (Conn syndrome); abnormal amounts of air, fluid, or stool; kidney stones; gallstones; foreign object located; or growths.

Extremity X-ray Test

14.12 If an extremity is injured, why would a healthcare provider not order an extremity X-ray?

The healthcare provider may not order an X-ray if the results of the X-ray would not alter treatment of the disorder.

14.13 What would you expect the healthcare provider to order if the extremities X-ray is inconclusive?

The healthcare provider may order a bone scan, CT scan, or MRI if the X-ray does not reveal a disorder.

14.14 If there is injury to a bone in the left leg, why might the healthcare provider order an extremities X-ray of both legs?

The healthcare provider may order X-rays of opposing extremities to compare extremities.

14.15 What can be assessed with an extremities X-ray ordered by the healthcare provider?

The test assesses for fracture, dislocation, tumors, deformities/degeneration, fluid around joints, growth, the underlying cause of pain in the extremity, alignment following treatment, infection, and foreign objects.

Spinal X-ray Test

14.16 Why would a healthcare provider not order a spinal X-ray for a strained back?

Strained back muscles or ligaments are not visible on an X-ray.

14.17 What are the four types of spinal X-rays?

The four types of spinal X-rays are:
1. Cervical spine X-ray: 7 vertebrae in the cervical area of the spine
2. Thoracic spine X-ray: 12 vertebrae in the thoracic area of the spine
3. Lumbosacral spine X-ray: 5 vertebrae in the lumbar area of the spine and 5 vertebrae in the sacrum area
4. Sacrum/coccyx X-ray: 5 vertebrae in the sacrum area and 4 vertebrae in the coccyx area

14.18 Why is a spinal X-ray ordered by the healthcare provider?

The spinal X-ray assesses for fracture, dislocation, tumors, deformities/degeneration, curvature of the spine, bone spurs, the underlying cause of weakness, pain, or numbness, and alignment following treatment.

Mammogram

14.19 If a mammogram shows signs of a mass or cyst, what would you expect the healthcare provider to order?

A breast ultrasound might be ordered to determine if a mass is a cyst or solid mass.

14.20 Is a mammogram used to diagnose breast cancer?

No. Suspicious masses are biopsied to determine if the mass is cancerous.

14.21 What would you tell a pregnant woman who wants a mammogram?

A mammogram is not normally performed if the patient is pregnant. If the mammogram must be performed, a lead apron is placed over the patient's abdomen.

14.22 Which has the higher degree of accuracy: a digital mammogram or an X-ray mammogram?

A digital mammogram is considered to have the same accuracy as an X-ray mammogram.

14.23 What would you say to a pregnant woman who wants to have a mammogram a few weeks after giving birth?

A mammogram is not performed if the patient is breast-feeding.

14.24 What must be assessed before the patient is given a mammogram?

Assess if the patient:
- Is pregnant
- Is breast-feeding
- Has breast implants
- Removed all powders, deodorant, ointments, or perfume from the breast, since these may appear on the X-ray image
- Was scheduled within 2 weeks after the end of the patient's menstrual period to reduce tenderness of the patient's breasts
- Had any previous breast biopsies; identify their locations

14.25 What might an abnormal mammogram reveal?

An abnormal mammogram might reveal signs of a cyst, signs of a solid mass, or signs of calcification.

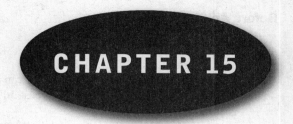

CHAPTER 15

Computed Tomography (CT) Scan

15.1 Definition

A *computed tomography* (CT) scan makes detailed images of structures within the body using a doughnut-shaped X-ray machine. As the patient lies within the scanner, an X-ray beam rotates around the patient, creating an image that represents a thin slice of the patient. Each rotation takes less than a second. All slices are stored on a computer. The computer is used to reassemble slices of the patient, enabling the healthcare provider to identify any abnormalities. Typically, the healthcare provider will print the image of any slices that indicate an abnormality, which are then saved with the patient's chart. The patient may be administered contrast material, such as iodine dye. The contrast material makes structures within the patient's body stand out on the computer by differentiating them in white, black, and shades of gray. Contrast material is administered intravenously or into joints or cavities of the body. The patient may also be asked to ingest other kinds of contrast material. A CT scan may be used for staging cancer to assess if the cancer has spread to other sites in the body. CT scans are also used to identify masses or tumors, as well as fluid and the infection process. CT scans guide the healthcare provider when performing a procedure such as a biopsy.

15.2 Full Body CT Scan

A full body CT scan creates an image of the patient's entire body. A healthcare provider orders a full body CT scan if:

- It is suspected that the patient may have disorders throughout the body.
- The healthcare provider is unable to narrow the disorder to specific areas of the body, such as if the patient is involved in a severe motor vehicle accident.

Typically, a healthcare provider orders a CT scan for a specific part of the body rather than ordering a full body scan. A full CT scan is time consuming and usually provides more information than is necessary for the healthcare provider to diagnose the patient's disorder. Some healthcare providers feel that a full body scan identifies benign growths and other disorders that do not adversely affect the patient and could lead to additional tests and surgery that are unnecessary. The result of a CT scan is commonly compared to the results of a positron emission tomography (PET) to identify cancer. Determine if the patient is allergic to shellfish or iodine. Contrast material may contain iodine and other substances that could cause the patient to have an allergic reaction. Also determine if the patient will be administered a sedative to relax him or her during the CT scan. If so, the make sure the patient does not drive following the CT scan until the sedative has worn off.

Why the Test Is Performed

The test assesses for growths, obstructions, inflammation or infection, foreign objects, bleeding, fluid collection, and pulmonary embolism.

Before Administering the Test

Assess if the patient:

- Has allergies (to shellfish, iodine)
- Is breastfeeding; since contrast material can pass to the baby in breast milk, the patient should be prepared to use formula instead of breast milk for 2 days following the CT scan if contrast material is administered
- Has heart disorder, asthma, thyroid disorder, kidney disorder, or diabetes
- Takes Glucophage
- Has taken Pepto-Bismol four days prior to the CT scan

Determine if the patient:

- Is claustrophobic
- Can lie still during the test

How the Test Is Performed

- Depending on the area or region of the body that is being scanned, the patient may be administered an enema or asked not to eat after midnight prior to the CT scan.
- If contrast material is required for the test, then the patient is administered the contrast material before the test. The method for administering the contrast material depends on the nature of the CT scan:
  - Approximately 40 minutes before the test, the patient may be asked to ingest contrast material.
  - Contrast material may be administered in a vein or in a cavity such as the bladder or rectum immediately before the test.
- The patient removes jewelry and clothes and is given a gown to wear during the test.
- The patient lies on the CT scanner table.
- The patient must lie still during the test.
- The patient will be in the CT room alone.
- The CT scan technician is in the next room observing through a window.
- The patient and the CT scan technician are able to converse during the test using an intercom.
- The CT scanner table moves into the opening of the CT scanner.
- The CT scanner moves around the patient when taking images of the patient.
- The patient hears a clicking sound as the CT scanner moves.
- The CT scan can take up to two hours.
- A radiologist who is a medical doctor interprets the results of the CT scan and writes a report that is given to the patient's healthcare provider.
- For 24 hours following the CT scan, the patient is asked to drink large amounts of water and other fluids to flush the contrast material from his or her body.

Teach the Patient

Explain why the CT scan is being administered, what the CT scan test does, and why contrast material may be administered. Explain that the contrast material may leave a metallic taste and that the patient may feel flushed when the contrast material is administered intravenously. Also explain that the healthcare provider may ask the patient to stop taking Glucophage several days before the CT scan, since there might be a reaction with contrast material, and that some patients may be allergic to the contrast material. It should be explained to the patient that the healthcare team is ready to take measures to reverse any adverse reaction to the contrast material. Inform the patient that the healthcare provider may ask the patient to stop breastfeeding for 2 days following the CT scan if contrast material is administered, that the patient will be asked to drink a large amount of water for 24 hours following the CT scan if contrast material is administered, and that the healthcare provider may administer a sedative prior to the test if the patient is unable to relax during the test. If a sedative is administered, the patient should arrange for someone else to drive him or her home following the test.

Understanding the Test Results

The result is available within 2 days.

- Normal:
  - Normal size organs and blood vessels
  - No blockages
  - No bleeding
  - No abnormal fluid collection
  - No growths
  - No inflammation
- Abnormal:
  - Abnormal size of organs and blood vessels
  - Blockages
  - Bleeding
  - Abnormal fluid collection
  - Growths
  - Inflammation

15.3   CT Scan of the Head

The CT scan of the head produces sliced images of the patient's skull and brain. The patient's head is placed into the CT scanner as the CT scanner takes sliced images of the patient's skull, brain, and other parts of the patient's head. The healthcare provider may order a perfusion CT. A perfusion CT is used to determine the blood supply to areas of the brain. Contrast material is administered intravenously. Areas of the brain that receive blood are highlighted on the computer image by the contrast material. Areas without blood flow are not highlighted.

Why the Test Is Performed

The test assesses for growths, obstructions, inflammation or infection, foreign objects, bleeding, fluid collection, headache, vertigo, vision problem, broken bones, the result of facial surgery, temporomandibular disorder, Paget's disease, stroke, and reasons for a change in the patient's level of consciousness. The test also provides baseline images before surgery.

Before Administering the Test

- See Full Body CT Scan
- Assess if the patient has removed glasses, contact lenses, and hearing aids

How the Test Is Performed

- See Full Body CT Scan.
- The CT scan of the head takes approximately 30 minutes.

Teach the Patient

See Full Body CT Scan. Explain that contrast material may be administered intravenously and flow throughout blood vessels in the brain, showing the areas of the brain that are receiving blood and those not receiving blood.

Understanding the Test Results

The result is available within 2 days.

- Normal:
  - Normal size skull, brain, ventricle, blood vessels, eyes, ears, sinuses
  - No blockages
  - No bleeding
  - No abnormal fluid collection
  - No foreign objects
  - No ischemia
- Abnormal:
  - Abnormal size skull, brain, ventricle, blood vessels, eyes, ears, sinuses
  - Blockages
  - Inflammation
  - Growth
  - Fluid collection
  - Foreign objects

15.4   CT Scan of the Spine

The CT scan of the spine creates images of the cervical spine, thoracic spine, and lumbosacral spine. All 33 vertebrae and discs are pictured, along with the cerebrospinal fluid (CSF). During the scan, the CT scanner can be tilted to follow the curvature of the spine. Depending on the purpose of the scan, the healthcare provider may require that contrast material be administered intrathecally into the spinal canal.

Why the Test Is Performed

The test assesses for growths, obstructions, narrowing of the spinal canal, deformities, fractures, inflammation and infection, bone compression, osteoporosis, and congenital defects.

Before Administering the Test

- See Full Body CT scan

How the Test Is Performed

- See Full Body CT Scan.
- The healthcare provider may order a CT myelogram.
- A CT myelogram requires that a sample of cerebrospinal fluid be removed for microscopic examination before contrast material is administered.
- Contrast material is then administered in the intrathecal space around the spinal cord.
- If a CT myelogram is performed, the patient lies on his or her stomach. An area of the lumbar spine is anesthetized and contrast material is injected.
- The CT table is tilted to help distribute the contrast material throughout the spine.
- After a CT myelogram, the patient is asked to keep his or her head raised to prevent seizures and headaches.

Teach the Patient

See Full Body CT Scan. Tell the patient to contact his or her healthcare provider if the patient experiences a severe headache or one that lasts more than a day following the CT scan, a temperature of 101.1° or greater, numbness, pain, or weakness in the extremities, irritability, difficult bowel movements, or trouble urinating.

Explain that the patient should keep his or her head raised following the CT scan to avoid headaches, may experience nausea and vomiting following the CT scan, and in rare situations the patient may experience a seizure following the CT scan. In that situation the patient should seek emergency medical help immediately.

Understanding the Test Results

The result is available within 2 days.

- Normal:
    - Normal size vertebrae, discs, and spinal canal
    - No blockages
    - No inflammation or infection
- Abnormal:
    - Abnormal size vertebrae, discs, and spinal canal
    - Blockages
    - Inflammation or infection
    - Osteoporosis, arthritis
    - Spinal stenosis
    - Growths

Solved Problems

Computed Tomography Scan

15.1 Describe how a CT scan works.

As the patient lies within the scanner, an X-ray beam rotates around the patient, creating an image that represents a thin slice of the patient. Each rotation takes less than a second. All slices are stored on a computer. The computer is used to reassemble slices of the patient, enabling the healthcare provider to identify any abnormalities.

15.2 Are all slices of the patient's CT scan retained in the patient's chart?

Typically, the healthcare provider will print the image of any slices that indicate an abnormality, which are then saved with the patient's chart.

15.3 Why would contrast material be administered during a CT scan?

The contrast material makes structures within the patient's body stand out on the computer by differentiating them in white, black, and shades of gray.

15.4 Why is a CT scan used in the treatment of cancer?

A CT scan may be used for staging cancer to assess if the cancer has spread to other sites in the body. CT scans are also used to identify masses or tumors as well as fluid and the infection process.

15.5 How is contrast material administered?

Contrast material is administered intravenously or into joints or cavities of the body. The patient may also be asked to ingest other kinds of contrast material.

Full Body CT Scan

15.6 Why might a healthcare provider order a full body CT scan?

A healthcare provider orders a full body CT scan if it is suspected that the patient may have disorders throughout the body or if the healthcare provider is unable to narrow the disorder to specific areas of the body, such as if the patient is involved in a severe motor vehicle accident.

15.7 Why would a healthcare provider not order a full body CT scan?

Typically, a healthcare provider orders a CT scan for a specific part of the body rather than ordering a full body scan. A full body CT scan is time consuming and usually provides more information than is necessary for the healthcare provider to diagnose the patient's disorder.

15.8 What is a drawback of a full body CT scan?

Some healthcare providers feel that a full body scan identifies benign growths and other disorders that do not adversely affect the patient and could lead to additional tests and surgery that are unnecessary.

15.9　How is a full body CT scan used to identify cancer?

The result of a CT scan is commonly compared to the results of a positron emission tomography (PET) to identify cancer.

15.10　What would you assess before administering the full body CT scan?

Assess if the patient:
- Has allergies (to shellfish, iodine)
- Is breastfeeding; since contrast material can pass to the baby in breast milk, the patient should be prepared to use formula instead of breast milk for 2 days following the CT scan, if contrast material is administered
- Has heart disorder, asthma, thyroid disorder, kidney disorder, or diabetes
- Takes Glucophage
- Has taken Pepto-Bismol 4 days prior to the CT scan

Determine if the patient:
- Is claustrophobic
- Can lie still during the test

15.11　What should you teach the patient who is undergoing a full body CT scan?

Explain why the CT scan is being administered, what the CT scan test does, and why contrast material may be administered. Explain that the contrast material may leave a metallic taste and that the patient may feel flushed when the contrast material is administered intravenously. Also explain that the healthcare provider may ask the patient to stop taking Glucophage several days before the CT scan, since there might be a reaction with contrast material, and that some patients may be allergic to the contrast material. The patient should know that the healthcare team is ready to take measures to reverse any adverse reaction to the contrast material. Inform the patient that the healthcare provider may ask the patient to stop breast-feeding for 2 days following the CT scan if the contrast material is administered, and that the patient will be asked to drink a large amount of water for 24 hours following the CT scan. Also inform the patient that the healthcare provider may administer a sedative prior to the test if the patient is unable to relax during the test. If a sedative is administered, the patient should arrange for someone else to drive him or her home following the test.

15.12　What might be detected in a full body CT scan?

A full body CT scan might detect abnormal sizes of organs and blood vessels, blockages, bleeding, abnormal fluid collection, growths, or inflammation.

CT Scan of the Head

15.13　What is a perfusion CT?

A perfusion CT is used to determine the blood supply to areas of the brain.

15.14　What is administered to the patient during a perfusion CT?

Contrast material is administered intravenously.

15.15　How does the healthcare provider know which areas of the brain are receiving blood?

Areas of the brain that receive blood are highlighted on the computer image by the contrast material. Areas without blood flow are not highlighted.

15.16　Why might the head CT scan be ordered?

A head CT scan might be ordered to assess for growths, obstructions, inflammation or infection, foreign objects, bleeding, fluid collection, headache, vertigo, vision problems, broken bones, the result of facial surgery, temporomandibular disorder, Paget's disease, stroke, or reasons for a change in the patient's level of consciousness.

15.17　Why is a head CT scan ordered before brain surgery?

A head CT scan provides baseline images before surgery.

15.18   What might be revealed during a head CT scan?

A head CT scan might reveal abnormal sizes of the skull, brain, ventricle, blood vessels, eyes, ears, sinuses, blockages, inflammation, growth, fluid collection, or foreign objects.

CT Scan of the Spine

15.19   What images are created in a CT scan of the spine?

The CT scan of the spine creates images of the cervical spine, thoracic spine, and lumbosacral spine.

15.20   Where is contrast material administered during a CT scan of the spine if ordered by the healthcare provider?

Depending on the purpose of the scan, the healthcare provider may require that contrast material be administered intrathecally into the spinal canal.

15.21   Why is the CT scan of the spine ordered?

A CT scan of the spine is ordered to assess for growths, obstructions, narrowing of the spinal canal, deformities, fractures, inflammation and infection, bone compression, osteoporosis, and congenital defects.

15.22   What is required for a CT myelogram?

A CT myelogram requires that a sample of cerebrospinal fluid be removed for microscopic examination before contrast material is administered.

15.23   How is the CT myelogram performed?

If a CT myelogram is performed, the patient lies on his or her stomach. An area of the lumbar spine is anesthetized and contrast material is injected. The CT table is tilted to help distribute the contrast material throughout the spine.

15.24   What would you ask the patient to do following a CT myelogram?

After a CT myelogram, the patient is asked to keep his or her head raised to prevent seizures and headaches.

15.25   What would you explain to the patient before the spinal CT scan?

Tell the patient to contact his or her healthcare provider if the patient experiences:
- A severe headache or one that lasts more than a day following the CT scan
- A temperature of 101.1°F or greater
- Numbness, pain, or weakness in the extremities
- Irritability
- Difficult bowel movements or trouble urinating

Explain that the patient:
- Should keep his or her head raised following the CT scan to avoid headaches
- May experience nausea and vomiting following the CT scan
- May in rare situations experience a seizure following the CT scan and that in this situation the patient should seek emergency medical help immediately

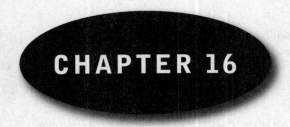

CHAPTER 16

Ultrasound Scan

16.1   Definition

An *ultrasound scan* creates an image of organs and structures inside the body using sound waves. High-frequency sound waves are transmitted by a transducer that is placed on the patient's skin. Sound waves penetrate the skin, bounce off of organs and structures in the patient's body, and are detected by the transducer. Sound waves detected by the transducer are translated into an image that appears on the ultrasound screen. The healthcare provider can then measure organs and structures that appear on the image to determine any abnormality. Images can be printed and included in the patient's chart or the images can be stored on a computer. An ultrasound can detect a growth but cannot differentiate between a malignant or benign growth, which is determined by a biopsy. An ultrasound can differentiate between a solid growth and a fluid-filled cyst. An ultrasound scan is commonly ordered instead of a CT scan or MRI because it is less expensive and in many situations provides the healthcare provider with sufficient information to assist in reaching a diagnosis.

16.2   Benign Prostatic Hyperplasia Ultrasound

The benign prostatic hyperplasia ultrasound is used to assist the healthcare provider diagnose benign prostatic hyperplasia. Middle-aged men might experience the urgency to void, hesitancy waiting for the urinary stream, or a weak urinary stream. These may be signs of an enlarged prostate that places pressure on the bladder and blocks the urinary stream. Noncancerous enlarged prostate is referred to as benign prostatic hyperplasia (BPH) or hypertrophy. The benign prostatic hyperplasia ultrasound is also used to help guide the healthcare provider when taking a biopsy of the prostate, which is commonly performed if the patient's prostate-specific antigen (PSA) level is elevated. The healthcare provider may also evaluate the bladder and the kidneys while performing the benign prostatic hyperplasia ultrasound to determine urinary retention and kidney stones that may block urinary flow. The benign prostatic hyperplasia ultrasound cannot determine if urinary flow is blocked by the prostate.

Why the Test Is Performed

The test assesses the size of the prostate, urinary retention, and a urinary blockage. It also guides the healthcare provider when taking a biopsy of the prostate.

Before Administering the Test

- Assess if the patient can lie still during the test.

How the Test Is Performed

- The ultrasound transducer is either inserted into the rectum (transrectal ultrasound [TRUS]) or placed on the patient's abdomen (transabdominal ultrasound).

- An image of the prostate, kidneys, and bladder appears on the screen.
- The healthcare provider estimates the size of the prostate and determines if there is any urinary retention or blockage.

Teach the Patient

Explain why the ultrasound is being taken, that clear gel will be placed on the ultrasound site to increase the conduction of sound, that the patient will not feel any pain, and that the patient must lie still during the test.

Understanding the Test Results

The test takes 30 minutes and the results are ready immediately if the test is performed by the healthcare provider or within a few hours if a technician performs the test.

- Normal:
  - Prostate is an acceptable size
  - Kidneys show no obstruction
  - No urine or an acceptable volume of urine in the bladder
- Abnormal:
  - Enlarged prostate
  - Enlarged kidneys
  - Kidney obstruction
  - Enlarged bladder
  - Significant volume of urine in the bladder

16.3 Transvaginal Ultrasound and Hysterosonogram

The transvaginal ultrasound or the hysterosonogram enables the healthcare provider to assess ovarian follicle development and the endometrium. When a woman has difficulty conceiving, the healthcare provider may perform a transvaginal ultrasound or a hysterosonogram. A hysterosonogram is also known as a sonohysterogram. This assessment may help the healthcare provider determine when to perform intrauterine insemination. The transvaginal ultrasound is the preferred method, rather than the transabdominal ultrasound, for assessing the uterine lining and follicle growth. The transvaginal ultrasound may not display scars or small tumors.

Why the Test Is Performed

The test assesses the uterus, fallopian tubes, ovaries, the endometrial cavity, uterine lining, and ovarian follicle development. The test is also used to schedule intrauterine insemination and to guide the healthcare provider when removing follicles.

Before Administering the Test

Assess if the patient can lie still during the test and has an empty bladder prior to the test.

How the Test Is Performed

- The patient may be required to have an empty bladder prior to the scan, or a full bladder depending on what is being examined.
- The ultrasound transducer is inserted into the vagina.
- The healthcare provider performs the ultrasound scan from within the vagina.
- With a hysterosonogram, the uterus is filled with fluid prior to insertion of the transducer into the vagina.

Teach the Patient

Explain why the ultrasound is being taken, that the patient must have an empty bladder before the scan, that the patient will not feel any pain, that the patient must lie still during the test, that the transducer is inserted into the vagina, and that the uterus will be filled with fluid if the healthcare provider orders a hysterosonogram.

Understanding the Test Results

The test takes 30 minutes and the results are ready immediately if the test is performed by the healthcare provider or within a few hours if a technician performs the test.

- Normal:
  - No growths
  - No scar tissue
  - The uterus is a normal shape
  - The fallopian tubes are not blocked
  - Ovaries are a normal size
  - The endometrial cavity is a normal shape
  - Uterine lining is a normal size
- Abnormal:
  - Few follicles
  - Uterine fibroids
  - Ovarian cysts
  - Hydrosalpinx (an old infection that causes the fallopian tubes to fill with fluid and enlarge or dilate)
  - Thick uterine lining
  - Deformed uterine lining
  - Enlarged uterus
  - Abnormal fallopian tubes

16.4 Testicular Ultrasound

The testicular ultrasound displays an image of the patient's testicles and scrotum. Also displayed is the *epididymis*, which is the coiled tube behind the testicle that collects sperm. The testicular ultrasound also displays an image of the *vas deferens*, which is the tube that connects the prostate gland to the testicles. A healthcare provider may order a testicular ultrasound if the patient shows signs and symptoms of testicular abnormalities or infertility.

Why the Test Is Performed

The test assesses the testicles, epididymis, vas deferens, scrotum, spermatic cord, and for hydrocele and spermatocele. The test also guides the healthcare provider when performing a testicular biopsy.

Before Administering the Test

- Assess if the patient:
  - Can lie still during the test
  - Has open skin in the scrotum
- A consent form must be signed if the patient is undergoing a testicular biopsy.
- The patient must remove all clothes from the waist down.
- Towels are used to lift the scrotum.
- Wipe the conductive gel from the patient's skin when the test is completed.

How the Test Is Performed

- A conductive gel is placed on the transducer or on the scrotum.

- The transducer is placed on the scrotum and moved around to capture the image.
- The patient may be asked to hold his breath for a few seconds while the image is being taken.

Teach the Patient

Explain why the ultrasound is being taken, that the patient will not feel any pain, that the patient must lie still during the test, that the patient will have to remove all clothes from the waist down, and that towels are used to lift the scrotum. Inform the patient that conductive gel is placed on the scrotum and that it will be wiped off after the test is completed, that the transducer is placed on and moved around the scrotum, and that a consent form must be signed if the patient is undergoing a testicular biopsy.

Understanding the Test Results

The test takes 30 minutes and the results are ready immediately if the test is performed by the healthcare provider or within a few hours if a technician performs the test.

- Normal:
  - No growths
  - The testicles are a normal shape
  - The epididymis does not show inflammation or blockage
  - The spermatic cord is not twisted
  - There is not fluid in the scrotum
- Abnormal:
  - There is a growth on one or both testicles
  - There is inflammation, infection, or blockage in the epididymis
  - The spermatic cord is twisted
  - There is fluid in the scrotum

16.5   Abdominal Ultrasound

An abdominal ultrasound is ordered to view upper abdominal organs and structures. Viewed are the liver, gallbladder, spleen, pancreas, and kidneys. It is also ordered to help the healthcare provider assess the abdominal aorta. The *abdominal aorta* is the artery located in the back of the chest and abdomen that supplies blood to the legs, abdomen, and organs in the lower portion of the body. The healthcare provider may order an ultrasound of specific organs or structures within the abdomen if the abdominal ultrasound shows an abnormal condition in the abdomen.

Why the Test Is Performed

The test assesses the liver, gallbladder, bile ducts, spleen, pancreas, kidneys, and abdominal aorta. The test also guides the healthcare provider when taking a biopsy or when performing a paracentesis.

Before Administering the Test

- Assess if the patient:
  - Can lie still during the test
  - Has ingested barium for an upper GI test two days prior to the ultrasound scan
  - Has had a barium enema for a lower GI test two days prior to the ultrasound scan
  - Has removed jewelry from the abdominal area
  - Has eaten a fat free dinner up to 12 hours before the test
  - Has not eaten 12 hours before the ultrasound scan
  - Has drunk six glasses of water one hour before the ultrasound scan
  - Has an open wound in the abdominal area
  - Is obese

- A consent form must be signed if the patient is undergoing a biopsy
- The patient must remove all clothes from the waist down
- Wipe the conductive gel from the patient's skin when the test is completed

How the Test Is Performed

- The patient removes jewelry from the abdominal area.
- The patient should eat a fat free dinner the night before the test.
- The patient should avoid eating 12 hours before the test to prevent gas from building up in the intestines.
- The patient may be asked to drink six glasses of water one hour before the test.
- The patient removes all clothes from the waist down.
- A conductive gel is placed on the abdomen.
- The transducer is placed on the abdomen and moved around to capture the image.
- The healthcare provider may push on the abdomen to move organs within the abdominal cavity to get a clearer view of other organs.
- The patient may be asked to change position during the test.
- The patient may be asked to hold his or her breath for a few seconds.

Teach the Patient

Explain why the ultrasound is being taken, that the patient will not feel any pain, that the patient must lie still during the test, and that the patient will have to remove all clothes from the waist down. The patient will need to remove jewelry from the abdominal area, eat a fat free dinner the night before the test, and avoid eating 12 hours before the test. The patient may be asked to drink six glasses of water one hour before the test. The healthcare provider may push on the abdomen to move organs within the abdominal cavity to get a clearer view of other organs. Inform the patient that he or she may be asked to change position during the test and/or may be asked to hold his or her breath for a few seconds. Conductive gel is placed on the abdomen and it will be wiped off after the test is completed. The transducer is placed on and moved around the abdomen. A consent form must be signed if the patient is undergoing a biopsy.

Understanding the Test Results

The test takes 60 minutes and the results are ready immediately if the test is performed by the healthcare provider or within a few hours if a technician performs the test.

- Normal:
  - No growths
  - All organs are normal shape
  - No inflammation or blockage of the bile ducts
- Abnormal:
  - There is a growth on one or multiple organs
  - There is inflammation, infection, or blockage of the bile ducts
  - The aorta is enlarged
  - Fluid appears in the abdomen

16.6   Breast Ultrasound

The breast ultrasound creates an image of all areas of the breast, including portions of the breast that are near the chest. A breast ultrasound is sometimes performed on younger women whose breast tissues are dense, preventing details of the breast to be assessed on a mammogram. A mammogram typically does not show images of the breast that are near the chest. A healthcare provider frequently orders a breast ultrasound to assess a lump identified by either palpation or from a mammogram. The breast ultrasound can distinguish between a solid mass and a cyst. If it is a solid mass, then the healthcare provider performs a biopsy to determine if the mass is benign or malignant. A breast ultrasound does not replace an annual mammogram.

Why the Test Is Performed

The test assesses a mass found through palpation or by a mammogram, the breast of a younger woman whose breasts are dense, silicone breast implants, and breast pain. The test also guides the healthcare provider when taking a biopsy or when draining a cyst.

Before Administering the Test

- Assess if the patient:
  - Can lie still during the test
  - Has removed jewelry from the breast area
  - Has an open wound in the breast area
- A consent form must be signed if the patient is undergoing a biopsy or a cyst drainage
- The patient must remove all clothes above the waist
- Wipe the conductive gel from the patient's skin when the test is completed

How the Test Is Performed

- The patient removes jewelry from the breast area.
- The patient removes all clothes above the waist.
- A conductive gel is placed on the transducer on the breast.
- The transducer is placed on the breast and moved around to capture the image.

Teach the Patient

Explain why the ultrasound is being performed, that the patient will not feel any pain, that the patient must lie still during the test, and that the patient will have to remove all clothes from the waist up. The patient will need to remove jewelry from the breast area, conductive gel from the transducer may remain on the breast and will be wiped off after the test is completed. Explain that the transducer is placed on and moved around the breast, and a consent form must be signed if the patient is undergoing a biopsy or drainage of a cyst.

Understanding the Test Results

The test takes 30 minutes and the results are ready immediately if the test is performed by the healthcare provider or within a few hours if a technician performs the test.

- Normal:
  - No mass found
  - Normal shaped breasts
  - No inflammation
- Abnormal:
  - There is a cyst
  - There is a solid mass
  - There is inflammation or infection

16.7   Cranial Ultrasound

A cranial ultrasound creates images of the brain and ventricles. An ultrasound cannot penetrate bone. A cranial ultrasound is performed on babies up to 18 months old whose cranium has yet to form. A cranial ultrasound is commonly used in premature newborns to assess complications of premature birth. A cranial ultrasound is also performed on adults during brain surgery to visualize any masses in the brain. The ultrasound is able to capture the image because a portion of the patient's cranium is removed during surgery, enabling the ultrasound to penetrate brain tissue.

Why the Test Is Performed

The test assesses: (for babies) why the baby has an abnormally large head, for encephalitis, meningitis, hydrocephalus, periventricular leukomalacia (PVL), intraventricular hemorrhage (IVH), and (for adults) brain mass.

Before Administering the Test

Assess if the:

- Baby can lie still during the test
- Parent can hold the baby still during the test
- Baby's cranium has closed

How the Test Is Performed

- For babies:
  - Feed the baby near the time of the ultrasound scan so that the baby is still and comfortable during the scan.
  - Place the baby on his or her back or have the parent hold the baby.
  - The transducer is placed on and moved around the fontanels.
- For adults:
  - A portion of the cranium is removed in surgery.
  - The transducer is placed on and moved around the exposed brain.

Teach the Patient

Explain why the ultrasound is being performed, that the patient will not feel any pain, and that the patient must lie still during the test and that the parent can hold the baby during the test. Conductive gel is placed on the fontanels and it will be wiped off after the test is completed. The transducer is placed on and moved around the fontanels. Explain to adults that the test will be conducted during surgery.

Understanding the Test Results

The test takes 30 minutes and the results are ready immediately.

- Normal:
  - No mass or cyst found
  - Normal shaped brain
  - No inflammation
  - No bleeding
  - There is no excessive cerebrospinal fluid (CSF)
- Abnormal:
  - There is a mass or cyst
  - There is inflammation or infection
  - There is bleeding
  - There is excessive cerebrospinal fluid (CSF)

16.8   Doppler Ultrasound

A Doppler ultrasound is used to assess blood flow through blood vessels. There are four types of Doppler ultrasounds:

1. **Continuous Wave Doppler**: It produces a pulsating audible sound reflecting pulsating blood through a blood vessel.
2. **Duplex Doppler**: It produces an image of the blood vessel, along with a computer generated graph that indicates the speed and direction of blood flow.

3. **Color Doppler**: It produces an image of the blood vessel with the speed and direction of the blood flow represented by colors on the image.
4. **Power Doppler**: It is similar to the color Doppler. However, the power Doppler is five times as sensitive in detecting blood flow.

Why the Test Is Performed

The test assesses for narrow blood vessels, blood clots (deep vein thrombosis), atherosclerosis, and stroke. The test also maps veins for use as grafts.

Before Administering the Test

Assess if the patient:

- Can lie still during the test
- Has smoked cigarettes, chewed tobacco, or otherwise ingested nicotine two hours before the test. Nicotine constricts blood vessels resulting in a false test result.
- Can perform the Valsalva's maneuver
- Is obese, since this can interfere with the test
- Has arrhythmias which may alter blood flow through unobstructed blood vessels

How the Test Is Performed

- The patient removes all jewelry around the site of the blood vessel.
- The patient will remove all clothes around the blood vessel.
- A conductive gel is placed on the skin that covers the blood vessel.
- The transducer is placed over and moved around the blood vessel.
- If the extremities are being tested, the healthcare provider may test both extremities to compare the results.
- Furthermore, the test may be performed with the patient lying and sitting.
- The healthcare provider may also place a blood pressure cuff on the extremities during the test.
- The patient may be asked to perform the Valsalva's maneuver by pinching his nose, closing his mouth, and then exhaling.
- If arteries in the neck are being tested, the patient will place his head on a pillow.

Teach the Patient

Explain why the ultrasound is being performed, that the patient will not feel any pain, and that the patient must lie still during the test. Explain that conductive gel is placed on the skin over the blood vessel and will be wiped off after the test is completed. The transducer is placed on and moved around the skin over the blood vessel. Inform the patient that he or she should avoid smoking, chewing tobacco, or otherwise ingesting nicotine 2 hours before the test. Also inform the patient that the healthcare provider may ask the patient to perform the Valsalva's maneuver, and arrhythmias may provide a false test result.

Understanding the Test Results

The test takes 60 minutes and the results are ready immediately.

- Normal:
  - No blood clots
  - Normal blood flow and pulse
- Abnormal:
  - Blockage in blood flow
  - Abnormal pulse
  - Abnormal shape of blood vessels

16.9   Fetal Ultrasound

A fetal ultrasound produces an image (sonogram) of the fetus, the placenta, and amniotic fluid during pregnancy. The healthcare provider orders a fetal ultrasound to determine the size, position, and sex of the fetus and to identify any abnormalities prior to birth. There are two types of fetal ultrasound tests:

1. **Transabdominal ultrasound**: The ultrasound transducer is placed on the patient's abdomen.
2. **Transvaginal ultrasound**: The ultrasound transducer is covered in a latex sheath and inserted into the vagina.

Verify that the patient is not allergic to latex if the healthcare provider is performing a transvaginal ultrasound. A normal fetal ultrasound does not rule out fetal abnormalities or problems with the placenta and amniotic fluid.

Why the Test Is Performed

The test assesses the progress of the pregnancy, gestational age of the fetus, fetal defects, number of fetuses, placenta, amniotic fluid, fetal position, and cervix. The test also detects ectopic pregnancy.

Before Administering the Test

Assess if the patient:

- Can lie still during the test
- Has a full bladder if a transabdominal ultrasound is being performed
- Is allergic to latex if a transvaginal ultrasound is being performed
- Is obese

How the Test Is Performed

- Transabdominal ultrasound:
  - The patient removes all jewelry from around the abdomen.
  - The patient will remove all clothes around the abdomen.
  - In early pregnancy, the patient needs a full bladder and must drink a large volume of water and avoid urinating until the test is completed.
    - The water moves the intestines away from the uterus.
    - If the patient is unable to fill her bladder, the healthcare provider may order the insertion of a urinary catheter through her urethra and fill the bladder with sterile water.
  - In late pregnancy, the patient does not need a full bladder since the intestines are repositioned by fetal growth.
  - The patient lies on her back.
  - A conductive gel is placed on the abdomen.
  - The transducer is placed over and moved around the abdomen.
  - If the patient becomes short of breath, the healthcare provider may raise the head of the bed or place the patient on her side.
- Transvaginal ultrasound:
  - The patient does not need a full bladder for this test.
  - The patient lies on her back with hips raised.
  - Verify before the test that the patient is not allergic to latex.
  - The healthcare provider places a transducer covered with a latex sheath into the vagina to capture the image.

Teach the Patient

Explain why the ultrasound is being taken, that the patient will not feel any pain, that the patient must lie still during the test, and that the patient will require a full bladder. If the patient is unable to drink a sufficient volume of water, a urinary catheter will be inserted and sterile water will be placed into her bladder (transabdominal). The patient will not urinate until after the test is concluded (transabdominal). Inform the patient that conductive gel is placed on the skin over the abdomen and that it will be wiped off after the test is completed (transabdominal), that the transducer is placed on and moved around the abdomen (transabdominal), and that the ultrasound transducer may be covered in a latex sheath and inserted into her vagina (transvaginal). If she feels short of breath during the test, the head of the bed will be raised or she will be repositioned on her side (transvaginal). A normal fetal ultrasound does not rule out abnormalities with the fetus, placenta, or amniotic fluid.

Understanding the Test Results

The test takes 60 minutes or less and the results are ready immediately.

- Normal:
  - Expected fetal gestation
  - Normal placenta
  - Expected volume of amniotic fluid
  - No birth defects
- Abnormal:
  - Underdeveloped or abnormally developed fetus
  - Unexpected fetal position
  - Placenta previa
  - Molar pregnancy
  - Suspected birth defect noticed
  - Unexpected volume of amniotic fluid

16.10   Pelvic Ultrasound

A pelvic ultrasound creates images of the bladder, ovaries, uterus, cervix, fallopian tubes, prostate gland, and seminal vesicles. There are three types of pelvic ultrasound tests:

1. **Transabdominal ultrasound**: the transducer is moved along the abdomen.
2. **Transrectal ultrasound**: the transducer is inserted into the rectum.
3. **Transvaginal ultrasound**: the transducer is covered with a latex sheath and inserted in the vagina.

Verify that the patient is not allergic to latex before a transrectal or transvaginal ultrasound is performed.

Why the Test Is Performed

The test assesses the cause of urinary disorders, the bladder, assesses for growths, pelvic inflammatory disease (PID), placement of intrauterine device (IUD), the size of pelvic organs and structures, the fetal position, and for the cause of infertility. The test also guides the healthcare provider when performing a biopsy.

Before Administering the Test

Assess if the patient:

- Has ingested contrast material 2 days before the ultrasound
- Can lie still during the test
- Has a full bladder (transabdominal)
- Is allergic to latex (transrectal or transvaginal)
- Has removed jewelry and clothes from below the waist
- Signed a consent form, if the ultrasound is used for a biopsy
- Has been given an enema an hour before the test (transrectal)
- Can lie on his or her left side and bend his or her knees (transrectal)
- Has not drunk fluids four hours before the test (transvaginal)
- Is obese

How the Test Is Performed

- Transabdominal ultrasound:
  - The patient removes all jewelry from below the waist.
  - The patient will remove all clothes from below the waist.
  - The patient will be required to fill his or her bladder to push the intestines away from the pelvic organs. If the patient is unable to drink water, the healthcare provider will insert a catheter into the patient's bladder and infuse sterile water.
  - The patient will be required to sign a consent form if the ultrasound is used to guide the healthcare provider in taking a biopsy.
  - The patient lies on his or her back.
  - A conductive gel is placed on the abdomen.
  - The transducer is placed over and moved around the abdomen.
- Transrectal ultrasound:
  - The patient is given an enema an hour before the test.
  - Verify that the patient is not allergic to latex.
  - A latex sheath is placed over the ultrasound transducer.
  - The patient lies on his or her left side with knees bent.
  - The ultrasound transducer is lubricated and then inserted into the patient's rectum to capture the image.
- Transvaginal ultrasound:
  - The patient avoids drinking fluids four hours before the test.
  - The patient lies on her back with hips raised.
  - Verify before the test that the patient is not allergic to latex.
  - The healthcare provider places a transducer covered with a latex sheath into the vagina to capture the image.

Teach the Patient

Explain why the ultrasound is being performed, that the patient will not feel any pain, that the patient must lie still during the test, that the patient cannot ingest contrast material 2 days before the test, and that the patient will require a full bladder. If the patient is unable to drink a sufficient volume of water, a urinary catheter will be inserted and sterile water will be placed into his or her bladder (transabdominal). The patient will be given an enema an hour before the test (transrectal) and will not urinate until after the test is concluded (transabdominal). The patient must avoid drinking 4 hours before the test (transvaginal).

Inform the patient that conductive gel is placed on the skin over the abdomen and that it will be wiped off after the test is completed (transabdominal). The transducer is placed on and moved around the abdomen (transabdominal) and the ultrasound transducer may be covered in a latex sheath and inserted into the rectum or vagina (transrectal or transvaginal). If she feels short of breath during the test, the head of the bed will be raised or she will be repositioned on her side if the transvaginal procured is used.

Understanding the Test Results

The test takes 30 minutes or less and the results are ready immediately.

- Normal:
  - Pelvic organs are normal size
  - No growth
  - No blockages
  - Intrauterine device is in the expected position
- Abnormal:
  - Unexpected size of one or more pelvic organs
  - Growths are seen

- Inflammation and infection noticed
- Unexpected fluid
- Blockage found
- Intrauterine device is not in the expected position

Solved Problems

Ultrasound Scan

16.1 How does an ultrasound scan work?

High-frequency sound waves are transmitted by a transducer that is placed on the patient's skin. Sound waves penetrate the skin, bounce off of organs and structures in the patient's body, and are detected by the transducer. Sound waves detected by the transducer are translated into an image that appears on the ultrasound screen.

16.2 Can an ultrasound scan identify a malignant growth?

An ultrasound can detect a growth but cannot differentiate between a malignant or benign growth, which is determined by a biopsy.

16.3 Can an ultrasound scan identify a cyst?

An ultrasound can differentiate between a solid growth and a fluid-filled cyst.

Benign Prostatic Hyperplasia Ultrasound

16.4 What is a benign prostatic hyperplasia?

Middle-aged men might experience the urgency to void, hesitancy waiting for the urinary stream, or a weak urinary stream. These may be signs of an enlarged prostate that places pressure on the bladder and blocks the urinary stream. Noncancerous enlarged prostate is referred to as benign prostatic hyperplasia (BPH) or hypertrophy.

16.5 When might the benign prostatic hyperplasia ultrasound be ordered by the healthcare provider?

The benign prostatic hyperplasia ultrasound is used to help guide the healthcare provider when taking a biopsy of the prostate, which is commonly performed if the patient's prostate-specific antigen (PSA) level is elevated.

16.6 What else can be assessed when performing a benign prostatic hyperplasia ultrasound?

The healthcare provider may also evaluate the bladder and kidneys while performing the benign prostatic hyperplasia ultrasound to determine urinary retention and kidney stones that may block urinary flow.

16.7 What should you teach the patient about the benign prostatic hyperplasia ultrasound scan?

Explain why the ultrasound is being taken, that clear gel will be placed on the ultrasound site to increase the conduction of sound, that the patient will not feel any pain, and that the patient must lie still during the test.

Transvaginal Ultrasound and Hysterosonogram

16.8 Why might the healthcare provider order the transvaginal ultrasound and hysterosonogram?

When a woman has difficulty conceiving, the healthcare provider may perform a transvaginal ultrasound or a hysterosonogram.

16.9 What is a drawback of the transvaginal ultrasound?

The transvaginal ultrasound may not display scars or small tumors.

16.10 What can the healthcare provider assess with a transvaginal ultrasound or a hysterosonogram?

The healthcare provider can assess the uterus, fallopian tubes, ovaries, endometrial cavity, uterine lining, and ovarian follicle development with a transvaginal ultrasound or a hysterosonogram. These tests can also help the healthcare provider to schedule intrauterine insemination and guide the healthcare provider when removing follicles.

16.11 What should you assess before the patient is administered the transvaginal ultrasound or a hysterosonogram?

Assess if the patient:
- Can lie still during the test
- Has an empty bladder prior to the test

16.12 How is the transvaginal ultrasound or a hysterosonogram performed?

The patient may be required to have an empty bladder prior to the scan or a full bladder, depending on what is being examined. The ultrasound transducer is inserted into the vagina. The healthcare provider performs the ultrasound scan from within the vagina. With a hysterosonogram, the uterus is filled with fluid prior to insertion of the transducer into the vagina.

16.13 What should you teach the patient about the transvaginal ultrasound or a hysterosonogram?

Explain why the ultrasound is being taken, that the patient must have an empty bladder before the scan, that the patient will not feel any pain, that the patient must lie still during the test, that the transducer is inserted into the vagina, and that the uterus will be filled with fluid if the healthcare provider orders a hysterosonogram.

16.14 What might be revealed by the transvaginal ultrasound or a hysterosonogram?

The transvaginal ultrasound or a hysterosonogram can reveal few follicles, uterine fibroids, ovarian cysts, hydrosalpinz, thick uterine lining, deformed uterine lining, enlarged uterus, or abnormal fallopian tubes.

Testicular Ultrasound

16.15 What is displayed by a testicular ultrasound?

The testicular ultrasound displays an image of the patient's testicles and scrotum. Also displayed is the epididymis, which is the coiled tube behind the testicle that collects sperm. The testicular ultrasound also displays an image of the vas deferens, which is the tube that connects the prostate gland to the testicles.

16.16 What must you assess before the testicular ultrasound is administered?

- Assess if the patient:
  - Can lie still during the test
  - Has open skin in the scrotum
- A consent form must be signed if the patient is undergoing a testicular biopsy.
- The patient must remove all clothes from the waist down.
- Towels are used to lift the scrotum.
- Wipe the conductive gel from the patient's skin when the test is completed.

16.17 How is the testicular ultrasound performed?

- A conductive gel is placed on the transducer or on the scrotum.
- The transducer is placed on the scrotum and moved around to capture the image.
- The patient may be asked to hold his breath for a few seconds while the image is being taken.

Abdominal Ultrasound

16.18 What is viewed by an abdominal ultrasound?

An abdominal ultrasound is ordered to view upper abdominal organs and structures. Viewed are the liver, gallbladder, spleen, pancreas, and kidneys. It is also ordered to assist the healthcare provider assess the abdominal aorta.

16.19   Why is the abdominal ultrasound ordered by the healthcare provider?

The abdominal ultrasound assesses the liver, gallbladder, bile ducts, spleen, pancreas, kidneys, and abdominal aorta. The test also guides the healthcare provider when taking a biopsy or when performing a paracentesis.

16.20   What should you assess before the abdominal ultrasound is performed?

Assess if the patient:
- Can lie still during the test
- Has ingested barium for an upper GI test two days prior to the ultrasound scan
- Has had a barium enema for a lower GI test two days prior to the ultrasound scan
- Has removed jewelry from the abdominal area
- Has eaten a fat free dinner the night before the test
- Has not eaten 12 hours before the ultrasound scan
- Has drunk six glasses of water an hour before the ultrasound scan
- Has an open wound in the abdominal area
- Is obese

A consent form must be signed if the patient is undergoing a biopsy. The patient must remove all clothes from the waist down. Wipe the conductive gel from the patient's skin when the test is completed.

16.21   What might be an abnormal result of the abdominal ultrasound?

An abnormal result of an abdominal ultrasound might be a growth on one or multiple organs, inflammation, infection or blockage of the bile ducts, enlarged aorta, or fluid appearing in the abdomen.

Breast Ultrasound

16.22   Why might a breast ultrasound be performed on younger women?

A breast ultrasound is sometimes performed on younger women whose breast tissues are dense, preventing details of the breast to show on a mammogram.

16.23   Why would a breast ultrasound be ordered following a mammogram?

A healthcare provider frequently orders a breast ultrasound to assess a lump identified by either palpation or from a mammogram. The breast ultrasound can distinguish between a solid mass and a cyst. If it is a solid mass, then the healthcare provider performs a biopsy to determine if the mass is benign or malignant.

16.24   What should you teach a patient who is to undergo a breast ultrasound?

Explain why the ultrasound is being taken, that the patient will not feel any pain, that the patient must lie still during the test, that the patient will have to remove all clothes from the waist up, that the patient will need to remove jewelry from the breast area, that conductive gel is placed on the breast and that it will be wiped off after the test is completed, that the transducer is placed on and moved around the breast, and that a consent form must be signed if the patient is undergoing a biopsy or drainage of a cyst.

16.25   Is a breast ultrasound an alternative to a mammogram?

A breast ultrasound does not replace an annual mammogram.

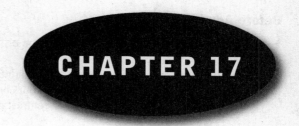

CHAPTER 17

Magnetic Resonance Imaging (MRI) Tests

17.1 Definition

Magnetic resonance imaging (MRI) uses pulsating radio waves in a magnetic field to produce an image of the inside of the patient's body. The patient lies on his or her back on a table. A coil is placed around the area of the patient that is being scanned and a belt is placed around the patient to detect breathing. The table moves into the magnetic field and the belt triggers the MRI scan so that breathing does not interfere with capturing the image. A snapping noise is produced while the MRI scans the patient. The patient may listen to music through headphones to block out the snapping noise.

There are two types of MRI machines: closed MRI and open MRI. In the closed MRI, the patient's body is entirely enclosed in the machine, while in the open MRI only a portion of the patient's body is enclosed in the machine. The healthcare provider may order that contrast material be administered to the patient prior to the MRI. The contrast material may be ingested or administered intravenously and highlights areas of the body that are being studied. The MRI produces digital images that are displayed on a computer screen and can be stored for further review by the patient's healthcare team. The MRI creates images that are more detailed than images produced by a CT scan, X-ray, or ultrasound.

No metal objects can be on or inside the patient during an MRI, including credit cards. Information on the credit card might be erased by the MRI magnetic field. An X-ray may be ordered to determine if there is any metal inside the patient before the MRI is administered, especially if the patient was in an accident where metal fragments might be embedded throughout the body. Dental fillings are usually permitted, although the patient is likely to feel tingling in his or her mouth during the MRI. The patient may experience skin irritation if the patient has iron pigment tattoos.

17.2 Abdominal MRI

An abdominal MRI produces detailed images of organs, structures, and tissues contained within the abdomen. The healthcare provider may order that the patient be administered contrast material prior to the MRI to highlight parts of the abdomen on the MRI image. Contrast material enables the healthcare provider to identify any subtle abnormalities that may exist in the abdomen.

Why the Test Is Performed

The test assesses the size of abdominal organs and structures, existence of a growth, blockages, existence of fluid within the abdomen, inflammation, and blood flow.

Before Administering the Test

- Determine if the patient has any metal on or inside his or her body.
- Assess if the patient:
  - Has eaten or drunk before the MRI is administered. Some MRI studies require that the patient refrain from eating or drinking 12 hours before the test is administered.
  - Is allergic to shellfish, iodine, or contrast material
  - Is pregnant
  - Is claustrophobic
  - Has kidney disease
  - Is wearing any medicine patches
  - Can lie still during the test

How the Test Is Performed

- The patient is assessed for any metal that might be on or inside his or her body.
- The healthcare provider determines if the presence of any metal may require cancellation of the MRI.
- An assessment is made to determine if the patient can be administered contrast material over a two-minute period, if required for the MRI.
- Contrast material is either ingested or administered via IV, causing a flushing feeling in the patient.
- Contrast material may or may not be used if the patient is allergic to shellfish and iodine or if the patient has kidney abnormalities or sickle cell anemia, depending on the type of contrast material that the healthcare provider plans to use for the test.
- An assessment is made to determine if the patient is claustrophobic. If so, then the healthcare provider may administer a sedative to the patient or schedule the test be performed using an open MRI.
- The patient removes all clothes and wears a gown during the MRI.
- The patient may be given headphones to reduce the sound of the tapping noise created by the MRI.
- The patient may be administered glucagon to reduce intestinal movement during the test.
- The patient lies on his or her back on the MRI table.
- A coil is placed on the patient's abdomen.
- A belt is placed on the patient to detect the patient's breathing patterns.
- The table is moved into the MRI machine as images are taken of the abdomen.
- Images are viewed during and after the MRI is completed to assist the healthcare provider reach a diagnosis.

Teach the Patient

Explain why the MRI is being performed, what the patient will experience during the MRI, that no metal can be on or inside the patient during the MRI, and that the patient will not feel any pain during the procedure, although the patient may feel a tingling sensation if he or she has metal fillings in his or her teeth. The patient may be administered a sedative if he or she is claustrophobic, and some patients who are allergic to shellfish and iodine may also be allergic to contrast material. If the patient is allergic to contrast material, the healthcare provider will discuss the risk and benefits of administering the contrast material with the patient. If the patient agrees that the benefits outweigh the risk, then the healthcare provider may administer medication that counteracts the allergic reaction of the contrast material. The patient may be asked to drink contrast material or the contrast material may be administered via IV, causing a flushing feeling. The patient may be asked to refrain from eating or drinking 12 hours before the MRI.

Understanding the Test Results

The test takes 60 minutes and the results are ready immediately if the test is performed by the healthcare provider or within a few hours if a technician performs the test.

- Normal:
  - Normal size of abdominal organs and structures
  - No growths

- ○ No blockage
- ○ No fluid within the abdomen
- ○ No inflammation
- ○ Normal blood flow
- Abnormal:
  - ○ Unusual size of abdominal organs and structures
  - ○ The existence of a growth
  - ○ A blockage is identified
  - ○ Fluid exists within the abdomen
  - ○ Inflammation or infection is present
  - ○ Unusual blood flow

17.3   Breast MRI

A breast MRI produces detailed images of the breast that provide more information to the healthcare provider than a breast ultrasound or traditional mammography. Healthcare providers typically order a breast MRI when other tests such as a mammography indicate an abnormality. If the abnormality is inflammation, a growth, or blood flow to breast tissues, the healthcare provider may administer contrast material to enhance the image of those areas of the breast. Women who are positive for the BRCA1 or BRCA2 gene or whose family members developed breast cancer before the age of 50 are considered high risk for developing breast cancer and may be recommended to receive an annual breast MRI to detect early signs of breast cancer. The healthcare provider may also order an annual breast MRI for women who normally have dense breast tissue. MRI is better suited to examine dense breast tissue than an ultrasound test.

Why the Test Is Performed

The test assesses for infection, the existence of a growth, inflammation, blood flow, women who are at a high risk for breast cancer, women who normally have dense breast tissue, breast cancer treatment, and breast implants.

Before Administering the Test

- Determine if the patient has any metal on or inside his or her body
- Assess if the patient:
  - ○ Is allergic to shellfish, iodine, or contrast material
  - ○ Is pregnant
  - ○ Is claustrophobic
  - ○ Has kidney disease
  - ○ Is wearing any medicine patches
  - ○ Can lie still during the test

How the Test Is Performed

- The patient is assessed for any metal that might be on or inside his or her body.
- The healthcare provider determines if the presence of any metal may require cancellation of the MRI.
- An assessment is made to determine if the patient can be administered contrast material over a two minute period, if required for the MRI.
- Contrast material is either ingested or administered via IV, causing a flushing feeling in the patient.
- Contrast material may not be used if the patient is allergic to shellfish and iodine or if the patient has kidney abnormalities or sickle cell anemia.
- An assessment is made to determine if the patient is claustrophobic.
- If so, then the healthcare provider may administer a sedative to the patient or schedule the test to be performed using an open MRI.
- The patient removes all clothes and wears a gown during the MRI.
- The patient may be given headphones to reduce the sound of the tapping noise created by the MRI.

- The patient lies on his or her back on the MRI table.
- A coil is placed on the patient's chest area.
- A belt is placed on the patient to detect the patient's breathing patterns.
- The table is moved into the MRI machine as images are taken of the breasts.
- Images are viewed during and after the MRI is completed to assist the healthcare provider reach a diagnosis.

Teach the Patient

Explain why the MRI is being performed, what the patient will experience during the MRI, that no metal can be on or inside the patient during the MRI, and that the patient will not feel any pain during the procedure, although the patient may feel a tingling sensation if she has metal fillings in her teeth. The patient may be administered a sedative if she is claustrophobic. Some patients who are allergic to shellfish and iodine may also be allergic to contrast material. If the patient is allergic to contrast material, the healthcare provider will discuss the risk and benefits of administering the contrast material with the patient. If the patient agrees that the benefits outweigh the risk, then the healthcare provider may administer medication that counteracts the allergic reaction of the contrast material. The contrast material may be administered via IV, causing a flushing feeling.

Understanding the Test Results

The test takes 60 minutes and the results are ready immediately if the test is performed by the healthcare provider or within a few hours if a technician performs the test.

- Normal:
  - No growths
  - No blockage
  - No infection
  - No inflammation
  - Normal blood flow
  - Breast implant correctly positioned
- Abnormal:
  - The existence of a growth
  - Breast implants improperly positioned
  - Inflammation or infection is present
  - Unusual blood flow or blockage

17.4   Head MRI

An MRI of the head is ordered to produce images of the brain and blood vessels that supply the brain. It is ordered to determine the underlying cause of headache, assess for head injury, or determine if the patient has abnormal blood flow or a disorder that affects the brain. Unlike an ultrasound, the head MRI is a closed procedure and does not require that the patient's skull be opened. There are three types of MRI used to assess the brain:

1. **Magnetic Resonance Spectroscopy**: Assesses changes in brain chemistry caused by disease.
2. **Magnetic Resonance Angiogram (MRA)**: Assesses speed, direction, and flow of blood in the brain.
3. **Diffusion-perfusion Imaging**: Assesses inflammation, tumors, and stroke by evaluating the fluid content of the brain.

Healthcare providers may order an MRI with gadolinium containing contrast material. Gadolinium can cause nephrogenic fibrosing dermopathy in patients who have kidney failure.

Why the Test Is Performed

The test assesses for infection, the existence of a growth, inflammation, blood flow, stroke, suspected head injury, hydrocephaly, multiple sclerosis (MS), Alzheimer's disease, Parkinson's disease, and Huntington's disease.

Before Administering the Test

- Determine if the patient has any metal on or inside his or her body
- Assess if the patient:
  - Is allergic to shellfish, iodine, or contrast material
  - Is pregnant
  - Is claustrophobic
  - Has kidney disease
  - Is wearing any medicine patches
  - Can lie still during the test

How the Test Is Performed

- The patient is assessed for any metal that might be on or inside his or her body.
- The healthcare provider determines if the presence of any metal may require cancellation of the MRI.
- An assessment is made to determine if the patient can be administered contrast material, if required for the MRI.
- Contrast material is administered via IV, causing a flushing feeling in the patient.
- Contrast material may not be used if the patient is allergic to shellfish and iodine or if the patient has kidney abnormalities or sickle cell anemia.
- An assessment is made to determine if the patient is claustrophobic.
- If so, then the healthcare provider may administer a sedative to the patient or schedule the test be performed using an open MRI.
- The patient removes all clothes and wears a gown during the MRI.
- The patient may be given headphones to reduce the sound of the tapping noise created by the MRI.
- The patient lies on his or her back on the MRI table.
- A belt is placed on the patient to detect the patient's breathing patterns.
- The table is moved into the MRI machine as images are taken of the brain.
- Images are viewed during and after the MRI is completed to assist the healthcare provider in reaching a diagnosis.

Teach the Patient

Explain why the MRI is being taken, what the patient will experience during the MRI, that no metal can be on or inside the patient during the MRI, and that the patient will not feel any pain during the procedure, although the patient may feel a tingling sensation if the patient has metal fillings in his or her teeth. The patient may be administered a sedative if he or she is claustrophobic. Some patients who are allergic to shellfish and iodine may also be allergic to contrast material. If the patient is allergic to contrast material, the healthcare provider will discuss the risk and benefits of administering the contrast material with the patient. If the patient agrees that the benefits outweigh the risk, then the healthcare provider may administer medication that counteracts the allergic reaction of the contrast material. The contrast material may be administered via IV, causing a flushing feeling.

Understanding the Test Results

The test takes 60 minutes and the results are ready immediately if the test is performed by the healthcare provider or within a few hours if a technician performs the test.

- Normal:
  - No growth
  - No blockage
  - No infection
  - No inflammation
  - Normal blood flow
- Abnormal:
  - The existence of a growth

- ○ Inflammation or infection is present
- ○ Unusual blood flow or blockage

17.5   Knee MRI

A knee MRI produces detailed images of structures and tissues contained within the knee. This enables the healthcare provider to identify any abnormalities that may exist in the knee, including damage to tendons, ligaments, cartilage, and fluid. The healthcare provider may order a knee MRI to assess if the patient requires arthroscopy of the knee.

Why the Test Is Performed

The test assesses the knee structures and tissues, existence of a growth, for arthritis, tendons, ligaments, cartilage, meniscus, and if arthroscopy is required.

Before Administering the Test

- Determine if the patient has any metal on or inside his or her body
- Assess if the patient:
  - ○ Is allergic to shellfish, iodine, or contrast material
  - ○ Is pregnant
  - ○ Is claustrophobic
  - ○ Has kidney disease
  - ○ Is wearing any medicine patches
  - ○ Can lie still during the test
  - ○ Has had prior knee surgeries where metal devices might have been implanted in the knee

How the Test Is Performed

- The patient is assessed for any metal that might be on or inside his or her body.
- The healthcare provider determines if the presence of any metal may require cancellation of the MRI.
- An assessment is made to determine if the patient can be administered contrast material, if required for the MRI.
- Contrast material is administered via IV, causing a flushing feeling in the patient.
- Contrast material may not be used if the patient is allergic to shellfish and iodine or if the patient has kidney abnormalities or sickle cell anemia.
- An assessment is made to determine if the patient is claustrophobic.
- If so, then the healthcare provider may administer a sedative to the patient or schedule the test be performed using an open MRI.
- The patient removes all clothes and wears a gown during the MRI.
- The patient may be given headphones to reduce the sound of the tapping noise created by the MRI.
- The patient lies on his or her back on the MRI table.
- A coil is placed on the patient's knee.
- A belt is placed on the patient to detect the patient's breathing patterns.
- The table is moved into the MRI machine as images are taken of the knee.
- Images are viewed during and after the MRI is completed to assist the healthcare provider reach a diagnosis.

Teach the Patient

Explain why the MRI is being taken, what the patient will experience during the MRI, that no metal can be on or inside the patient during the MRI, and that the patient will not feel any pain during the procedure, although the patient may feel a tingling sensation if the patient has metal fillings in his or her teeth. The patient may be administered a sedative if he or she is claustrophobic. Some patients who are allergic to shellfish and iodine may also be allergic to contrast material. If the patient is allergic to contrast material, the healthcare provider will discuss the risk and benefits of administering the contrast material with the patient. If the patient agrees that the benefits outweigh the risk, then the healthcare provider may administer medication that counteracts the allergic reaction of the contrast material. The patient may be administered an IV, causing a flushing feeling.

Understanding the Test Results

The test takes 60 minutes and the results are ready immediately if the test is performed by the healthcare provider or within a few hours if a technician performs the test.

- Normal:
    - Normal structures and tissues in the knee
    - No growths
    - No blockage
    - No fluid within the knee
    - No inflammation
    - Normal blood flow
- Abnormal:
    - Unusual structures and tissues in the knee
    - The existence of a growth
    - A blockage is identified
    - Fluid exists within the knee
    - Inflammation or infection is present
    - Unusual blood flow

17.6   Shoulder MRI

The shoulder MRI is ordered to show the healthcare provider detailed images of inside the shoulder, including ligaments, cartilage, muscles, and the bone structure within the shoulder and fluid. These images are more detailed than can be achieved using ultrasound and CT scans and are commonly ordered to assess shoulder pain that is unexplained by other signs or symptoms.

Why the Test Is Performed

The test assesses the shoulder structures and tissues, existence of a growth, for arthritis, tendons, ligaments, cartilage, bones, muscles, rotator cuff disorders, and if arthroscopy is required.

Before Administering the Test

- Determine if the patient has any metal on or inside his or her body
- Assess if the patient:
    - Is allergic to shellfish, iodine, or contrast material
    - Is pregnant
    - Is claustrophobic
    - Has kidney disease
    - Is wearing any medicine patches
    - Can lie still during the test
    - Has had prior surgeries where metal devices might have been implanted in the shoulder or other parts of the body

How the Test Is Performed

- The patient is assessed for any metal that might be on or inside his or her body.
- The healthcare provider determines if the presence of any metal may require cancellation of the MRI.

- An assessment is made to determine if the patient can be administered contrast material, if required for the MRI.
- Contrast material is administered via IV, causing a flushing feeling in the patient.
- Contrast material may not be used if the patient is allergic to shellfish and iodine or if the patient has kidney abnormalities or sickle cell anemia.
- An assessment is made to determine if the patient is claustrophobic. If so, then the healthcare provider may administer a sedative to the patient or schedule the test be performed using an open MRI.
- The patient removes all clothes and wears a gown during the MRI.
- The patient may be given headphones to reduce the sound of the tapping noise created by the MRI.
- The patient lies on his or her back on the MRI table.
- A coil is placed on the patient's shoulder.
- A belt is placed on the patient to detect the patient's breathing patterns.
- The table is moved into the MRI machine as images are taken of the shoulder.
- Images are viewed during and after the MRI is completed to assist the healthcare provider reach a diagnosis.

Teach the Patient

Explain why the MRI is being taken, what the patient will experience during the MRI, that no metal can be on or inside the patient during the MRI, and that the patient will not feel any pain during the procedure, although the patient may feel a tingling sensation if the patient has metal fillings in his or her teeth. The patient may be administered a sedative if he or she is claustrophobic. Some patients who are allergic to shellfish and iodine may also be allergic to contrast material. If the patient is allergic to contrast material, the healthcare provider will discuss the risk and benefits of administering the contrast material with the patient. If the patient agrees that the benefits outweigh the risk, then the healthcare provider may administer medication that counteracts the allergic reaction of the contrast material. The patient may be administered an IV, causing a flushing feeling.

Understanding the Test Results

The test takes 60 minutes and the results are ready immediately if the test is performed by the healthcare provider or within a few hours if a technician performs the test.

- Normal:
  - Normal structures and tissues in the shoulder
  - No growth
  - No blockage
  - No fluid within the shoulder
  - No inflammation
  - Normal blood flow
- Abnormal:
  - Unusual structures and tissues in the shoulder
  - The existence of a growth
  - A blockage is identified
  - Fluid exists within the shoulder
  - Inflammation or infection is present
  - Unusual blood flow
  - Rotator cuff disorders
  - Ligament and tendon tear or injury

17.7　Spinal MRI

The spinal MRI shows detailed images of the patient's spine. This includes the cervical spine, thoracic spine, and lumbosacral spine. The spinal MRI helps the healthcare provider assess if the patient has spinal disc disorders or spinal stenosis, as well as tumors and arthritis. The healthcare provider also orders a spinal MRI to assess unexplained spinal pain.

Why the Test Is Performed

The test assesses the spinal structures and tissues, ruptured disc, sciatica, spinal stenosis, growths, arthritis, and for damaged nerves.

Before Administering the Test

- Determine if the patient has any metal on or inside his or her body
- Assess if the patient:
  - Is allergic to shellfish, iodine, or contrast material
  - Is pregnant
  - Is claustrophobic
  - Has kidney disease
  - Is wearing any medicine patches
  - Can lie still during the test
  - Has had prior surgeries where metal devices might have been implanted in the spine or other parts of the body

How the Test Is Performed

- The patient is assessed for any metal that might be on or inside his or her body.
- The healthcare provider determines if the presence of any metal may require cancellation of the MRI.
- An assessment is made to determine if the patient can be administered contrast material, if required for the MRI.
- Contrast material is administered via IV, causing a flushing feeling in the patient.
- Contrast material may not be used if the patient is allergic to shellfish and iodine or if the patient has kidney abnormalities or sickle cell anemia.
- An assessment is made to determine if the patient is claustrophobic.
- If so, then the healthcare provider may administer a sedative to the patient or schedule the test be performed using an open MRI.
- The patient removes all clothes and wears a gown during the MRI.
- The patient may be given headphones to reduce the sound of the tapping noise created by the MRI.
- The patient lies on his or her back on the MRI table.
- A belt is placed on the patient to detect the patient's breathing patterns.
- The table is moved into the MRI machine as images are taken of the spine.
- Images are viewed during and after the MRI is completed to assist the healthcare provider reach a diagnosis.

Teach the Patient

Explain why the MRI is being taken, what the patient will experience during the MRI, that no metal can be on or inside the patient during the MRI, and that the patient will not feel any pain during the procedure, although the patient may feel a tingling sensation if the patient has metal fillings in his or her teeth. The patient may be administered a sedative if he or she is claustrophobic. Some patients who are allergic to shellfish and iodine may also be allergic to contrast material. If the patient is allergic to contrast material, the healthcare provider will discuss the risk and benefits of administering the contrast material with the patient. If the patient agrees that the benefits outweigh the risk, then the healthcare provider may administer medication that counteracts the allergic reaction of the contrast material. The patient may be administered an IV, causing a flushing feeling.

Understanding the Test Results

The test takes 60 minutes and the results are ready immediately if the test is performed by the healthcare provider or within a few hours if a technician performs the test.

- Normal:
  - Normal structures and tissues in the spine
  - No growths
  - No blockage
  - No inflammation
  - Normal blood flow
  - No damaged nerves
- Abnormal:
  - Unusual structures and tissues in the spine
  - The existence of a growth
  - A blockage is identified
  - Inflammation or infection is present
  - Ruptured disc
  - Sciatica
  - Spinal stenosis
  - Arthritis

Solved Problems

Magnetic Resonance Imaging

17.1   What does an MRI use to produce an image?

Magnetic resonance imaging (MRI) uses pulsating radio waves in a magnetic field to produce an image of the inside of the patient's body.

17.2   Can a patient listen to music through headphones while undergoing an MRI?

The patient may listen to music through headphones to block out the snapping noise.

17.3   What are the two types of MRI machines?

These are the closed MRI and open MRI. In the closed MRI, the patient's body is entirely enclosed in the machine, while only a portion of the patient's body is enclosed in an open MRI machine.

17.4   What is the benefit of an MRI over a CT scan, X-ray, or ultrasound?

The MRI creates images that are more detailed than images produced by a CT scan, X-ray, or ultrasound.

17.5   What might happen if a credit card is on a patient during an MRI?

Information on the credit card might be erased by the MRI magnetic field.

17.6   What might a healthcare provider do if a patient who was involved in an accident involving metal fragments requires an MRI?

An X-ray may be ordered to determine if there is any metal inside the patient before the MRI is administered, especially if the patient was in an accident where metal fragments might be embedded throughout the body.

17.7   How would you respond if a patient refuses an MRI because she has metallic dental fillings?

Dental fillings are usually permitted, although the patient is likely to feel tingling in his or her mouth during the MRI.

17.8   How would you respond if a patient refuses an MRI because she has tattoos?

The patient may experience skin irritation if the patient has iron pigment tattoos.

Abdominal MRI

17.9   How would organs be highlighted on an abdominal MRI?

The healthcare provider may order that the patient be administered contrast material prior to the MRI to highlight parts of the abdomen on the MRI image. Contrast material enables the healthcare provider to identify any subtle abnormalities that may exist in the abdomen.

17.10   Why might an abdominal MRI be ordered by a healthcare provider?

The test assesses the size of abdominal organs and structures, existence of a growth, blockages, existence of fluid within the abdomen, inflammation, and blood flow.

17.11   What must you assess before the patient is administered the abdominal MRI?

Determine if the patient has any metal on or inside his or her body. Assess if the patient:
- Has eaten or drunk before the MRI is administered. Some MRI studies require that the patient refrain from eating or drinking 12 hours before the test is administered.
- Is allergic to shellfish, iodine, or contrast material
- Is pregnant
- Is claustrophobic
- Has kidney disease
- Is wearing any medicine patches
- Can lie still during the test

17.12   What might the healthcare provider do to reduce intestinal movement during the abdominal MRI?

The patient may be administered glucagon to reduce intestinal movement during the test.

17.13   Why is a belt placed on the patient to detect the patient's breathing patterns during an abdominal MRI?

Images are taken in coordination with the patient's breathing patterns.

17.14   What should you teach a patient who is undergoing an abdominal MRI?

Explain why the MRI is being taken; what the patient will experience during the MRI; that no metal can be on or inside the patient during the MRI; that the patient will not feel any pain during the procedure, although the patient may feel a tingling sensation if the patient has metal fillings in his or her teeth, and that the patient may be administered a sedative if he or she is claustrophobic. Some patients who are allergic to shellfish and iodine may also be allergic to contrast material. If the patient is allergic to contrast material, the healthcare provider will discuss the risk and benefits of administering the contrast material with the patient.

   If the patient agrees that the benefits outweigh the risk, then the healthcare provider may administer medication that counteracts the allergic reaction of the contrast material. The patient may be asked to drink contrast material or the contrast material may be administered with an IV, causing a flushing feeling. The patient may be asked to refrain from eating or drinking 12 hours before the MRI.

17.15   What might be revealed in abnormal findings of an abdominal MRI?

Abnormal findings of an abdominal MRI might reveal unusual size of abdominal organs and structures, the existence of a growth, a blockage, fluid existing within the abdomen, inflammation or infection, or unusual blood flow.

Breast MRI

17.16   When might a breast MRI be ordered by a healthcare provider?

Healthcare providers typically order a breast MRI when other tests such as a mammography indicate an abnormality.

17.17   When will a healthcare provider use contrast material in a breast MRI?

If the abnormality is inflammation, a growth, or blood flow to breast tissues, the healthcare provider may administer contrast material to enhance the image of those areas of the breast.

17.18   When might a healthcare provider recommend to a patient to undergo an annual breast MRI?

Women who are positive for the BRCA1 or BRCA2 gene or whose family members developed breast cancer before the age of 50 are considered high risk for developing breast cancer and may be recommended for annual breast MRI to detect early signs of breast cancer. The healthcare provider may also order an annual breast MRI for women who normally have dense breast tissue. A MRI is better suited to examine dense breast tissue than an ultrasound test.

17.19 What conditions might a breast MRI be used to detect?

A breast MRI might be used to detect infection, the existence of a growth, inflammation, blood flow, breast cancer treatment, and breast implants. A breast MRI is very useful for women at a high risk for breast cancer and women who normally have dense breast tissue.

17.20 What should be assessed before administering a breast MRI?

Determine if the patient has any metal on or inside her body. Assess if the patient:
- Is allergic to shellfish, iodine, or contrast material
- Is pregnant
- Is claustrophobic
- Has kidney disease
- Is wearing any medicine patches
- Can lie still during the test

17.21 Why might a patient who is allergic to shellfish and iodine agree to an MRI with contrast material?

Some patients who are allergic to shellfish and iodine may also be allergic to contrast material. If the patient is allergic to contrast material, the healthcare provider will discuss the risk and benefits of administering the contrast material with the patient. If the patient agrees that the benefits outweigh the risk, then the healthcare provider may administer medication that counteracts the allergic reaction of the contrast material.

17.22 Why might a patient be administered a sedative before undergoing a breast MRI?

The patient may be administered a sedative if she is claustrophobic.

Head MRI

17.23 Why might a head MRI be ordered by a healthcare provider?

A head MRI might be ordered to determine the underlying cause of headache, assess for head injury, or determine if the patient has abnormal blood flow or a disorder that affects the brain.

17.24 What types of MRI are used to assess the brain?
- Magnetic Resonance Spectroscopy: Assesses changes in brain chemistry caused by disease.
- Magnetic Resonance Angiogram (MRA): Assesses speed, direction, and flow of blood in the brain.
- Diffusion-Perfusion Imaging: Assesses inflammation, tumors, and stroke by evaluating the fluid content of the brain.

17.25 What is the potential risk of using gadolinium containing contrast material in a brain MRI?

Gadolinium can cause nephrogenic fibrosing dermopathy in patients who have kidney failure.

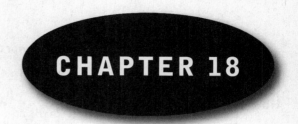

CHAPTER 18

Positron Emission Tomography (PET) Scan

18.1   Definition

A *positron emission tomography* (PET) scan is a nuclear medicine test that creates a roadmap of blood flow in the patient's body. The healthcare provider can visualize abnormal blood flow to the patient's tissues and organs. A radioactive chemical called a tracer and a special camera that detects the tracer inside the patient's body are the keys to a PET scan. The healthcare provider administers the tracer into the patient's veins prior to the scan. The tracer gives off positrons, which are very small charged particles that can be detected by the PET scan camera. The PET scan camera takes a series of images, each capturing the position of positrons in the body. These images are stored and replayed on a computer screen. Images show the tracer containing blood as the blood makes its way into organs and tissues, giving the healthcare provider a clear picture of blood flow within the body.

18.2   PET Scan

The PET scan is ordered to study blood flow and metabolic activity within a patient's body. Healthcare providers frequently combine results from the PET scan with the CT scan results to obtain a thorough understanding of how well tissues and organs are being infused with blood. Sometimes a CT scan is performed along with a PET scan. The tracer contains low level radiation that will rarely lead to tissue damage. The tracer is flushed from the patient's body in 24 hours following the scan. It is rare that a patient will have an allergic reaction to the tracer. The healthcare provider may order a single photon emission computed tomography (SPECT) to determine if a patient with chest pain is at risk for cardiac arrest.

Why the Test Is Performed

The test assesses blood flow to organs and tissues, metabolic activity or organs, for stroke and transient ischemic attack (TIA), multiple sclerosis, Parkinson's disease, Alzheimer's disease, epilepsy, coronary artery disease, and the presence of cancer and if the cancer has metastasized.

Before Administering the Test

- The patient will likely be asked to withhold medications 24 hours before the PET scan
- The healthcare provider may ask the patient to decrease his or her dose of insulin if the patient is a diabetic
- Assess if the patient:
  - Has ingested caffeine or alcohol 24 hours before the PET scan
  - Eaten eight hours before the PET scan

○ Is pregnant
○ Is breastfeeding
○ If the patient signed a consent form prior to the PET scan
○ Can lie still during the test

How the Test Is Performed

- The patient is administered the tracer intravenously.
- The patient lies on a table.
- The patient may be given a blindfold or earplugs to wear during the scan.
- Electrocardiogram electrodes are placed on the patient, if the patient's heart is being studied.
- The PET scan camera moves around the patient.
- The patient might be asked to tell a story or read during the scan, if the patient's brain is being studied.
- The healthcare provider or PET scan technician is outside the PET scan room and is able to speak to the patient through an intercom and see the patient through a window.
- The patient must drink lots of fluid for a full day to flush the tracer from the patient's body.

Teach the Patient

Explain why the PET scan is being performed, what the patient will experience during the PET scan, that the patient will not feel any pain during the procedure, and that the patient may be administered a sedative if he or she is claustrophobic. The patient must refrain from ingesting alcohol, caffeine, and tobacco for 24 hours prior to the PET scan. The patient may be asked to stop taking or reduce the dose of medication prior to the PET scan. Inform the patient that the PET scan may not be administered if the patient is pregnant or breastfeeding, and that the healthcare provider may administer a sedative prior to the PET scan if the patient is anxious and unable to lie still for the test. Explain to the patient that the healthcare provider may ask the patient to tell a story or read during the PET scan and EKG electrodes may be attached to the patient's body during the test.

Understanding the Test Results

The test takes 3 hours and the results are ready immediately if the test is performed by the healthcare provider or within a few hours if a technician performs the test.

- Normal:
  ○ Normal blood flow
  ○ No growth
  ○ No blockage
  ○ Normal metabolic activity
- Abnormal:
  ○ Unexpected blood flow
  ○ The existence of a growth
  ○ A blockage is identified
  ○ Unusual metabolic activity

Solved Problems

A Positron Emission Tomography Scan

18.1 What does a positron emission tomography scan produce?

A positron emission tomography (PET) scan is a nuclear medicine test that creates a roadmap of blood flow in the patient's body.

18.2 What is a tracer?

A radioactive chemical called a tracer is used in a PET scan.

18.3 How does a tracer work?

The tracer gives off positrons, which are very small charged particles.

18.4 How does a PET scan camera work?

The PET scan camera detects positrons given off by a tracer using the positrons to create an image.

18.5 What images are created by the PET scan camera?

Images show the tracer containing blood as the blood makes its way into organs and tissues, giving the healthcare provider a clear picture of blood flow within the body.

18.6 Why might a healthcare provider order a PET scan?

The PET scan is ordered to study blood flow and metabolic activity within a patient's body.

18.7 How would you respond if the patient is concerned that the tracer will cause tissue damage?

The tracer contains low level radiation that will rarely lead to tissue damage.

18.8 Does the tracer remain in the patient following the PET scan?

The tracer is flushed from the patient's body in 24 hours following the scan.

18.9 How would you respond if the patient says she might have an allergic reaction to the tracer?

It is rare that a patient will have an allergic reaction to the tracer.

18.10 What might the healthcare provider order if the patient with chest pain is at risk for cardiac arrest when a PET scan is ordered?

The healthcare provider may order a single photon emission computed tomography (SPECT) test to determine if a patient with chest pain is at risk for cardiac arrest.

18.11 What is being assessed by the PET scan?

The PET scan assesses blood flow to organs and tissues, metabolic activity or organs, stroke and transient ischemic attack (TIA), multiple sclerosis, Parkinson's disease, Alzheimer's disease, epilepsy, coronary artery disease, and the presence of cancer and if the cancer has metastasized.

18.12 What might the healthcare provider request for a patient who takes regular medication before he or she receives a PET scan?

The patient will likely be asked to withhold medications 24 hours before the PET scan.

18.13 What might the healthcare provider request for a patient who is a diabetic before he or she receives a PET scan?

The healthcare provider may ask the patient to decrease the dose of insulin he or she is taking.

18.14 What would you do if the patient said he had two cups of coffee the morning of his PET scan?

Notify the healthcare provider, because the patient should not ingest caffeine within 24 hours of the PET scan.

18.15 How many hours before a PET scan should the patient refrain from eating?

The patient should refrain from eating 8 hours before the PET scan.

18.16 Why might a patient be administered a sedative before a PET scan?

The healthcare provider may administer a sedative prior to the PET scan if the patient is anxious and unable to lie still for the test.

18.17 How would you respond if the patient who is scheduled for a PET scan says she is afraid of pain during the scan?

The patient will not feel any pain during the procedure.

18.18 If the patient who is scheduled for a PET scan tells you he is claustrophobic, how would you respond?

The patient may be administered a sedative if he is claustrophobic.

18.19 Why might the healthcare provider attach an EKG to the patient during a PET scan?

The EKG is used to monitor the patient's heart if the healthcare provider is also studying the patient's heart.

18.20 How is the tracer inserted into the patient?

The patient is administered the tracer intravenously.

18.21 Where are the images from a PET scan viewed?

These images are stored and replayed on a computer screen.

18.22 What might a healthcare provider do to obtain a thorough understanding of how well tissues and organs are being infused with blood?

Healthcare providers frequently combine results from the PET scan with the CT scan results to obtain a thorough understanding of how well tissues and organs are being infused with blood.

18.23 What should you assess in a female patient before the PET scan is administered?

Assess if the patient is pregnant or breastfeeding.

18.24 What is an important behavior that should be assessed before an elderly patient is administered a PET scan?

The most important behavior that should be assessed is that the elderly patient can lie still during the PET scan.

18.25 How is the tracer flushed from the patient following the PET scan?

The patient must drink lots of fluid for a full day to flush the tracer from his or her body.

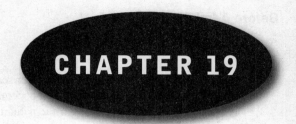

CHAPTER 19

Cardiovascular Tests and Procedures

19.1   Definition

Cardiovascular tests are performed to determine if the blood is adequately pumping and flowing throughout the patient's body. These tests measure:

- Cardiac contraction
- The risk for coronary artery disease
- Blockage to coronary arteries and blood vessels to the extremities

When a blockage is identified, the healthcare provider can perform one of several procedures to restore blood flow. The blockage might be surgically removed. The blockage might be pressed against the wall of the blood vessel and held in place by a stent. The healthcare provider may surgically bypass the blocked blood vessels, using a vein from the patient's leg or by using an artificial blood vessel.

19.2   Cardiac Blood Pool Scan

The cardiac blood pool scan measures the percentage of the patient's blood that is pumped in a cardiac contraction. This measures how well the heart is contracting. This is referred to as the ejection fraction. The healthcare provider administers radioactive material called a tracer into the patient's vein. A gamma camera is used to monitor the tracer as the blood flows throughout the patient's heart. The healthcare provider can use one of two types of cardiac blood pool scans to estimate the ejection fraction:

- **Multigated Acquisition (MUGA) Scan**: This is also known as a gated scan. Each contraction of the heart triggers the gamma camera to take a picture of the heart, which is stored in a computer. These images are then placed on a computer screen showing cardiac contractions. The healthcare provider may perform the MUGA scan twice, first without medication and the second after giving the patient nitroglycerin. Nitroglycerin dilates arteries and veins, reducing the amount of blood that must be pumped by the heart, which decreases the amount of oxygen required of the heart because the heart works less. The impact of the decreased cardiac workload should be reflected in the MUGA scan.
- **First-Pass Scan**: This captures images of the blood going through the heart and lungs for the first time.

The MUGA scan is not used on children and does not provide information about heart valves and thickness of cardiac walls. The first-pass scan is used on children to assess existence of congenital heart disease. The cardiac blood pool scan is not performed if the patient is pregnant.

Why the Test Is Performed

The test assesses cardiac blood flow and ventricle contractions.

Before Administering the Test

Assess if the patient:

- Has any allergies
- Has recently undergone radioactive tracer scans
- Has an implant in the chest, such as a pacemaker
- Is wearing comfortable clothes, if the patient will be asked to exercise
- Can lie still on his or her back
- Has recently had a barium enema
- If the patient is pregnant. The cardiac blood pool scan is not performed if the patient is pregnant
- Has not eaten four hour before the scan.
- Has not ingested caffeine six hours before the scan
- Has not smoked six hours before the scan
- Has provided the healthcare provider with all medications that the patient takes. Digoxin and nitrate medication can affect the scan results.

How the Test Is Performed

- The patient is administered the radioactive tracer in a vein.
- Multigated Acquisition (MUGA) scan:
  - A sample of blood is taken.
  - The radioactive tracer is mixed with the blood sample.
  - The blood sample is then re-injected into the patient's vein.
- It takes 4 hours for the patient's red blood cells to absorb the entire tracer.
- The patient may be able to leave the healthcare facility during this period.
- The patient is asked to remove dentures and jewelry before the scan is performed.
- The patient will remove his or her clothes.
- The patient lies on a table.
- An electrocardiogram is attached to the patient.
- The patient must lie still each time a picture is taken, which can take 5 minutes.
- The gamma camera is positioned close to the patient's chest and is repositioned during the scan.
- The patient may be asked to change position or leave the table to perform exercises and then return to the table to continue the scan.
- The patient may be administered nitroglycerin.
- The patient will drink lots of fluid for 2 days following the scan to flush the tracer from his or her body.
- The MUGA scan takes 3 hours to complete and the first-pass scan takes 1 hour to complete.

Teach the Patient

Explain why the scan is being performed, what the patient will experience during the scan, that the patient will not feel any pain during the procedure except for a pinch from the needle used to administer the tracer, and that the patient must tell the healthcare provider of any allergies, if he or she has recently undergone radioactive tracer scans, has an implant in the chest such as a pacemaker, or has recently had a barium enema. The patient cannot eat 4 hours before the scan, ingest caffeine 6 hours before the scan, or smoke 6 hours before the scan. The patient must tell the healthcare provider of all medications that the patient takes.

Understanding the Results

The MUGA scan takes 3 hours and the first-pass scan takes 1 hour. Results are ready within a week of the scan.

- Normal:
  - Ejection fraction 55% to 65%
  - Normal blood flow through the heart
  - Cardiac structures are normal and contracting normally

- Abnormal:
  - ○ Less than 55% ejection fraction
  - ○ Inadequate cardiac contractions
  - ○ Abnormal cardiac structures
  - ○ Improper blood flow through the heart

19.3 Cardiac Calcium Scoring

Calcium scoring determines the level of calcium containing plaque on the coronary artery walls using a computed tomography (CT) scan. Coronary arteries supply blood to cardiac muscles. Restricted coronary arteries decrease blood and oxygen supply to cardiac muscles. Blood flow through the coronary arteries becomes restricted by a plaque buildup on the coronary artery wall. Plaque contains calcium. Cardiac images of thin sections of the heart are taken using the CT scan and are stored in a computer and reviewed by the healthcare provider to assess signs of coronary artery disease. A patient can have a high cardiac calcium score without having coronary artery disease. Healthcare providers use a variety of assessment methods to determine if the patient has coronary artery disease.

Why the Test Is Performed

The test assesses the buildup of plaque containing calcium on the walls of the coronary arteries and for coronary artery disease.

Before Administering the Test

Assess if the patient:

- Is claustrophobic
- Can lie still on his or her back
- Has removed jewelry
- Has ingested caffeine
- Has smoked

How the Test Is Performed

- The patient removes all jewelry.
- The patient will remove clothes above the waist.
- The patient lies on a table.
- An electrocardiogram is attached to the patient.
- The patient may be administered medication to decrease cardiac contraction if the patient's heart rate is greater than 90 beats per minute.
- The patient may be administered a sedative if the patient feels claustrophobic being inside the CT machine.
- The patient will be alone in the CT room, but can communicate with the CT technician using an intercom.
- The patient must lie still on a table.
- The table slides into the CT scanner (see Chapter 15).
- The patient is asked to hold his or her breath and lie still for 30 seconds while images are taken by the CT machine.

Teach the Patient

Explain why the scan is being performed, what the patient will experience during the scan, and that the patient will not feel any pain during the procedure except for a pinch from the needle used to administer the sedative, if necessary. The patient should not ingest caffeine or smoke before the test. The patient will be administered a sedative if the patient feels claustrophobic being in the CT machine.

Understanding the Results

The cardiac calcium scoring test takes 30 minutes. Results are ready within a week of the scan.

- Normal:
  - Score 0 = No plaque, means 5% chance of developing coronary artery disease.
  - Score < 11 = 10% chance of developing coronary artery disease.
- Abnormal:
  - Score 11 to 100 = Plaque was found. Patient has mild coronary artery disease.
  - Score 101 to 400 = Plaque was found. Patient has coronary artery disease and possibly a blockage of one or more coronary arteries.
  - Score > 400 = Plaque was found. Patient has coronary artery disease and there is a 90% chance that there is a blockage of one or more coronary arteries.

19.4   Electrocardiogram

An electrocardiogram (EKG/ECG) records electrical activity of the heart on paper. Electrical activity causes the contraction of the heart, resulting in blood being pumped throughout the body. Any disruption of the electrical activity might cause the heart to perform less than normally, which appears on the electrocardiogram paper tracing. Telemetry is a type of electrocardiogram that is used in a healthcare facility to constantly monitor the patient's cardiac activity. Cardiac electrical activity is transmitted by a transmitter worn by the patient connected to a telemetry monitor at the nurse's station. An alarm is sounded whenever there is abnormal cardiac activity. A telemetry nurse interprets the tracing on the telemetry monitor and prints the tracing while taking appropriate action.

The *Holter monitoring electrocardiogram*, sometimes referred to as an ambulatory electrocardiogram, is a type of portable electrocardiogram that is attached to the patient for 24 hours. The Holter monitoring electrocardiogram is worn on the patient's waist or around his or her shoulder, enabling the healthcare provider to detect abnormal electrical activity of the patient's heart during activities of daily living such as when the patient exercises and is sleeping. Holter monitoring can be continuously recorded or intermittently recorded. There are two types of intermittent Holter monitoring:

1. **Event monitor**: The patient presses a button whenever a cardiac symptom occurs, causing the Holter monitor to record cardiac activity.
2. **Loop recorder**: The Holter monitor constantly records cardiac electrical activity. The patient presses a button whenever a cardiac symptom occurs.

Why the Test Is Performed

The test assesses:

- The cause of chest pain, palpitations, and other symptoms
- The effects of medication on the heart
- Signs and symptoms of heart disease
- The performance of a pacemaker

Before Administering the Test

Assess if the patient:

- Can lie still on his or her back
- Has removed jewelry

How the Test Is Performed

- The patient will remove his or her clothes in the area where the electrocardiogram leads are attached to the patient.
- The patient lies on a table.

- An electrocardiogram is attached to the patient.
- The patient lies still.

Teach the Patient

Explain why the electrocardiogram is being performed, what the patient will experience during the procedure, that the patient will not feel any pain during the procedure, and that the patient will be required to remove jewelry.

Understanding the Results

The EKG/ECG test takes an hour. Results are ready immediately.

- Normal:
  - Expected electrical activity on the trace paper
- Abnormal:
  - Unexpected electrical activity on the trace paper

19.5   Cardiac Perfusion Scan

The cardiac perfusion scan determines if the heart is receiving sufficient blood supply. The cardiac perfusion scan is commonly performed to determine the volume of blood in cardiac muscle during stress and at rest. Before the test, the patient is administered a radioactive tracer into his or her vein. A camera scans the patient's heart while at rest and stores the image in a computer. The patient's heart is then placed under stress by using medication or asking the patient to exercise. The patient's heart is then scanned by the camera and images are stored in the computer. The healthcare provider then compares the images to determine if the heart is receiving sufficient blood supply.

Why the Test Is Performed

The test assesses the underlying cause of chest pain and the results of angioplasty and bypass surgery.

Before Administering the Test

Assess if the patient:

- Can lie still on his or her back
- Has allergies
- Has taken Viagra, Cialis, or Levitra within two days of the procedure. This can cause the patient's blood pressure to fall if the patient is administered nitroglycerin during the procedure.
- Is taking anticoagulants such as coumadin, aspirin, or heparin
- Is taking Trental or Persantine
- Is pregnant
- Is breast-feeding. If so, the patient must discard breast milk collected two days following the test, since the breast milk will contact the radioactive tracer.
- Has eaten or drunk three hours before the test
- Has avoided ingesting caffeine, alcohol, and tobacco one day before the test
- Has removed jewelry
- Can exercise
- Recently had a heart attack or myocarditis
- Has a pacemaker
- Has an electrolyte imbalance

How the Test Is Performed

- The patient removes all jewelry.
- The patient will remove his or her clothes above the waist.

- The patient lies on a table.
- An electrocardiogram is attached to the patient.
- Radioactive tracer is administered into the patient's vein.
- The camera is placed close to the patient's chest.
- The patient must remain still when the image is taken.
- The camera is moved and the patient is asked to exercise using a treadmill or stationary bike. While exercising, the patient's blood pressure is monitored with an electrocardiogram.
- If the patient is unable to exercise, medication is administered to simulate the stress of exercise on the patient's heart.
- The patient lies on the table.
- Radioactive tracer is administered into the patient's vein.
- The camera is placed close to the patient's chest.
- The patient remains still when the image is taken.
- The patient can resume normal activity following the test.

Teach the Patient

Explain why the test is being performed, what the patient will experience during the procedure, and that the patient might feel flushed, nauseous, dizzy, or have a headache if medication is administered to place the patient's heart under stress. The patient will not feel any pain during the procedure except for a pinch from the needle used to administer the trace material. The patient should not drink or eat three hours before the procedure and should tell the healthcare provider if taking Viagra, Cialis, Levitra, coumadin, aspirin, heparin, Trental, or Persantine. The patient should tell the healthcare provider during the test if he or she experiences fatigue, chest pain, shortness of breath, aching in the lower extremities, or lightheadedness while the test is in progress. The patient will be required to remove jewelry, may resume normal activities following the test, and should call for emergency medical care if he or she experiences difficulty breathing or chest pains after leaving the healthcare facilities following the test.

Understanding the Results

The test takes 1 hour. Results are ready within a week.

- Normal:
  - Normal blood volume in the cardiac muscle
- Abnormal:
  - Decreased blood volume in the cardiac muscle

19.6   Ankle-Brachial Index

The ankle-brachial index (ABI) evaluates circulation in the lower extremity for peripheral arterial disease. This may also be performed to determine how well blood is flowing to the extremities after procedures or surgery. The ankle-brachial index is determined by measuring the patient's blood pressure in both ankles and arms while the patient is resting. The patient may be asked to exercise. If so, the same blood pressures are taken and compared to the resting blood pressure.

Why the Test Is Performed

The test assesses for peripheral arterial disease and risk for stroke.

Before Administering the Test

Assess if the patient:

- Is able to have his or her blood pressure taken in both arms and legs
- Can lie on his or her back

- Can walk on a treadmill
- Is wearing comfortable clothes
- Has been diagnosed with arterial disease

How the Test Is Performed

- The patient lies on a table.
- Blood pressure is taken in both arms and legs.
- The ankle-brachial index is calculated as: ABI = ankle blood pressure/brachial blood pressure.

Teach the Patient

Explain why the test is being performed, what the patient will experience during the scan, that the patient will not feel any pain during the test, and that the patient should wear comfortable clothes since he or she will be walking on the treadmill.

Understanding the Results

The test takes less than 1 hour. Results are ready immediately.

- Normal:
  - An index of 1 or 1.1 indicates that blood pressure in the arms and ankles are approximately the same. Peripheral blood flow is unobstructed.
- Abnormal:
  - 0.98: Narrowing of peripheral blood flow
  - 0.80: Intermittent claudication
  - 0.25: High risk for peripheral arterial disease (PAD)

19.7 Echocardiogram

An echocardiogram is an ultrasound scan of the patient's heart. Sound waves are transmitted by a transducer through the patient's chest to the heart. Sound waves echo off of the heart and are detected by the transducer, creating an image of the heart. Images are stored on a computer, enabling the healthcare provider to play back images showing the beating heart. There are four types of echocardiograms:

1. **Stress echocardiogram**: Two sets of images of the heart are captured. The first set of images is of the resting heart. The second set of images is taken when the heart is under stress, either following exercise or stressed by medication.
2. **Transthoracic echocardiogram (TTE)**: This creates a set of views that illustrate the beating heart, which is the most common type of echocardiogram.
3. **Transesophageal echocardiogram (TEE)**: Under local anesthesia, the transducer is inserted down the patient's esophagus, enabling the generation of a clear image of the heart, since images are not obscured by bones. This is commonly used to assess for vegetation on the heart valves.

Why the Test Is Performed

The test assesses cardiac function, cardiac abnormalities, for pericardial effusion, for valve abnormalities and vegetations, and for ejection fraction.

Before Administering the Test

Assess if the patient:

- Can lie on his or her back
- Can swallow (transesophageal echocardiogram)

- Can walk on a treadmill or pedal a stationary bicycle (stress echocardiogram)
- Is wearing comfortable clothes
- Has lung disease
- Has large breasts
- Has not eaten or drunk for 6 hours before the test
- Has dentures
- Has transportation home, if the patient is to receive a sedative
- Signed a consent form
- Has difficulty breathing
- Has removed jewelry
- Has removed clothes above the waist

How the Test Is Performed

- The patient removes clothes above the waist.
- The patient removes jewelry above the waist.
- The patient lies on a table.
- The patient is attached to an electrocardiogram.
- Stress echocardiogram:
  ○ The patient is given a baseline EKG.
  ○ The patient is asked to pedal a stationary bicycle or walk on a treadmill while another EKG is taken.
  ○ If the patient is unable to exercise, the healthcare provider will administer dobutamine to the patient to chemically stress the patient's heart.
  ○ The patient is asked to lie on the table.
  ○ The patient may be administered saline through a vein to help the healthcare provider assess the patient's cardiac function.
  ○ If the healthcare provider is unable to obtain a clear view of the heart, the healthcare provider may administer contrast material in the patient's vein. If so, the patient will be placed on a mechanical ventilator to assist the patient's respiration.
  ○ Conductive gel is placed on the left side of the patient's chest.
  ○ A transducer is moved along the patient's chest; the transducer generates sound waves through the body and receives reflected sound waves.
  ○ The healthcare provider asks the patient to change position, breathe slowly, or hold his or her breath at different times during the test.
  ○ Reflected sound waves create an image of the heart on a computer screen.
- Transesophageal echocardiogram:
  ○ A saline or heparin lock is inserted into the patient's arm.
  ○ The patient is administered medication that decreases saliva and stomach secretions.
  ○ The patient is administered a sedative. The patient remains conscious during the test.
  ○ The patient's blood oxygen level is measured using the pulse oximeter during the test.
  ○ The healthcare provider sprays an anesthetic in the back of the patient's throat to decrease the patient's gag reflex.
  ○ The patient's head is titled forward.
  ○ A mouth guard is inserted into the patient's mouth to protect the patient's teeth.
  ○ A transducer-probe is inserted down the patient's esophagus as the patient swallows. The transducer-probe remains in place for 20 minutes.
  ○ The healthcare provider will suction excess saliva.
  ○ The patient is asked not to swallow during the test.
  ○ The transducer sends and receives sound waves and generates an image of the patient's heart.
  ○ The transducer-probe is removed once all images of the heart are captured.
  ○ The patient is not permitted to ingest anything until the gag reflex is restored when the anesthetic wears off.

Teach the Patient

Explain why the test is being performed, how the test is performed, what the patient will experience during the test, and that the patient will not feel any pain during the test. The patient should wear comfortable clothes since he or she will be walking on the treadmill or pedaling a stationary bicycle (stress echocardiogram). The patient will need to remove jewelry and clothes from the waist up. The patient should refrain from eating and drinking six hours before the test. The patient should remove all dentures prior to the test. The patient will not be able to drive for 12 hours following the test if a sedative is administered to the patient. The conductive gel will be wiped off of the patient following the test.

The patient's heart rate may increase for 15 minutes and then return to normal in 3 minutes following administration of dobutamine, if the patient is undergoing a stress echocardiogram and is unable to exercise. The patient can request to take a break during the test if he or she feels uncomfortable. The patient may experience an unusual feeling in the throat if the patient is receiving a transesophageal echocardiogram. The patient may feel sleepy or experience blurred vision, trouble speaking, or a dry mouth following the test. These should resolve shortly following the test. Although the patient is awake during the test, the patient probably will not remember the test itself. The patient may experience hoarseness or a sore throat following a transesophageal echocardiogram. Lozengers and gargling with warm salt water will provide relief.

The patient should avoid drinking alcohol for a day following the transesophageal echocardiogram. The patient may experience nausea. Prior to the test, the patient and the healthcare provider should arrange for a signal that the patient can give the healthcare provider to indicate that the patient is uncomfortable during a transesophageal echocardiogram. The patient should call his or her healthcare provider if he or she experiences chest pains, difficulty swallowing, difficulty speaking, experiences a fast heartbeat, or difficulty breathing following the test.

Understanding the Results

The transthoracic echocardiogram, stress echocardiogram, and Doppler echocardiogram take 1 hour to perform. The transesophageal echocardiogram takes 2 hours to perform. Results are available in 1 week.

- Normal:
  - Normal cardiac function
  - No cardiac growth
  - No fluid buildup around the heart
  - Normal ejection fraction
- Abnormal:
  - Unexpected cardiac function
  - Cardiac growth
  - Fluid buildup around the heart
  - Heart valve vegetations or other valve abnormalities
  - Abnormal ejection fraction

19.8   Pericardiocentesis

The healthcare provider may perform a pericardiocentesis to remove the excess fluid, thereby restoring normal cardiac contraction. There are disorders that cause pericardial effusion, which results in excess fluid building up in the *pericardium* (sac around the heart). As a result, the patient may experience cardiac tamponade, which inhibits cardiac contraction and is a life threatening emergency. Pericardial effusion can be caused by inflammation of the pericardium, virus, bacteria or fungi infection, blood from an injury, or disorders such as kidney failure, hypothyroidism, or rheumatoid arthritis. Sometimes pericardiocentesis is performed in the emergency department.

Why the Test Is Performed

The test is performed to remove excess fluid from the pericardium, restore cardiac contraction, and assess the source of pericardial effusion.

Before Administering the Test

Assess if the patient:

- Can lie on his or her back
- Can respond to direction during the procedure
- Has taken anticoagulation (coumadin, heparin) or antiplatelets (aspirin, clopidogrel) medicines
- Has allergies
- Has recently been administered antibiotics
- Has not eaten or drunk 12 hours before the test
- Signed a consent form
- Has removed jewelry
- Has removed clothes above the waist

How the Test Is Performed

- A blood test is taken prior to the procedure to determine if the patient has anticoagulation problems.
- The patient removes clothes above the waist.
- The patient removes jewelry above the waist.
- The patient angles his or her back on a table.
- A saline or heparin lock is inserted into the patient's arm.
- The patient is attached to an electrocardiogram.
- The patient is administered a sedative.
- The insertion site is cleaned with an antiseptic.
- The patient is administered a local anesthetic at the insertion site.
- A needle is inserted either between the patient's left ribs or below the sternum and into the pericardium, guided by an echocardiogram.
- The patient may be asked to remain still or hold his or her breath while the needle is inserted.
- A catheter is slid over the needle into the pericardium and the needle is removed.
- The fluid is drained from the catheter.
- The catheter is removed once fluid is drained.
- Pressure is applied to the site for five minutes to stop bleeding.
- A chest X-ray is taken of the patient to assure there is no collateral damage, such as a collapsed lung.
- The patient may remain in the healthcare facility for observation.

Teach the Patient

Explain why the procedure is being performed, how the procedure is performed, what the patient will experience during the procedure, that the patient will not feel any pain during the procedure, and that the patient might experience an irregular heartbeat during the procedure. The patient will need to remove jewelry and clothes from the waist up and should refrain from eating and drinking 12 hours before the test. The patient may feel pressure as the needle is inserted.

The patient may remain in the healthcare facilities for observation following the procedure. The patient should tell the healthcare provider if he or she experiences chest pain or shortness of breath either during or after the procedure. After returning home, the patient should call for emergency medical help if the patient experiences chest pain, trouble breathing, sweating, lightheadedness, and signs of shock. The patient should call his or her healthcare provider if the patient vomits blood, is short of breath, has a fever, or feels dizzy.

Understanding the Results

The procedure takes 30 minutes. However, the fluid may drain for several hours following the procedure. Results from analyses of the fluid removed from the pericardium are available within a week.

- Normal:
  - Less than or equal to 50 mL of fluid drained
  - Normal clear/pale yellow fluid

- ○ No bacteria
- ○ No abnormal cells
- ○ Less than 500 white blood cells present in the fluid
- Abnormal:
  - ○ Greater than 50 ml of fluid drained
  - ○ Fluid appears cloudy
  - ○ Bacteria cells found in the fluid
  - ○ Abnormal cells found in the fluid
  - ○ More than 500 white blood cells present in the fluid

19.9　Venogram

A venogram is used by healthcare providers to assess the function of valves in the vein and if there is a deep vein thrombosis (DVT). A venogram produces an X-ray image of blood flowing through the patient's veins. There are several types of venograms:

- Extremities
- Pelvis
- Kidneys

Why the Test Is Performed

The test assesses blood flow through veins and valves in veins. It identifies thrombosis and sites for filters.

Before Administering the Test

Assess if the patient:

- Has signed a consent
- Can lie still on his or her back
- Has allergies
- Is pregnant
- Is taking coumadin, heparin, or aspirin
- Has avoided eating or drinking for 4 hours before the test
- Has emptied his or her bladder before the test
- Has removed jewelry
- Has kidney disorder
- Has asthma
- Has diabetes

How the Test Is Performed

- The patient removes all jewelry.
- The patient will remove his or her clothes.
- The patient must not eat 4 hours before the test.
- The patient can drink clear fluids up to 4 hours before the test, but must not drink after 4 hours.
- The patient is asked to empty his or her bladder.
- The patient lies on a table that may tilt during the test.
- For extremities, an elastic band is placed around the extremity that is being examined to fill the vein with blood.
- The patient may be administered a local anesthetic at the insertion site.
- Contrast material is inserted into the patient's vein.
- For kidneys:
  - ○ A catheter is inserted into the femoral vein in the groin and guided into the vein in the patient's kidney.

- ○ The contrast material is administered through the catheter. The catheter is removed once the test is completed.
- ○ The contrast material may also be administered into the inferior vena cava.
- X-ray images are taken of the area that is being studied.
- After the test is completed, saline is inserted into the vein to help flush the contrast material.
- The patient may be administered heparin to prevent a blood clot following the test.
- A dressing is placed on the insertion site.
- The patient is asked to drink a lot of water to flush the contrast material from his or her body.

Teach the Patient

Explain why the test is being performed, what the patient will experience during the test, that the patient will not feel any pain during the test except for a pinch when the contrast material is inserted into the vein, and that the patient may feel pins and needles in the arm or leg that is being studied, but this dissipates quickly following the test. The patient will have to sign a consent form, must empty his or her bladder before the test, will be required to rest in bed for 3 hours if a kidney venogram is performed, and should drink lots of water for a day following the procedure to flush the contrast material from his or her body. The patient should call his or her healthcare provider if after the test the patient feels pain or experiences swelling in the area that was studied or if he or she experiences a fever.

Understanding the Results

A venogram takes 1 hour or less to perform.

- Normal:
  - ○ Normal blood flow
  - ○ No growth in the kidney
- Abnormal:
  - ○ Blockage of blood flow
  - ○ Varicose veins
  - ○ Growth in the kidney

Solved Problems

Cardiac Blood Pool Scan

19.1   What does a cardiac blood pool scan measure?

The cardiac blood pool scan measures the percentage of the patient's blood that is pumped in a cardiac contraction.

19.2   What is an ejection fraction?

An ejection fraction is the percentage of the patient's blood that is pumped in a cardiac contraction.

19.3   How does a cardiac blood pool scan work?

The healthcare provider administers radioactive material called a tracer into the patient's vein. A gamma camera is used to monitor the tracer as the blood flows throughout the patient's heart.

19.4   What is a multigated acquisition scan?

A multigated acquisition (MUGA) scan is also known as a gated scan. Each contraction of the heart triggers the gamma camera to take a picture of the heart, which is stored in a computer. These images are then placed on the computer screen, showing cardiac contractions. The healthcare provider may perform the MUGA scan twice, first without medication and the second after giving the patient nitroglycerin. Nitroglycerin dilates arteries and veins, reducing the amount of blood that must be pumped by the heart, which decreases the amount of oxygen required of the heart because the heart works less. The impact of the decreased cardiac workload should be reflected in the MUGA scan.

19.5   What is a first pass scan?

The first-pass scan captures images of the blood going through the heart and lungs for the first time. The first-pass scan is used on children to assess the existence of congenital heart disease.

19.6   Why might a healthcare provider order a PET scan?

The PET scan is ordered to study blood flow and metabolic activity within a patient's body.

19.7   Why might a cardiac blood pool scan be ordered by the healthcare provider?

The cardiac blood pool scan assesses cardiac blood flow and ventricle contractions.

19.8   What must you assess before the cardiac blood pool scan is administered?

Assess if the patient:
- Has any allergies
- Has recently undergone radioactive tracer scans
- Has an implant in the chest, such as a pacemaker
- Is wearing comfortable clothes, if the patient will be asked to exercise
- Can lie still on his or her back
- Has recently had a barium enema
- If the patient is pregnant. The cardiac blood pool scan is not performed if the patient is pregnant.
- Has not eaten 4 hours before the scan
- Has not ingested caffeine 6 hours before the scan
- Has not smoked 6 hours before the scan
- Has provided the healthcare provider with all medications that the patient takes. Digoxin and nitrate medication can affect the scan results.

19.9   What is an abnormal finding of the cardiac blood pool scan?

An abnormal finding of the cardiac blood pool scan is less than 55% ejection fraction, inadequate cardiac contractions, abnormal cardiac structures, or improper blood flow through the heart.

Cardiac Calcium Scoring

19.10   What is cardiac calcium scoring?

Calcium scoring determines the level of calcium containing plaque on the coronary artery walls.

19.11   How would you respond to a patient who is concerned that she might have a high cardiac calcium score?

A patient can have a high cardiac calcium score without having coronary artery disease. Healthcare providers use a variety of assessment methods to determine if the patient has coronary artery disease.

19.12   What would you assess before the cardiac calcium score test is administered?

Assess if the patient:
- Is claustrophobic
- Can lie still on his or her back
- Has removed jewelry
- Has ingested caffeine
- Has smoked

19.13   What is an abnormal cardiac calcium score?

- Score 11 to 100 = Plaque was found. Patient has mild coronary artery disease.
- Score 101 to 400 = Plaque was found. Patient has coronary artery disease and possibly a blockage of one or more coronary arteries.
- Score > 400 = Plaque was found. Patient has coronary artery disease and there is a 90% chance that there is a blockage of one or more coronary arteries.

Electrocardiogram

19.14   What is telemetry?

Telemetry is a type of electrocardiogram that used in a healthcare facility to constantly monitor the patient's cardiac activity. Cardiac electrical activity is transmitted by a transmitter worn by the patient connected to a telemetry monitor at the nurse's station. An alarm is sounded whenever there is abnormal cardiac activity. A telemetry nurse interprets the tracing on the telemetry monitor and prints the tracing while taking appropriate action

19.15   What is a Holter monitoring electrocardiogram?

The Holter monitoring electrocardiogram, sometimes referred to as an ambulatory electrocardiogram, is a type of portable electrocardiogram that is attached to the patient for 24 hours. The Holter monitoring electrocardiogram is worn on the patient's waist or around his or her shoulder enabling the healthcare provider to detect abnormal electrical activity of the patient's heart during activities of daily living such as when the patient exercises and is sleeping.

19.16   What is an event monitor?

An event monitor is the button the patient presses whenever a cardiac symptom occurs, causing the Holter monitor to record cardiac activity.

19.17   What is a loop recorder?

A loop recorder is the Holter monitor constantly recording cardiac electrical activity. The patient presses a button whenever a cardiac symptom occurs.

19.18   Why is an electrocardiogram ordered by the healthcare provider?

An electrocardiogram assesses the cause of chest pain, palpitations, and other symptoms, the effects of medication on the heart, signs and symptoms of heart disease, and the performance of a pacemaker.

19.19   What should you assess before the ECG is administered?

Assess if the patient:
- Can lie still on his or her back
- Has removed jewelry

Cardiac Perfusion Scan

19.20   Why is a cardiac perfusion scan ordered by the healthcare provider?

The cardiac perfusion scan assesses the underlying cause of chest pain and the results of angioplasty and bypass surgery.

19.21   What does the cardiac perfusion scan measure?

The cardiac perfusion scan is used to determine if the heart is receiving sufficient blood supply. The cardiac perfusion scan is commonly performed to determine the volume of blood in cardiac muscle during stress and at rest.

19.22   What must be assessed before the patient undergoes the cardiac perfusion scan?

Assess if the patient:
- Can lie still on his or her back
- Has allergies
- Is taking Viagra, Cialis, or Levitra within two days of the procedure. This can cause the patient's blood pressure to fall if the patient is administered nitroglycerin during the procedure
- Is taking anticoagulants such as coumadin, aspirin, or heparin
- Is taking trental or persantine
- Is pregnant
- Is breastfeeding. If so, the patient must discard breast milk collected 2 days following the test, since the breast milk will contact the radioactive tracer
- Has eaten or drunk 3 hours before the test

- Has avoided ingesting caffeine, alcohol, and tobacco one day before the test
- Has removed jewelry
- Can exercise
- Recently had a heart attack or myocarditis
- Has a pacemaker
- Has an electrolyte imbalance

19.23 What should you teach the patient before the patient undergoes the cardiac perfusion scan?

Explain why the test is being performed, what the patient will experience during the procedure, that the patient might feel flushed, nauseous, dizzy, or have a headache if medication is administered to place the patient's heart under stress, and that the patient will not feel any pain during the procedure except for a pinch from the needle used to administer the trace material. The patient should not drink or eat 3 hours before the procedure and should tell the healthcare provider if the patient takes Viagra, Cialis, Levitra, coumadin, aspirin, heparin, trental, or persantine. The patient should tell the healthcare provider during the test if the patient experiences fatigue, chest pain, shortness of breath, aching in the lower extremities, or lightheadedness while the test is in progress. The patient will be required to remove jewelry, may resume normal activities following the test, and should call for emergency medical care if he or she experiences difficulty breathing or chest pains after leaving the healthcare facilities following the test.

Ankle-Brachial Index

19.24 What is assessed by the ankle-brachial index?

The ankle-brachial index (ABI) evaluates circulation in the lower extremities for peripheral arterial disease.

19.25 What should you assess before the patient undergoes the ankle-brachial index test?

Assess if the patient:
- Is able to have blood pressure taken in both arms and legs
- Can lie on his or her back
- Can walk on a treadmill
- Is wearing comfortable clothes
- Has been diagnosed with arterial disease

CHAPTER 20

Lung Tests and Procedures

20.1 Definition

Tests and procedures performed on lungs help the healthcare provider determine if the patient has lung disease and how to treat the disease, if is exists. The lungs exchange carbon dioxide and oxygen on the hemoglobin in red blood cells. In order to do so effectively, the lungs must be able to expand and retract and blood must freely flow to the lungs. When the patient experiences signs and symptoms of lung disorder and disease, the healthcare provider tests the lungs and orders procedures to evaluate the respiratory system. The healthcare provider can examine the respiratory tract using a bronchoscopy and remove samples of suspicious tissue for microscopic examination.

The capacity and function of the lungs are measured using several pulmonary function tests. Blood flow to the lungs is monitored by a lung scan and by performing a pulmonary angiogram to identify restriction or blockage of blood flow to the lungs. This is also performed using CT imaging. The patient may experience difficulty breathing when excess fluid builds in the plural space, inhibiting the expansion of the lung. A thoracentesis is sometimes performed, which removes the excess fluid. Diseases such as lung cancer can destroy part or the entire lung, requiring the healthcare provider to surgically remove a portion (wedge resection), lobes of the lung (lobectomy), or the entire lung (puneumonectomy).

20.2 Lung Scan

A lung scan is performed to detect pulmonary emboli that impede blood flow in the lungs. There are three types of lung scans:

1. **Perfusion Scan**: In a perfusion scan, the patient is injected with a radioactive tracer into a blood vessel. An image is taken of the lungs as the tracer circulates to the lungs. Pulmonary emboli are suspected in areas of the lung where the tracer is not seen.
2. **Ventilation Scan**: In a ventilation scan, the patient inhales gas that contains a radioactive tracer. An image is taken of the lungs. Pulmonary emboli are suspected in areas of the lung that are not receiving the tracer.
3. **V/Q Scan**: A V/Q scan consists of both the perfusion scan and the ventilation scan. The ventilation scan is performed first. This is the most commonly performed lung scan.

Why the Test Is Performed

The test assesses blood flow to the lungs.

Before Administering the Test

Assess if the patient:

- Has signed a consent form
- Takes anticoagulants such as coumadin, aspirin, heparin, or Plavix

- Is pregnant
- Can lie still on his or her back
- Has pulmonary disease
- Has cardiac disease
- Can hold his or her breath for 10 seconds, if the ventilation scan is performed
- Has taken Pepto-Bismol or barium prior to the procedure

How Is the Test Performed

- The patient will remove his or her clothes.
- The patient lies on a table.
- Perfusion scan:
  - The radioactive trace is injected into the patient's arm.
- Ventilation scan:
  - A mask is placed over the patient's mouth and nose.
  - The patient is asked to take a deep breath to inhale a mixture of oxygen and tracer gas and hold his or her breath for 10 seconds as the image is taken.
- The scanning camera is placed over the patient's chest.
- The patient must remain still when each image is taken.
- The scanning camera may be repositioned during the procedure.
- The patient may be repositioned during the procedure.

Teach the Patient

Explain why the procedure is being performed, that the patient will need to sign a consent form, what the patient will experience during the procedure, and that the patient will not feel any pain during the procedure except for a pinch from the needle used to administer the tracer, if the perfusion scan is performed. Inform the patient that he or she must tell the healthcare provider if taking anticoagulants, he or she may be asked to change position during the procedure, and that he or she might have swelling at the injection site that is relieved by placing warm compresses on the site. The patient should promptly flush the toilet and wash hands thoroughly with soap and water after using the toilet following the procedure, since the tracer exits the body in urine and stool. The patient should discard any breast milk up to 2 days following the procedure if the patient is breastfeeding.

Understanding the Results

The lung scan takes about 30 minutes to perform. The results are usually known immediately.

- Normal:
  - Normal blood flow throughout the lungs
- Abnormal:
  - Obstructed blood flow in a portion of the lungs
  - A pulmonary emboli identified

20.3　Pulmonary Function Tests

Pulmonary function tests assess how well the patient's lungs perform. These tests are:

- **Gas Diffusion Tests**: Measure the amount of gases that cross the alveoli per minute. These include arterial blood gases and the carbon monoxide diffusing capacity.
- **Spirometry Test**: Measures the volume and capacity of the lungs.
- **Exercise Stress Test**: Measures the effect exercise has on the lungs.
- **Body Plethysmograph Test**: Measures the volume and capacity of the lungs.
- **Inhalation Challenge Test**: Assesses the patient's airway responses to allergens.

Why the Test Is Performed

The test assesses the function of the patient's lungs and monitors the progress of lung therapy.

Before Administering the Test

Assess if the patient:

- Has not eaten a large meal 8 hours before the test
- Is able to have his or her nose pinched
- Is able to breathe through a mouthpiece
- Is able to breathe normally
- Is able to follow directions during the test
- Has removed dentures, if the dentures prevent a tight seal around the patient's mouth
- Has not smoked 6 hours before the test
- Has not ingested caffeine 6 hours before the test
- Has not exercised 6 hours before the test
- Is wearing comfortable clothes, if the patient is taking the exercise stress test
- Has taken medication that affects the respiratory tract
- Has taken a sedative before the test
- Has cardiovascular disease
- Has allergies
- Is not pregnant

How Is the Test Performed

- A nose clip may be placed on the patient's nose to prevent the patient from breathing through his nose, depending on the test that is being performed.
- A mouthpiece connected to the measuring device is placed in the patient's mouth.
- Gas Diffusion Test:
  - Arterial Blood Gases:
    - A needle is inserted into an artery in the patient's arm.
    - A sample of blood is removed from an artery.
    - Pressure is placed on the site for approximately 5 minutes to stop any bleeding.
    - A bandage is then placed over the site.
  - Carbon Monoxide Diffusing Capacity:
    - A mask is connected to a container of a mixture of air and a small amount of carbon monoxide.
    - The patient breathes the gas mixture.
    - A mouthpiece connected to the measuring device is placed in the patient's mouth.
    - The patient exhales. The amount of carbon monoxide in the patient's breath is measured by the device. This is referred to as the diffusing capacity of the patient's lungs.
- Spirometry Test
  - A nose clip is placed on the patient's nose to prevent the patient from breathing through his or her nose.
  - A mouthpiece connected to the spirometery is placed in the patient's mouth.
  - The patient inhales, and then exhales with force to measure the forced vital capacity (FVC). The exhaled air flow is also measured halfway through the exhale to measure the forced expiratory flow 25% to 75%. The peak exhale flow is measured, which is referred to as the peak expiratory flow (PEF).
  - The patient inhales, then exhales with force. The amount of air exhaled is measured each second for three seconds to determine the forced expiratory volume (FEV).
  - The patient is asked to take a deep breath and then exhale to measure the maximum voluntary ventilation (MVV).

- The patient is asked to take a deep breath and then slowly exhale to measure the slow vital capacity (SVC) and the total lung capacity (TLC).
- The patient is asked to take a normal breath and exhale to measure the functional residual capacity (FRC).
- The patient is asked to inhale normally and then exhale with force (RV). The amount exhaled is subtracted from the functional residual capacity (FRC) to calculate the expiratory reserve volume (ERV).
- The patient's expiratory reserve volume (ERF) is calculated by subtracting the reserve volume from the functional residual capacity (FRC).
- Exercise Stress Test:
  - The patient undergoes a spirometry test.
  - The patient exercises.
  - The patient undergoes another spirometry test.
  - Results of both spirometry tests are compared to assess the patient's lung function before and after exercising.
- Inhalation Challenge Test:
  - The patient undergoes a spirometry test.
  - The patient places a face mask over his or her nose and mouth.
  - The face mask is attached to a nebulizer.
  - An allergen is gradually added to the mixture in the nebulizer.
  - The patient inhales a fine mist that contains the allergen from the nebulizer.
  - The patient is monitored for bronchospasm that may be triggered by the allergen.
  - The patient undergoes another spirometry test.
  - The results of both spirometry tests are compared to determine the effect that the allergen had on the patient.
- Body Plethysmography Test:
  - The patient sits inside an airtight plethysmograph booth.
  - The booth is filled with a mixture of oxygen and helium or 100% oxygen.
  - Instruments attached to the booth measure pressure changes within the booth as the patient breathes.

Teach the Patient

Explain why the procedure is being performed, what the patient will experience during the procedure, and that the patient will not feel any pain during the test except if the patient undergoes the arterial blood gas test, during which the patient will feel a pinch when the needle is inserted into the patient's arm. The patient should avoid taking a sedative prior to the test. The patient may be asked to stop taking respiratory medication 24 hours before the test and may be able to resume taking medication after the test. The patient may be given instructions during the test, should not eat a big meal 8 hours before the test, and should wear comfortable clothes the day of the test, especially if the patient is undergoing an exercise stress test.

Explain that the patient should promptly flush the toilet and wash hands thoroughly with soap and water after using the toilet following the procedure, since the tracer exits in the body in urine and stool. The patient should discard any breast milk up to two days following the procedure, if the patient is breastfeeding. The patient should also tell the healthcare provider if he or she feels lightheaded when breathing rapidly during the test. The patient will be given time to adjust his or her breathing, which normally relieves the lightheadedness.

Understanding the Results

The lung scan takes about 30 minutes to perform. The results are usually known immediately.

- Normal:
  - Normal for age, height, sex, weight, and race
- Abnormal:
  - Decreased pulmonary function based on the patient's age, height, sex, weight, and race

Solved Problems

Lung Tests and Procedures

20.1 What does a healthcare provider use to examine the respiratory tract?

The healthcare provider can examine the respiratory tract using a bronchoscopy.

20.2 What is the purpose of a pulmonary function test?

The capacity and function of the lungs are measured using several pulmonary function tests.

20.3 What is a thoracentesis?

The patient may experience difficulty breathing when excess fluid builds in the plural space, inhibiting the expansion of the lung. A thoracentesis is sometimes performed, which removes the excess fluid.

Lung Scan

20.4 Why might the healthcare provider order a lung scan?

A lung scan is performed to detect pulmonary emboli that impede blood flow in the lungs.

20.5 What is a perfusion scan?

In a perfusion scan, the patient is injected with a radioactive tracer into a blood vessel. An image is taken of the lungs as the tracer circulates to the lungs. Pulmonary emboli are suspected in areas of the lung where the tracer is not seen.

20.6 How is a ventilation scan administered?

In a ventilation scan, the patient inhales gas that contains a radioactive tracer. An image is taken of the lungs. Pulmonary emboli are suspected in areas of the lung that are not receiving the tracer.

20.7 What is a V/Q scan?

A V/Q scan consists of both the perfusion scan and the ventilation scan. The ventilation scan is performed first. This is the most commonly performed lung scan.

20.8 What should you assess before the patient undergoes a lung scan?

Assess if the patient:
- Has signed a consent form
- Takes anticoagulants such as coumadin, aspirin, heparin, or Plavix
- Is pregnant
- Can lie still on his or her back
- Has pulmonary disease
- Has cardiac disease
- Can hold his or her breath for 10 seconds, if the ventilation scan is performed
- Has taken Pepto-Bismol or barium prior to the procedure

20.9 What should you teach the patient who is undergoing a lung scan?

Explain why the procedure is being performed, that the patient will need to sign a consent form, what the patient will experience during the procedure, and that the patient will not feel any pain during the procedure except for a pinch from the needle used to administer the tracer, if the perfusion scan is performed. The patient must tell the healthcare provider if the patient is taking anticoagulants, may be asked to change position during the procedure, and might have swelling at the injection site, which is relieved by placing warm compresses on the site.

20.10 Why should a patient who has undergone a lung scan discard breast milk?

The patient should discard any breast milk up to 2 days following the procedure if the patient is breastfeeding, because it may contain the tracer that was administered during the lung scan.

20.11 What should the patient do when toileting following a lung scan?

The patient should promptly flush the toilet and wash hands thoroughly with soap and water after using the toilet following the procedure, since the tracer exits the body in urine and stool.

20.12   How would you respond if the patient asks how long it takes to complete the lung scan?

The lung scan takes about 30 minutes to perform.

20.13   How would you respond if the patient who has undergone a ventilation scan questions why he has to use precautions when toileting following the scan?

The patient is asked to take a deep breath to inhale a mixture of oxygen and tracer gas and hold his breath for 10 seconds as the image is taken. The tracer is radioactive.

20.14   How would you respond if the patient is concerned about tissue damage caused by the tracer used in the lung scan?

Explain that a very low dose of radiation is used that causes practically no tissue damage. The benefits of undergoing the lung scan outweigh the risk of tissue damage.

Pulmonary Function Tests

20.15   What is an exercise stress test?

An exercise stress test measures the effect exercise has on the lungs.

20.16   How would you explain a gas diffusion test to a patient?

A gas diffusion test measures the amount of gasses that cross the alveoli per minute. These include arterial blood gases and the carbon monoxide diffusing capacity.

20.17   What does a body plethysmograph test measure?

A body plethysmograph test measures the volume and capacity of the lungs.

20.18   Why might a healthcare provider administer a spirometry test?

A spirometry test measures the volume and capacity of the lungs.

20.19   Why is the inhalation challenge test administered?

The inhalation challenge test assesses the patient's airway responses to allergens.

20.20   What should you assess before the patient is administered a pulmonary function test?

Assess if the patient:
- Has not eaten a heavy meal 8 hours before the test
- Is able to have his or her nose pinched
- Is able to breathe through a mouthpiece
- Is able to breathe normally
- Is able to follow directions during the test
- Has removed dentures, if the dentures prevent a tight seal around the patient's mouth
- Has not smoked 6 hours before the test
- Has not ingested caffeine 6 hours before the test
- Has not exercised 6 hours before the test
- Is wearing comfortable clothes, if the patient is taking the exercise stress test
- Has taken medication that affects the respiratory tract
- Has taken a sedative before the test
- Has cardiovascular disease
- Has allergies
- Is not pregnant

20.21   How is carbon monoxide diffusing capacity measured?

- A mask is connected to a container of a mixture of air and a small amount of carbon monoxide.
- The patient breathes the gas mixture.
- A mouthpiece connected to the measuring device is placed in the patient's mouth.
- The patient exhales. The amount of carbon monoxide in the patient's breath is measured by the device. This is referred to as the diffusing capacity of the patient's lungs.

20.22   How is the spirometry test administered?

- A nose clip is placed on the patient's nose to prevent the patient from breathing through his or her nose.
- A mouthpiece connected to the spirometry is placed in the patient's mouth.
- The patient inhales, and then exhales with force to measure the forced vital capacity (FVC). The exhaled air flow is also measured halfway through the exhale to measure the forced expiratory flow 25% to 75%. The peak exhale flow is measured, which is referred to as the peak expiratory flow (PEF).
- The patient inhales, then exhales with force. The amount of air exhaled is measured each second for three seconds to determine the forced expiratory volume (FEV).
- The patient is asked to take a deep breath and then exhale to measure the maximum voluntary ventilation (MVV).
- The patient is asked to take a deep breath and then slowly exhale to measure the slow vital capacity (SVC) and the total lung capacity (TLC).
- The patient is asked to take a normal breath and exhale to measure the functional residual capacity (FRC).
- The patient is asked to inhale normally and then exhale with force (RV). The amount that is exhaled is subtracted from the functional residual capacity (FRC) to calculate the expiratory reserve volume (ERV).
- The patient's expiratory reserve volume (ERF) is calculated by subtracting the reserve volume from the functional residual capacity (FRC).
- The radioactive trace is injected into the patient's arm.

20.23   How is the exercise stress test administered?

- The patient undergoes a spirometry test.
- The patient exercises.
- The patient undergoes another spirometry test.
- Results of both spirometry tests are compared to assess the patient's lung function before and after exercising.

20.24   How is the inhalation challenge test administered?

- The patient undergoes a spirometry test.
- The patient places a face mask over his or her nose and mouth.
- The face mask is attached to a nebulizer.
- An allergen is gradually added to the mixture in the nebulizer.
- The patient inhales a fine mist that contains the allergen from the nebulizer.
- The patient is monitored for bronchospasm that may be triggered by the allergen.
- The patient undergoes another spirometry test.
- The results of both spirometry tests are compared to determine the effect that the allergen had on the patient.

20.25   How is the body plethysmograph test administered?

- The patient sits inside an airtight plethysmograph booth.
- The booth is filled with a mixture of oxygen and helium or 100% oxygen.
- Instruments attached to the booth measure pressure changes within the booth as the patient breathes.

CHAPTER 21

Women's Health Tests and Procedures

21.1　Definition

Women's health tests and procedures are administered to assess the health of the female patient. Female patients routinely undergo breast and cervical examinations for signs of cysts, growths, abnormal tissue, structural abnormalities, and infection. When a mammogram reveals a suspicious growth, the healthcare provider usually orders a breast ultrasound to closely examine the growth and then possibly a breast biopsy. If the tissue sample is cancerous, the healthcare provider may perform a mastectomy. A mastectomy may be performed even if there are not any signs of breast cancer. The patient may decide to have her breasts altered for therapeutic or cosmetic reasons. There are a number of tests used to examine the patient's vulva, vagina, cervix, uterus, and fallopian tubes. Many of these tests enable the healthcare provider to take a tissue sample or perform a biopsy on abnormal tissue. If the tissue sample is identified to be cancerous, the cancerous organ is removed.

21.2　Breast Cancer Gene Test (BRCA)

The breast cancer gene test determines if the patient's BRCA1 and BRCA2 genes are mutated. Scientists have discovered two genes called the breast cancer genes (BRCA1, BRCA2) that if mutated are associated with breast and ovarian cancer. A patient who carries this mutated gene and who has a family history of breast or ovarian cancer may have a higher than normal chance of developing cancer or ovarian cancer. The patient also has a chance of not developing these cancers. The presence of the breast cancer gene does not mean that the patient will develop breast or ovarian cancer. However, some patients may decide to have a prophylactic mastectomy and/or oophorectomy to lessen their risk of these cancers developing. Patients who test positive may also be advised to take tamoxifen to inhibit this gene. Male patients who have a family history of breast cancer and prostate cancer may also have this gene. These patients can also develop breast cancer and prostate cancer.

Why the Test Is Performed

The test assesses the patient's chances of developing breast cancer or ovarian cancer. It also provides information so the patient may decide to take preventive measures.

Before Administering the Test

Assess if the patient:

- Has signed a consent form
- Has taken anticoagulant medication such as Plavix, coumadin, heparin, or aspirin
- Has undergone genetic counseling to understand the significance of this test

How Is the Test Performed

- The healthcare provider removes a blood sample from a vein in the patient's arm.
- The blood sample is sent to the laboratory for examination.

Teach the Patient

Explain why the test is being performed, what the patient will experience during the test, that the patient will have to sign a consent form, and that the patient should undergo genetic counseling before the test is administered to fully understand the significance of the test. A negative result does not mean that the patient will not develop breast or ovarian cancer. A positive result does not mean that the patient will develop breast or ovarian cancer. It means there is a higher probability if the patient also has a strong history of breast or ovarian cancer. The patient should undergo genetic counseling if the test is positive or is uncertain she fully understands the significance of these results.

Understanding the Results

The procedure takes less than 1 hour. Results are ready within 2 weeks of the procedure. A normal result does not mean that the patient will not develop breast or ovarian cancer.

- Normal (negative):
  - The BRCA1 and BRCA2 genes are not mutated
- Uncertain (variant of uncertain significances VUS):
  - It is undetermined if the BRCA1 and BRCA2 genes are mutated
- Abnormal (positive):
  - One or both BRCA1 and BRCA2 genes are mutated
  - Positive for endometrial hyperplasia
  - Cancer cells were present in the sample

21.3   Breast Ultrasound

A breast ultrasound is performed to examine suspicious findings of a mammogram. Breast ultrasound technology can differentiate between a cyst and solid tissue. A breast ultrasound can examine areas of the breast that are difficult to view in a mammogram.

Why the Test Is Performed

The test determines if a lump in the breast is a cyst or a solid mass, assesses suspicious results from a mammogram, assesses the underlying cause of swelling and pain in the breast, guides the healthcare provider in taking a breast biopsy, and assesses breast implants.

Before Administering the Test

Assess if the patient:

- Can sit or lie on her back

How the Test Is Performed

- The patient removes her clothes from above the waist.
- The patient either sits or lies on a table.
- A conductive gel is placed on the ultrasound transducer.
- The ultrasound transducer is pressed on and moved around the breast.
- Images of breast tissue are displayed on a computer screen.
- Any conductive gel remaining on the breast is removed.

Teach the Patient

Explain why the procedure is being performed, what the patient will experience during the procedure, and that the patient may feel pain if she has a fibrocystic breast.

Understanding the Results

The procedure takes less than 1 hour. Preliminary results are immediate. Complete results are within 2 days.

- Normal:
  - Normal breast tissue
- Abnormal:
  - The lump is identified as a cyst
  - The lump is identified as a solid mass

21.4 Pap Smear

A Pap smear is a procedure the removes sample cells from the cervix to assess if there are any abnormal cells. The sample is sent to the laboratory for microscopic identification. Further examination is necessary if the sample is positive, indicating abnormal cells on the cervix. A negative Pap smear result does not mean that the patient is free from cervical cancer. It means that no abnormal cells were contained in the tissue sample. Abnormal cells might exist in areas of the cervix that were not sampled.

Why the Test Is Performed

The test assesses cervical tissue and identifies abnormal tissue that might be cancerous.

Before Administering the Test

Assess if the patient:

- Has taken anticoagulant medication such as Plavix, coumadin, heparin, or aspirin
- Can lie on her back
- Is pregnant
- Is using birth control
- Has undergone cervical surgery
- Is taking the test 8 to 12 days after her menstrual period
- Has not used a tampon 24 hours prior to the procedure
- Has not douched 24 hours prior to the procedure
- Has not administered vaginal medications 24 hours prior to the procedure
- Is not having her menstrual period
- Did not have a pelvic, cervix, or vaginal infection within 6 weeks prior to the procedure
- Has been the victim of rape. If so, the patient may not feel comfortable having a pelvic exam or a Pap smear performed.

How the Test Is Performed

- The patient removes her clothes below the waist.
- The patient lies on a table with her feet in stirrups.
- A speculum is placed into the vagina to spread the vaginal walls.
- The healthcare provider inserts a cytobrush to gather samples from several areas of the cervix and from the endocervical canal.
- The tissue sample is sent to the laboratory for identification.

Teach the Patient

Explain why the procedure is being performed and what the patient will experience during the procedure. Inform the patient not to use a tampon 24 hours prior to the procedure, not to douche 24 hours prior to the procedure, and not to use vaginal medications 24 hours prior to the procedure. The patient cannot have the procedure performed during her menstrual period and cannot have the procedure performed if she had a pelvic, cervix, or vaginal infection within six weeks prior to the procedure. There may be a small amount of vaginal bleeding following the procedure.

Understanding the Results

The procedure takes less than 30 minutes. Results are available within 2 weeks.

- Normal:
  - Normal cervical tissue
- Abnormal:
  - Abnormal cervical tissue
- Inconclusive:
  - The sample did not contain a sufficient amount of cells to make a determination if cells were normal

21.5   Vaginosis Tests

Vaginosis tests involve the healthcare provider taking a sample of vaginal discharge and sending the sample to a laboratory for examination to determine the cause of vaginosis. Vaginosis is the inflammation of the vulva and vagina, caused by an infection or a reaction to an irritant and results in a painful vaginal discharge and itching. The most common causes of vaginosis are:

- *Candida albicans*: This is a yeast infection that causes lumpy white discharge and itching.
- *Trichomonas vaginalis*: This causes a foamy yellow-green odorous vaginal discharge.
- *Bacterial vaginosis*: This causes a milky thick vaginal discharge that gives off a fishy odor.

There are four vaginosis tests:

1. **Whiff Test**: Potassium hydroxide solution is dropped on the sample. If a fishy order emanates, then the patient has bacterial vaginosis.
2. **KOH Slide**: The sample is mixed with potassium hydroxide solution. Only the yeast remains on the slide, indicating that the patient has a yeast infection.
3. **Wet Mount**: The sample is mixed with saline on a slide. The laboratory technician then identifies through microscopic examination the organism that is causing the infection.
4. **Vaginal pH**: The pH level of the sample is tested. A pH level greater than 4.5 indicates bacterial vaginosis.

Why the Test Is Performed

The test assesses the cause of vaginal itch, inflammation, and discharge, and identifies the treatment for vaginosis.

Before Administering the Test

Assess if the patient:

- Has taken anticoagulant medication such as Plavix, coumadin, heparin, or aspirin.
- Can lie on her back.
- Is pregnant.
- Is using birth control.
- Has undergone cervical surgery.
- Is taking the test 8 to 12 days after her menstrual period.

- Has not had sexual intercourse 24 hours before the procedure.
- Has not used a tampon 24 hours prior to the procedure.
- Has not douched 24 hours prior to the procedure.
- Has not administered vaginal medications 24 hours prior to the procedure.
- Is not having her menstrual period.
- Has been the victim of rape. If so, the patient may not feel comfortable having a sample of the discharge taken.

How the Test Is Performed

- The patient removes her clothes below the waist.
- The patient lies on a table with her feet in stirrups.
- A speculum is placed into the vagina to spread the vaginal walls.
- The healthcare provider inserts a swab to gather a sample of the discharge.
- The sample is sent to the laboratory for identification.

Teach the Patient

Explain why the procedure is being performed, what the patient will experience during the procedure, and that the patient will have to sign a consent form. Inform the patient not to use a tampon 24 hours prior to the procedure, not to douche 24 hours prior to the procedure, and not to use vaginal medications 24 hours prior to the procedure. The patient cannot have the procedure performed during her menstrual period and should not have sexual intercourse 24 hours before the procedure. There will be a small amount of vaginal bleeding following the procedure.

Understanding the Results

The procedure takes less than 30 minutes. Results are available within 2 days.

- Normal:
  - Normal vaginal discharge. No vaginosis.
- Abnormal:
  - Presence of a microorganism that is causing vaginosis.

21.6   Sperm Penetration Tests

Sperm penetration tests are performed when a woman is having difficulty becoming pregnant to determine if the sperm can move through the cervical mucus and into the fallopian tubes. There are two types of sperm penetration tests:

1. **Sperm Penetration Assay**: This test mixes sperm with hamster eggs to see if the sperm can penetrate the egg. The result is measured as a sperm capacitation index.
2. **Sperm Mucus Penetration**: This test determines if sperm can move through the cervical mucus.

Why the Test Is Performed

The test determines the underlying cause of infertility.

Before Administering the Test

Assess if the patient:

- Has ejaculated 2 days before the semen sample is taken
- Has ejaculated within 5 days before the semen sample is taken

- Has urinated before the semen sample was taken
- Washed his hands and penis before the semen sample was taken
- Did not use lubricants or condoms when collecting the semen sample
- Did not collect a semen sample after withdrawing from intercourse
- Placed the semen sample in a sterile cup
- Kept the sample at body temperature
- Kept the sample from direct sunlight
- Delivered the sample to the lab immediately
- Was ovulating during the test
- Has signed a consent form

How the Test Is Performed

- The patient signs a consent form.
- Sperm Penetration Assay:
  - Ejaculation should not occur for 2 days before the semen sample is taken.
  - Ejaculation should occur within 5 days before the semen sample is taken.
  - Before the semen sample is taken, the patient should urinate.
  - The patient's hands and penis should be washed.
  - Do not use lubricants or condoms when collecting the sample.
  - Do not collect a semen sample after withdrawing from intercourse.
  - Place the semen sample in a sterile cup.
  - Keep the sample at body temperature.
  - Keep the sample from direct sunlight.
  - Deliver the sample to the lab immediately.
  - The lab will mix the semen with hamster eggs to determine the sperm capacitation index.
- Sperm Mucus Penetration Test:
  - The woman must be ovulating in order to perform this test.
  - Determine if she is ovulating by collecting a urine sample in the mid- to late morning.
  - The woman should avoid drinking fluids before giving a urine sample.
  - The urine sample is analyzed for the presence of luteinizing hormone (LH). This hormone indicates that she is ovulating.
  - The woman is given a pelvic exam during which a sample of cervical mucus is collected.
  - The man provides a semen sample (see Sperm Penetration Assay above).
  - The cervical mucus and the semen samples are mixed in the lab to determine if sperm can move through the cervical mucus.

Teach the Patient

Explain why the procedure is being performed, what the patient will experience during the procedure, that the patient will not feel any pain during the procedure, that the patient must sign a consent form, and how to collect the semen sample.

Understanding the Results

The procedure takes less than 1 hour. Results are known within 2 days.

- Normal:
  - Sperm penetrated the hamster egg
  - Sperm moved through the cervical mucus
- Abnormal:
  - Sperm could not penetrate the hamster egg
  - Sperm could not move through the cervical mucus

Solved Problems

Breast Cancer Gene Test

21.1 What are BRCA1 and BRCA2?

Scientists have discovered two genes called the breast cancer genes (BRCA1, BRCA2), that if mutated are associated with breast and ovarian cancer.

21.2 What is the importance of the BRCA genes?

A patient who carries this mutated gene and who has a family history of breast or ovarian cancer may have a higher than normal chance of developing breast cancer or ovarian cancer.

21.3 What would you say if the patient told you she has the BRCA genes?

The presence of the breast cancer gene does not mean that the patient will develop breast cancer or ovarian cancer.

21.4 What might the healthcare provider recommend for a patient who tests positive for the BRCA genes?

Patients who test positive may be advised to take tamoxifen to inhibit this gene.

21.5 Can a male have the BRCA genes?

Male patients who have a family history of breast cancer and prostate cancer may also have this gene. These patients can also develop breast cancer and prostate cancer.

21.6 Does a patient who tests positive for the BRCA genes always develop breast cancer?

The patient also has a chance of not developing these cancers.

21.7 What precautionary procedures might a patient request if the patient tests positive for BRCA genes?

Some patients may decide to have a mastectomy and/or oophorectomy to prevent these cancers from developing.

21.8 What should be assessed before administering the BRCA test?
Assess if the patient:
- Has signed a consent form
- Has taken anticoagulant medication such as Plavix, coumadin, heparin, or aspirin
- Has undergone genetic counseling to understand the significance of this test

21.9 How is the BRCA test performed?

The healthcare provider removes a blood sample from a vein in the patient's arm. The blood sample is sent to the laboratory for examination.

Breast Ultrasound

21.10 Why might a breast ultrasound be ordered by a healthcare provider?

A breast ultrasound determines if a lump in the breast is a cyst or a solid mass, assesses suspicious results from a mammogram, assesses the underlying cause of swelling and pain in the breast, guides the healthcare provider in taking a breast biopsy, and assesses breast implants.

21.11 How is the breast ultrasound performed?

- The patient removes her clothes from above the waist.
- The patient either sits or lies on a table.
- A conductive gel is placed on the ultrasound transducer.
- The ultrasound transducer is pressed on and moved around the breast.
- Images of breast tissue are displayed on a computer screen.
- Any conductive gel remaining on the breast is removed.

21.12 What should you teach the patient about a breast ultrasound?

Explain why the procedure is being performed, what the patient will experience during the procedure, and that the patient may feel pain if she has a fibrocystic breast.

21.13 What are abnormal findings of a breast ultrasound?

Abnormal findings of a breast ultrasound are that a lump is identified as a cyst or as a solid mass.

Pap Smear

21.14 What is a Pap smear?

A Pap smear is a procedure the removes sample cells from the cervix to assess if there are any abnormal cells.

21.15 How would you respond to a patient when the patient says, "I'm free from cervical cancer because my Pap smear result is negative."?

A negative Pap smear result does not mean that the patient is free from cervical cancer. It means that no abnormal cells were contained in the tissue sample. Abnormal cells might exist in areas of the cervix that were not sampled.

21.16 Why might a Pap smear be ordered by a healthcare provider?

The test assesses cervical tissue and identifies abnormal tissue that might be cancerous.

21.17 What should be assessed before the Pap smear is administered?

Assess if the patient:
- Has taken anticoagulant medication such as Plavix, coumadin, heparin, or aspirin
- Can lie on her back
- Is pregnant
- Is using birth control
- Has undergone cervical surgery
- Is taking the test 8 to 12 days after her menstrual period
- Has not used a tampon 24 hours prior to the procedure
- Has not douched 24 hours prior to the procedure
- Has not administered vaginal medications 24 hours prior to the procedure
- Is not having her menstrual period
- Did not have a pelvic, cervical, or vaginal infection within six weeks prior to the procedure

21.18 Why is it important to know if the patient has ever been a victim of rape?

Assess if the patient has been the victim of rape. If so, the patient may not feel comfortable having a pelvic exam or a Pap smear performed.

21.19 How is a Pap smear performed?

- The patient removes her clothes below the waist.
- The patient lies on a table with her feet in stirrups.
- A speculum is placed into the vagina to spread the vaginal walls.
- The healthcare provider inserts a cytobrush to gather samples from several areas of the cervix and from the endocervical canal.
- The tissue sample is sent to the laboratory for identification.

21.20 What should you teach the patient who is going to have a Pap smear?

Explain why the procedure is being performed and what the patient will experience during the procedure. Inform the patient not to use a tampon 24 hours prior to the procedure, not to douche 24 hours prior to the procedure, and not to use vaginal medications 24 hours prior to the procedure. The patient cannot have the procedure performed during her menstrual period and cannot have the procedure performed if she had a pelvic, cervix, or vaginal infection within 6 weeks prior to the procedure. There may be a small amount of vaginal bleeding following the procedure.

21.21 Why might the Pap smear results be inconclusive?

The sample did not contain a sufficient amount of cells to make a determination if cells were normal.

Vaginosis Tests

21.22   What is vaginosis?

Vaginosis is the inflammation of the vulva and vagina caused by an infection or a reaction to an irritant, resulting in a painful vaginal discharge and itching.

21.23   What are the three most common causes of vaginosis?

- *Candida albicans*: This is a yeast infection that causes lumpy white discharge and itching.
- *Trichomonas vaginalis*: This causes a foamy yellow-green odorous vaginal discharge.
- *Bacterial vaginosis*: This causes a milky thick vaginal discharge that gives off a fishy odor.

21.24   What is the whiff test?

The whiff test is when potassium hydroxide solution is dropped on the sample. If a fishy order emanates, then the patient has bacterial vaginosis.

21.25   What is the vaginal pH test?

The vaginal pH test is when the pH level of the sample is tested. A pH level greater than 4.5 indicates bacterial vaginosis.

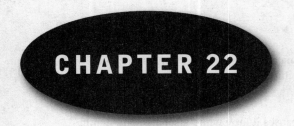

CHAPTER 22

Maternity Tests

22.1 Definition

Several tests might be performed during pregnancy and shortly after childbirth to assess the health of the fetus and newborn. In a high risk pregnancy, the healthcare provider might perform a chorionic villus sampling or amniocentesis early on to determine if the fetus has a genetic disorder or other health issues. Amniocentesis may be suggested in high risk pregnancies that have a high risk of birth defects. The risk for birth defects is confirmed by performing a cordocentesis where a sample of blood is taken from the umbilical cord while in the womb. Later in the pregnancy, the healthcare provider performs a biophysical profile of the fetus to determine the overall health of the fetus to assess:

- The fetal heart rate
- Breathing
- Body movements
- Muscle tone
- The volume of amniotic fluid

The mother may undergo a contraction stress test to determine if the fetus is healthy enough to survive the reduced oxygen levels that are common with natural childbirth. In some pregnancies, the woman might experience an incompetent cervix that could result in the cervix opening prior to the thirty-seventh week of gestation, causing a premature birth. In this situation, the healthcare provider is likely to perform a cervical cerclage, which temporarily closes the cervix until the mother enters labor. If the birth is premature, the healthcare provider may perform a cranial ultrasound to determine if there were complications caused by the premature birth. The newborn is typically administered the sweat test, which helps determine if the newborn has a high level of chloride in his or her sweat. This may be an indication of cystic fibrosis.

22.2 Biophysical Profile (BPP)

The biophysical profile test assesses the health of the fetus. This is commonly performed in the last trimester of the pregnancy. The healthcare provider may perform this test earlier and frequently in high risk pregnancies. The biophysical profile test consists of a non-stress test and a fetal ultrasound. Each element of the test is graded according to the following Table 22.1:

Why the Test Is Performed

The test assesses fetal movement, fetal heart rate, the volume of amniotic fluid, muscle tone, and breathing rate.

TABLE 22.1 Biophysical profile grading chart.

	NONSTRESS TEST	BREATHING MOVEMENT	BODY MOVEMENT	MUSCLE TONE	AMNIOTIC FLUID VOLUME
Normal (2 points)	2 or more heart rate increases with a rate of 15 minutes or greater while the fetus moves.	1 or more breathing movements of 60 seconds.	3 or more arm, leg, or body movements.	Flexed arms and legs. Head rests on chest. One or more extensions and flexion.	1 cm of amniotic fluid in the uterine cavity.
Abnormal (0 points)	1 or more heart rate increases or the rate is not 15 minutes or greater while the fetus moves.	Breathing movements of less than 60 seconds.	Less than 3 arm, leg, or body movements.	Arms, legs, and spine are extended. Open hand. Fetus not returning to normal position. Extension and flexion are slow.	Less than 1 cm of amniotic fluid in the uterine cavity.

Before Administering the Test

Assess if the patient:

- Can lie on her back
- Is able to lie still
- Is able to follow instructions
- Has not smoked two hours before the test
- Has a full bladder
- Is not hypoglycemic or hyperglycemic
- Is not using alcohol or narcotics

How the Test Is Performed

- The patient refrains from smoking two hours before the test.
- The patient must have a full bladder, except if patient is near term.
- If the patient is unable to fill her bladder, a urinary catheter is inserted into the urethra and saline will be infused into the bladder.
- The patient lies on a table with her abdomen exposed.
- Non-stress test:
  - Conductive gel is placed on her abdomen.
  - Two belts of the fetal monitor are placed on her abdomen to measure fetal heart rate and contractions.
  - The fetal monitor constantly records the fetus during the test. The results appear on a strip of paper.
  - The patient is asked to press a button connected to the fetal monitor each time the fetus moves and if there is a contraction.
  - The two belts of the fetal monitor are removed and the gel wiped from the patient's abdomen.
- Fetal ultrasound:
  - Conductive gel is applied to the patient's abdomen.
  - A transducer is pressed against and moved about the abdomen.
  - Images of the fetus appear on a computer screen.
  - Conductive gel is wiped off the abdomen.

Teach the Patient

Explain why the test is being performed, what the patient will experience during the test, that the patient will not feel any pain during the test, that the patient must not smoke 2 hours before the test, and that the patient must have a full bladder unless the patient is near term.

Understanding the Results

The procedure takes less than 30 minutes. Results are known immediately.

- Normal:
    - A score of 8 or greater.
- Undetermined:
    - A score of 5 to 8. The patient should be retested.
- Abnormal:
    - A score of less than 5. The healthcare provider will order different tests to further assess the fetus and mother.

22.3   Contraction Stress Test

The contraction stress test determines if the fetus will remain healthy during natural childbirth. A biophysical profile of the fetus assesses fetal breathing, movement, muscle tone, and the volume of amniotic fluid. If the biophysical profile indicates suspicious results, then the healthcare provider might perform a contraction stress test. Uterine contractions reduce oxygen to the fetus, which normally does not harm the fetus. Some fetuses can become negatively affected by the lower oxygen level, so the healthcare provider might decide on a caesarian birth.

During the contraction stress test a fetal heart monitor is attached to the mother while the mother is administered oxytocin. *Oxytocin* is a hormone that induces uterine contractions. The fetal heart rate is expected to decelerate during a contraction and accelerate following the contraction. If the heart rate does not accelerate, then the fetus may not remain healthy during natural childbirth. This test is not usually performed if the mother has had a past cesarean section, placenta previa, placenta abruptio, incompetent cervix, and premature rupture of the amniotic membrane. The test is also not usually performed if the patient has been administered magnesium sulfate or is pregnant with multiple fetuses.

Why the Test Is Performed

The test assesses the ability of the fetus to remain healthy during natural childbirth and the health of the placenta.

Before Administering the Test

Assess if the patient:

- Has signed a consent form
- Has any allergies
- Has taken anticoagulant medication such as Plavix, coumadin, heparin, or aspirin
- Can lie on her back
- Is able to lie still
- Is able to follow instructions
- Has not eaten or drunk 8 hours before the test
- Has not smoked 2 hours before the test
- Has emptied her bladder

How the Test Is Performed

- The patient refrains from eating or drinking 8 hours before the test.
- The patient refrains from smoking 2 hours before the test.

- The patient empties her bladder.
- The patient signs a consent form.
- The patient lies on the table with her back raised, lying slightly to the left side.
- The patient exposes her abdomen.
- Conductive gel is placed on the patient's abdomen.
- Two fetal monitor straps are placed on the abdomen to record contractions and the fetal heart rate.
- The patient's vital signs are monitored.
- A baseline of the fetal heart rate and contractions is measured for 10 minutes.
- A low dose of oxytocin is administered. The dose is increased until there are three contractions each lasting more than 45 seconds over a 10-minute period.
- The fetal monitor continually records the fetal heart rate and contractions during the test.
- The healthcare provider continues to monitor the fetal monitor until it shows the fetal heart and contractions have returned to the baseline values.

Teach the Patient

Explain why the test is being performed, what the patient will experience during the test, and that the patient will not feel any pain during the procedure except for a pinch from the needle used to administer the oxytocin. The patient cannot eat 12 hours before the open biopsy, cannot smoke 2 hours before the test, and should empty her bladder before the test.

Understanding the Results

The procedure takes less than 2 hours. Preliminary results are known immediately. Detailed results are known within a week. The contraction stress test may have a false positive result.

- Normal (negative):
  - The fetal heart rate returned to normal following the contractions
- Abnormal (positive):
  - The fetal heart rate showed late decelerations following the contractions
  - Contractions were hyperstimulated, lasting longer than 90 seconds.

22.4   Cranial Ultrasound

A cranial ultrasound is performed on premature newborns to assess complications that might have arisen during a premature birth. During a cranial ultrasound, images of the newborn's brain are captured, displayed on a computer screen, and stored in a computer. The healthcare provider might order several cranial ultrasounds weeks apart. Some complications such as intraventricular hemorrhage (IVH) can be detected during the first week of birth while other complications such as periventricular leukomalacia (PVL) might occur 8 weeks after birth. *Periventricular leukomalacia* is damaged tissue around the ventricles. A cranial ultrasound is not performed after the child is 18 months of age because the cranium is fully formed and the fontanel is closed.

Why the Test Is Performed

The test assesses for hydrocephalus, the risk of developing cerebral palsy, the cause of an enlarged head, for intraventricular hemorrhage, and for periventricular leukomalacia.

How the Test Is Performed

- A conduction gel is placed on the newborn's head.
- A transducer is moved across the newborn's head, capturing images that appear on a computer monitor.

Teach the Patient

Explain why the test is being performed, what the newborn will experience during the test, that the newborn will not feel any pain during the test, and that the mother can hold and feed the newborn during the test.

Before Administering the Test

- The mother can hold the newborn during the test.
- The newborn can be fed during the test.

Understanding the Results

The procedure takes less than 30 minutes. Preliminary results are known immediately. Detailed results are known within a week.

- Normal:
  - No complications found
- Abnormal:
  - Complications found

22.5 Amniocentesis

Amniocentesis is the removal of some amniotic fluid. Amniotic fluid contains cells shed by the fetus. At about the sixteenth week of gestation, the healthcare provider may perform amniocentesis. Fetal cells contain amniotic fluid, which is analyzed to determine if the fetus has a birth defect. Amniocentesis is also performed during the third trimester if there is a risk of premature birth to determine fetal lung development and to assess if the mother has *chorioamnionitis*, which is infection of the amniotic fluid. Amniocentesis is ordered if an integrated test is positive, indicating that the fetus has a high chance of having a birth defect. These tests include:

- Alpha-fetoprotein (AFP)
- Estriol
- Inhibin A
- Chorionic gonadotropin (hCG)

It is also ordered if parents are carriers of a genetic trait that is likely to be passed on to the fetus. These include:

- Cystic fibrosis
- Duchenne muscular dystrophy
- Sickle cell anemia
- Thalassemia
- Hemophilia
- Tay-Sachs disease

Amniocentesis is also performed to determine if the fetus is Rh-positive when the mother has the Rh factor. This tests the amniotic fluid for an increase in bilirubin levels after the twentieth week of gestation, which indicates that the fetal blood cells are being attacked by the mother's antibodies. Amniocentesis does not identify all birth defects. There are many birth defects that are not revealed by amniocentesis.

Why the Test Is Performed

The test assesses for birth defects, fetal lung development, chorioamnionitis, and Rh antibodies.

Before Administering the Test

Assess if the patient:

- Signed a consent form
- Has emptied her bladder

- Can lie on her back
- Is able to lie still

How the Test Is Performed

- The patient signs a consent form.
- The patient must have an empty bladder.
- The patient lies on a table with her abdomen exposed.
- The insertion site is cleaned with an antiseptic.
- The insert site is injected with a local anesthetic.
- Conductive gel is placed on the mother's abdomen.
- A fetal monitor is placed on the mother's abdomen to monitor the fetus during the procedure.
- The mother's vital signs are monitored during the procedure.
- The healthcare provider performs a fetal ultrasound to guide the insertion of the needle.
- A needle is passed through the abdomen into the uterus. The needle is removed and reinserted if the fetus moves close to the needle.
- Two tablespoons of amniotic fluid are drawn up from the needle into a syringe.
- The needle is removed.
- A bandage covers the insertion site.

Teach the Patient

Explain why the test is being performed, what the patient will experience during the test, that the patient will not feel any pain during the test except a pinch when the local anesthetic is administered, and that the patient should breathe slowly during the procedure to relax her abdominal muscle. The patient may feel a cramp in the abdomen, may feel pulling on her abdomen when amniotic fluid is removed, must sign a consent form, and must empty her bladder before the procedure. The patient should also avoid exercise for 24 hours following the test, should not have sexual intercourse for 24 hours following the test, and should not douche or use tampons for 24 hours following the test. The patient should call her healthcare provider if she notices fluid or blood discharge from the insertion site or if there is swelling and redness at the insertion site, or if she experiences fever, pain, or cramping of her abdomen.

Understanding the Results

The procedure takes less than 30 minutes. Results are known within 2 weeks. A normal result from amniocentesis does not rule out a birth defect.

- Normal:
  - No signs of birth defects
  - Fetal lungs are adequately developed
  - No signs of chorioamnionitis
- Abnormal:
  - Signs of birth defects
  - Fetal lungs are not adequately developed
  - The mother has chorioamnionitis

22.6   Cordocentesis

A cordocentesis is the sampling of fetal blood from the umbilical cord to determine if the fetus has a blood disorder or is Rh-positive. If amniocentesis or other tests reveal that the fetus might have anemia, the health provider may order a cordocentesis to confirm the finding, typically in the second trimester. The blood sample is also used to assess the oxygen level in fetal blood.

Why the Test Is Performed

The test assesses for fetal anemia, if the fetus is Rh-Positive, and the oxygen level in fetal blood.

Before Administering the Test

Assess if the patient:

- Signed a consent form
- Has emptied her bladder
- Can lie on her back
- Is able to lie still

How the Test Is Performed

- The patient signs a consent form.
- The patient must have an empty bladder.
- The patient lies on a table with her abdomen exposed.
- The insertion site is cleaned with an antiseptic.
- The insert site is injected with a local anesthetic.
- Conductive gel is placed on the mother's abdomen.
- A fetal monitor is placed on the mother's abdomen to monitor the fetus during the procedure.
- The mother's vital signs are monitored during the procedure.
- The healthcare provider performs a fetal ultrasound to guide insertion of the needle.
- A needle is passed through the abdomen into the umbilical cord.
- A small amount of blood is drawn up from the needle into a syringe.
- The needle is removed.
- A bandage covers the insertion site.
- The healthcare provider may administer medication to temporarily stop the fetus from moving and/or to prevent preterm labor and infection.

Teach the Patient

Explain why the test is being performed, what the patient will experience during the test, that the patient will not feel any pain during the test except a pinch when the local anesthetic is administered, that the patient should breathe slowly during the procedure to relax her abdominal muscle, and that the patient may feel a cramp in the abdomen. The patient must sign a consent form, must empty her bladder before the procedure, should avoid exercise for 24 hours following the test, should not have sexual intercourse for 24 hours following the test, and should not douche or use tampons for 24 hours following the test. The patient should call her healthcare provider if she notices fluid or blood discharge from the insertion site or if there is swelling and redness at the insertion site, or if she experiences fever, pain, or cramping of her abdomen.

Understanding the Results

The procedure takes less than 30 minutes. Results are known within 2 weeks.

- Normal:
  - Fetal blood is normal
- Abnormal:
  - Fetal anemia
  - The fetus is Rh-positive
  - Abnormal oxygen level in the fetal blood

22.7 Sweat Test

The sweat test measures the amount of chloride in sweat. The sweat test is administered to a newborn between the ages of 2 days and 5 months old to assess if the newborn might have cystic fibrosis. Newborns that have cystic fibrosis have increased sodium chloride in their sweat.

Why the Test Is Performed

The test assesses for cystic fibrosis.

Before Administering the Test

Assess if the patient:

- Is less than 4 weeks of age. Newborns less than 4 weeks of age usually do not produce enough sweat for the test.
- Is dehydrated
- Is ill
- Is taking steroids
- Has a rash

How the Test Is Performed

- The right arm or thigh is washed and dried.
- A small gauze pad is soaked with pilocarpine.
- Another small gauze pad is soaked with salt water.
- Both are placed on the skin.
- Electrodes are paced over the gauze pads.
- A mild current flows through the electrodes, forcing the medication into the skin. The newborn may feel a slight tingling.
- The gauze pads are removed after 10 minutes.
- The skin under the gauze pad that contains pilocarpine is reddened.
- The skin is cleaned with water and dried.
- The reddened skin is covered with a dry gauze pad.
- The dry gauze pad is covered with plastic to prevent evaporation.
- The dry gauze pad remains in place for 30 minutes to soak up sweat.
- The dry gauze pad is removed and placed in a collection bottle, which is sealed and sent to the laboratory, where the dry gauze is weighed to determine the amount of chloride and/or sodium that is on the gauze.
- The skin beneath the dry gauze is cleaned and dried.
- The skin remains reddened for less than 5 hours following the test.
- The healthcare provider may use the macroduct technique of collecting sweat, which uses a coil rather than gauze pads.

Teach the Patient

Explain why the test is being performed, what the newborn will experience during the test, that the newborn will not feel any pain during the test except for a slight tingle when the current is applied to the electrode, and that any reddened skin will return to normal color within 5 hours of the test.

Understanding the Results

The procedure takes less than 1 hour. Results are known within 2 days. An abnormal result indicates that the newborn may have cystic fibrosis. Further testing is necessary to diagnose cystic fibrosis.

- Normal:
  - Normal amount of chloride
- Borderline:
  - A high normal level of chloride
- Abnormal:
  - A high level of chloride

22.8   Chorionic Villus Sampling (CVS)

Chorionic villus sampling is a procedure where a sampling of chorionic villi is biopsied between the tenth and twelfth week of gestation and examined to determine if the fetus has a genetic disorder. The placenta contains chorionic villi, which are tiny growths that contain the same genetic material as the fetus. There are two methods used to biopsy the chorionic villus:

1. **Transabdominal**: A needle is inserted through the abdomen.
2. **Transcervical**: A needle is inserted through the cervix.

Chorionic villus sampling is performed earlier in gestation than amniocentesis.

Why the Test Is Performed

The test assesses for fetal genetic disorders.

Before Administering the Test

Determine if the patient:

- Has a full bladder
- Has signed a consent form
- Has allergies

How the Test Is Performed

- The patient signs a consent form.
- The patient lies on a table.
- The patient either removes her clothes below the waist or exposes her abdomen, depending on which biopsy method is used by the healthcare provider.
- Conductive gel is placed on her abdomen.
- A fetal monitor is attached to the abdomen to monitor the fetus.
- Transabdominal:
  - The insertion site is cleaned with an anesthetic.
  - A local anesthetic is administered to the insertion site.
  - An ultrasound transducer is pressed on and moved around the abdomen.
  - Images of the fetus and uterus are displayed on a computer screen.
  - A needle is inserted through the abdomen.
  - A sample of the chorionic villi is removed.
  - The needle is removed.
  - The insertion site is bandaged.
- Transcervical:
  - The patient places her feet in stirrups.
  - A speculum is inserted into the vagina to spread apart the vaginal wall.
  - The cervix is cleaned with an antiseptic soap.
  - An ultrasound transducer is pressed on and moved around the abdomen.
  - Images of the fetus and uterus are displayed on a computer screen.
  - A catheter is inserted through the cervix.
  - A sample of the chorionic villi is removed.
  - The needle is removed.

Teach the Patient

Explain why the test is being performed, what the patient will experience during the test, and that the patient will not feel any pain during the test except for a slight pinch when the local anesthetic is administered. The patient might feel cramping, may have vaginal spotting, or may have a small amount of amniotic fluid leakage following the procedure. The patient should call her healthcare provider if cramping, spotting, and leakage of amniotic fluid occurs 48 hours after the procedure, or if she experiences a fever, swelling at the insertion site, or is dizzy.

Understanding the Results

The procedure takes less than 1 hour. Results are known within 2 weeks.

- Normal:
  - Normal cells in the sample
- Abnormal:
  - Abnormal genetic material found

22.9 Karyotyping

Karyotyping determines the number and quality of chromosomes in a cell and is used to detect possible genetic disorders. Tissue samples for karyotyping are typically taken during the chorionic villus sampling or amniocentesis procedure.

Why the Test Is Performed

The test assesses for fetal genetic disorders.

Before Administering the Test

Assess if the patient:

- Has undergone genetic counseling

How the Test Is Performed

- The patient should undergo genetic counseling to understand the test and the results of the test.
- The sample is taken using chorionic villus sampling or amniocentesis.
- Chromosomes are removed from cells and examined under a microscope.

Teach the Patient

Explain why the test is being performed and why it is important to have genetic counseling to fully understand the test and the results.

Understanding the Results

The procedure takes less than 1 hour. Results are known within 2 weeks.

- Normal:
  - Normal number and quality of chromosomes
- Abnormal:
  - Abnormal number and quality of chromosomes

22.10 Cervical Cerclage (weak cervix)

A cervical cerclage is a procedure to close the cervix to assure that the cervix remains closed until after the thirty-seventh week of gestation. If the patient has an incompetent cervix, the cervix might open prior to the thirty-seventh week of gestation and could result in premature birth. The cervix must be manually opened before the patient goes into labor, otherwise the healthcare provider may perform a cesarean section.

Why the Test Is Performed

The test prevents premature opening of the cervix.

Before Administering the Test

Determine if the patient:

- Has signed a consent form
- Has any allergies
- Has taken anticoagulant medication such as Plavix, coumadin, heparin, or aspirin
- Can lie on her back
- Is able to lie still
- Has been treated for infection of the pelvis, cervix, or vagina
- Has not eaten or drunk for 12 hours before the procedure
- Does not have uterine contractions
- Does not have vaginal bleeding
- Does not have ruptured membranes

How the Test Is Performed

- The patient removes her clothes.
- The patient lies on a table with her feet in stirrups.
- A breathing tube is inserted into the patient's throat.
- The patient is connected to an EKG.
- The patient is connected to a pulse oximeter to measure the oxygen content of the patient's blood.
- A speculum is placed into the vagina to spread the vaginal walls.
- If the amnion (amniotic sac) is protruding:
  - A catheter is inserted through the cervix.
  - A bulb at the end of the catheter is inflated, pushing the amnion into the pelvis.
- Incisions are made in the cervix.
- Tape is tied through the incisions, closing the cervix, or stitches are placed to close the cervix.

Teach the Patient

Explain why the procedure is being performed, what the patient will experience during the procedure, and that the patient will have to sign a consent form. The patient should not eat or drink 12 hours before the procedure, should not exercise following the procedure, and should not perform any heavy lifting following the procedure. The patient should call her healthcare provider if she has a fever, an odorous discharge from the vagina, experiences heavy vaginal bleeding, or has abdominal pain.

Understanding the Results

The procedure takes less than 1 hour. Results are immediate.

- Normal:
  - The cervix is closed
- Abnormal:
  - The healthcare provider is unable to close the cervix

22.11 Galactosemia Test

The galactosemia test determines if certain enzymes are present in the newborn's blood. Newborns that have galactosemia may experience seizures, brain damage, and mental retardation if their bodies are unable to convert galactose, which is found in breast milk and formula, into glucose. These newborns lack three enzymes needed for this process. These enzymes can also be detected in a urine sample.

Why the Test Is Performed

The test screens for galactosemia.

Before Administering the Test

Assess if the patient:

- Has had a blood transfusion
- Has relatives with galactosemia; galactosemia is a genetic disorder

How the Test Is Performed

Heel Stick: Several drops of blood are collected from the heel of a newborn or baby. The heel is cleaned using alcohol. A sterile lancer is used to puncture the heel. Several drops of blood are collected in a small test tube. A gauze pad is pressed over the site until bleeding stops. A small bandage is applied.

Teach the Patient

Explain why the blood sample is taken, how the sample is taken, and that the newborn that has galactosemia must not ingest milk or milk by-products.

Understanding the Results

Test results are available within 2 days. The laboratory determines normal values based on calibration of testing equipment with a control test. Test results are reported as high, normal, or low based on the laboratory's control test.

- Normal (negative): The enzymes are present.
- Abnormal (positive): The enzymes are not present.

Solved Problems

Biophysical Profile

22.1 What does the biophysical profile test assess?

The biophysical profile test assesses the health of the fetus.

22.2 When is the biophysical profile test performed?

The biophysical profile test is commonly performed in the last trimester of the pregnancy.

22.3 What are components of a biophysical profile test?

The biophysical profile test consists of a non-stress test and a fetal ultrasound.

22.4 What is assessed by the biophysical profile test?

The biophysical profile test assesses fetal movement, fetal heart rate, the volume of amniotic fluid, muscle tone, and breathing rate.

22.5 What should you assess before administering the biophysical profile test?

Assess if the patient:
- Can lie on her back
- Is able to lie still
- Is able to follow instructions
- Has not smoked 2 hours before the test
- Has a full bladder
- Is not hypoglycemic or hyperglycemic
- Is not using alcohol or narcotics

22.6   How is the non-stress test portion of the biophysical profile test performed?

- Conductive gel is placed on the patient's abdomen.
- Two belts of the fetal monitor are placed on her abdomen to measure fetal heart rate and contractions.
- The fetal monitor constantly records the fetus during the test. The results appear on a strip of paper.
- The patient is asked to press a button connected to the fetal monitor each time the fetus moves and if there is a contraction.
- The two belts of the fetal monitor are removed and the gel is wiped from the patient's abdomen.

22.7   What would you anticipate the healthcare provider will do if the biophysical profile test has a score of 6?

The patient should be retested if the test has a score of 5 to 8.

Contraction Stress Test

22.8   Why does a healthcare provider order a contraction stress test?

The contraction stress test determines if the fetus will remain healthy during natural childbirth.

22.9   When might the contraction stress test be ordered?

If the biophysical profile indicates suspicious results, then the healthcare provider might perform a contraction stress test.

22.10   How would you explain the contraction stress test to a patient?

During the contraction stress test a fetal heart monitor is attached to the mother while the mother is administered oxytocin. Oxytocin is a hormone that induces uterine contractions. The fetus heart rate is expected to decelerate during a contraction and accelerate following the contraction. If the heart rate does not accelerate, then the fetus may not remain healthy during natural childbirth.

22.11   A patient who is pregnant with her second child wants the healthcare provider to order a contraction stress test. How would you respond to this patient?

Assess if the patient has had conditions that might prevent the test from being performed. This test is not usually performed if the mother has had a cesarean section, placenta previa, placenta abruptio, incompetent cervix, and premature rupture of the amniotic membrane in the past. It is also not usually performed if the mother has been administered magnesium sulfate or is pregnant with multiple fetuses.

22.12   What should you assess before the patient undergoes the contraction stress test?

Assess if the patient:
- Has signed a consent form
- Has any allergies
- Has taken anticoagulant medication such as Plavix, coumadin, heparin, or aspirin
- Can lie on her back
- Is able to lie still
- Is able to follow instructions
- Has not eaten or drunk 8 hours before the test
- Has not smoked 2 hours before the test
- Has emptied her bladder

22.13   A patient who is scheduled for a contraction stress test asks how the test is performed. How would you respond?

- The patient refrains from eating or drinking 8 hours before the test.
- The patient refrains from smoking 2 hours before the test.
- The patient empties her bladder.
- The patient signs a consent form.
- The patient lies on the table with her back raised, lying slightly to the left side.
- The patient exposes her abdomen.
- Conductive gel is placed on the patient's abdomen.
- Two fetal monitor straps are placed on the abdomen to record contractions and the fetal heart rate.

- The patient's vital signs are monitored.
- A baseline of the fetal heart rate and contractions is measured for 10 minutes.
- A low dose of oxytocin is administered. The dose is increased until there are three contractions, each lasting more than 45 seconds over a 10-minute period.
- The fetal monitor continually records the fetal heart rate and contractions during the test.
- The healthcare provider continues to monitor the fetal monitor, until it shows the fetal heart rate and contractions have returned to the baseline values.

22.14   What is a positive finding of the contraction stress test?

A positive finding of the contraction stress test is the fetal heart rate showed late decelerations following the contractions or the contractions were hyperstimulated, lasting longer than 90 seconds.

Cordocentesis

22.15   A patient overhears the healthcare provider talk about ordering a cordocentesis and asks you to explain this procedure. What would you say?

"A cordocentesis is the sampling of fetal blood from the umbilical cord to determine if the fetus has a blood disorder or is Rh-positive, and to assess the oxygen level in fetal blood."

22.16   How is a cordocentesis performed?

- The patient signs a consent form.
- The patient must have an empty bladder.
- The patient lies on a table with her abdomen exposed.
- The insertion site is cleaned with an antiseptic.
- The insertion site is injected with a local anesthetic.
- Conductive gel is placed on the mother's abdomen.
- A fetal monitor is placed on the mother's abdomen to monitor the fetus during the procedure.
- The mother's vital signs are monitored during the procedure.
- The healthcare provider performs a fetal ultrasound to guide insertion of the needle.
- A needle is passed through the abdomen into the umbilical cord.
- A small amount of blood is drawn up from the needle into a syringe.
- The needle is removed.
- A bandage covers the insertion site.
- The healthcare provider may administer medication to temporarily stop the fetus from moving and/or to prevent preterm labor and infection.

22.17   What should you teach a patient who is scheduled to undergo a cordocentesis?

Explain why the test is being performed, what the patient will experience during the test, that the patient will not feel any pain during the test except a pinch when the local anesthetic is administered, that the patient should breathe slowly during the procedure to relax her abdominal muscle, and that the patient may feel a cramp in the abdomen. The patient must sign a consent form, must empty her bladder before the procedure, should avoid exercise for 24 hours following the test, should not have sexual intercourse for 24 hours following the test, and should not douche or use tampons for 24 hours following the test. The patient should call her healthcare provider if she notices fluid or bloody discharge from the insertion site or if there is swelling and redness at the insertion site, or if she experiences fever, pain, or cramping of her abdomen.

Sweat Test

22.18   When is the sweat test administered?

The sweat test is administered to a newborn between the age of 2 days and 5 months old to assess if the newborn might have cystic fibrosis.

22.19   What is the rationale for administering the sweat test?

Newborns that have cystic fibrosis have increased sodium chloride in their sweat.

22.20 What should you assess before administering the sweat test?

Assess if the patient:

- Is less than 4 weeks of age. Newborns less than four weeks of age usually do not produce enough sweat for the test.
- Is dehydrated
- Is ill
- Is taking steroids
- Has a rash

22.21 How is the sweat test administered?

- The right arm or thigh is washed and dried.
- A small gauze pad is soaked with pilocarpine.
- Another small gauze pad is soaked with salt water.
- Both are placed on the skin.
- Electrodes are placed over the gauze pads.
- A mild current flows through the electrodes, forcing the medication into the skin. The newborn may feel a slight tingling.
- The gauze pads are removed after 10 minutes.
- The skin under the gauze pad that contains pilocarpine is reddened.
- The skin is cleaned with water and dried.
- The reddened skin is covered with a dry gauze pad.
- The dry gauze pad is covered with plastic to prevent evaporation.
- The dry gauze pad remains in place for 30 minutes to soak up sweat.
- The dry gauze pad is removed and placed in a collection bottle, which is sealed and sent to the laboratory where the dry gauze is weighed to determine the amount of chloride and/or sodium that is on the gauze.
- The skin beneath the dry gauze is cleaned and dried.
- The skin remains reddened for less than 5 hours following the test.
- The healthcare provider may use the macroduct technique of collecting sweat, which uses a coil rather than gauze pads.

22.22 What should you explain to the parents of the newborn who is undergoing the sweat test?

Explain why the test is being performed, what the newborn will experience during the test, that the newborn will not feel any pain during the test except for a slight tingle when current is applied to the electrode, and that any reddened skin will return to normal color within 5 hours of the test.

22.23 What should you tell parents of a newborn whose sweat test is abnormal?

An abnormal result indicates that the newborn may have cystic fibrosis. Further testing is necessary to diagnose cystic fibrosis.

Chorionic Villus Sampling

22.24 When is a CVS performed?

Chorionic villus sampling is a procedure where a sampling of chorionic villi is biopsied between the tenth and twelfth weeks of gestation.

22.25 Why is CVS performed?

Chorionic villus sampling is performed earlier in gestation than amniocentesis to determine if the fetus has a genetic disorder.

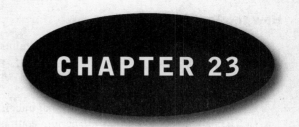

CHAPTER 23

Chest, Abdominal, and Urinary Tract Tests

23.1 Definition

Chest, abdominal, and urinary tract tests and procedures are performed to assess problems with several organs within the body. These include the upper gastrointestinal tract, thyroid gland, liver, gallbladder, kidney, spleen, urinary tract, stomach, duodenum, and bile and pancreatic ducts.

23.2 Upper Gastrointestinal (UGI) Series

The upper gastrointestinal series consists of a group of tests that assess the esophagus, stomach, and the duodenum. Prior to the series, the patient ingests barium contrast material and water. X-ray images of the esophagus, stomach, and duodenum are taken using a fluoroscope as the barium moves through the upper gastrointestinal tract. Images are displayed on a computer screen and stored for further review. If the healthcare provider sees anything suspicious, he or she might perform an endoscopy, wherein an endoscope is inserted down the esophagus and into the stomach and duodenum to directly view the upper gastrointestinal tract. The upper gastrointestinal series is also performed during a full gastrointestinal series, which also involves examination of the lower gastrointestinal tract.

Why the Test Is Performed

The test assesses the cause of stomach pain and indigestion and the cause of malabsorption syndrome.

Before Administering the Test

Assess if the patient:

- Has signed a consent form
- Has any allergies
- Has taken anticoagulant medication such as Plavix, coumadin, heparin, or aspirin
- Can lie on his or her back or stomach
- Is able to lie still
- Is able to follow instructions
- Has eaten a lower fiber diet during the 3 days before the test
- Has not eaten or drunk 6 hours before the test
- Has taken a laxative 12 hours before the test
- Has removed dentures before the test
- Is able to swallow the barium contrast material

How the Test Is Performed

- 12 hours before the test the patient is administered a laxative
- The patient signs a consent form
- The patient removes his or her clothes.
- The patient lies on his or her back.
- An X-ray of the upper gastrointestinal tract is taken.
- The patient sits and drinks the barium contrast material.
- A series of X-rays are taken.
- The patient may be asked to drink additional amounts of barium contrast material during the test. After each swallow additional X-rays are taken.

Teach the Patient

Explain why the procedure is being performed, what the patient will experience during the procedure, and that the patient will not feel any pain during the procedure. The patient should eat a lower fiber diet for 3 days before the test, must not eat or drink 12 hours before the test, should take a laxative 12 hours before the test, and will be swallowing the barium contrast material several times during the test. Barium contrast material is sweet flavored. The patient might feel bloated and/or nauseous following the test. Feces will appear white for 3 days following the test. The healthcare provider may administer a stool softener following the test to prevent constipation from the barium contrast material. The patient should call his or her healthcare provider if he or she has not had a bowel movement within 3 days following the test.

Understanding the Results

The procedure takes less than 1 hour. Preliminary results are known immediately. Comprehensive results are ready within 2 weeks of the procedure.

- Normal:
  - Normal structure of the upper gastrointestinal tract
- Abnormal:
  - Abnormal structure of the upper gastrointestinal tract

23.3 Esophagus Test Series

The esophagus test series consists of two tests that assess the esophagus and esophageal sphincters:

1. **Esophageal Manometry**: Measures esophageal muscle contractions.
2. **Esophageal Acidity Test**: Measures the pH of the esophagus.

Why the Test Is Performed

The test assesses the cause of GERD and chest pain.

Before Administering the Test

Assess if the patient:

- Has signed a consent form
- Has not eaten or drunk for 12 hours before the test
- Has not smoked or ingested alcohol 24 hours before the test
- Does not have esophageal varices
- Does not have heart failure
- Has taken anticoagulant medication such as Plavix, coumadin, heparin, or aspirin
- Can lie on his or her back
- Can swallow
- Has not taken Prevacid, Prilosec, Protonix, Nexium, Aciphex, Zantac, Pepcid, Axid, Tagamet, or antacids prior to and during the test

- Has not taken corticosteroids
- Has not taken blood pressure medication
- Has not taken medication to treat bladder and intestinal muscle spasms
- Has not taken medication for Parkinson's disease
- Has not taken theophylline

How the Test Is Performed

- The patient signs a consent form.
- The patient removes his or her clothes.
- The patient lies on a table with his or her head slightly raised.
- Esophageal manometry:
  - The patient swallows a transducer that is attached to a tube.
  - The tube contains pressure-sensing holes.
  - The patient is asked to swallow several times during the test. Pressure in the esophagus is measured with each swallow.
  - A graph depicting the pressure is recorded and assessed by the healthcare provider.
- Esophageal acidity test (Bravo Wireless):
  - The patient swallows a capsule that contains a transmitter. The transmitter measures the acidity of the patient's stomach and transmits it to a receiver carried by the patient.
  - The patient keeps a diary of his or her activities.
  - The patient is asked to press a button on the pager when experiencing a symptom.
  - The transmitter passes as a bowel movement within a week.
- Esophageal acidity test (Non-Wireless):
  - An anesthetic is sprayed in the back of the patient's throat and in the patient's nose.
  - A tube containing a probe that measures acidity is passed through the patient's nose and down the esophagus.
  - The probe remains in place for 24 hours. It records the acidity level in the esophagus as the patient goes about his or her normal daily activities.
  - The patient keeps a diary of his or her activities and symptoms.
  - The patient must avoid activities that may cause the monitor to become wet.
  - The probe is removed after 24 hours and the results are analyzed by the healthcare provider.

Teach the Patient

Explain why the procedure is being performed, what the patient will experience during the procedure, and that the patient will not feel any pain during the procedure. The patient should not eat or drink 12 hours before the test, should not smoke or ingest alcohol 24 hours before the test, and should not take Prevacid, Prilosec, Protonix, Nexium, Aciphex, Zantac, Pepcid, Axid, Tagamet, or antacids prior to and during the test.

Understanding the Results

The procedure takes less than 1 hour. The esophageal acidity test takes 24 hours. Results are known within 2 weeks of the test.

- Normal:
  - Normal structure and function of the esophagus or normal pH level
- Abnormal:
  - Abnormal structure or function of the esophagus or acidic pH level

23.4 Gallbladder Scan

The gallbladder scan assesses the function of the gallbladder. The gallbladder scan is used to identify blockages in the bile ducts. A radioactive tracer is injected in the patient's vein. The tracer is removed from the blood by the liver, which places the tracer into bile that flows into the gallbladder and into the duodenum. A camera takes an image of the tracer as the tracer flows through the liver to the duodenum.

Why the Test Is Performed

The test assesses the gallbladder and the cause of upper right abdominal pain.

Before Administering the Test

Assess if the patient:

- Has signed a consent form
- Has not eaten or drunk for 12 hours before the test
- Has allergies
- Is pregnant
- Has recently had a barium test performed within 4 days prior to the test
- Has taken anticoagulant medication such as Plavix, coumadin, heparin, or aspirin
- Has taken Pepto-Bismol

How the Test Is Performed

- The patient signs a consent form.
- The patient removes his or her clothes.
- The patient lies on a table.
- The injection site is cleaned.
- The patient is injected with the radioactive tracer.
- The camera is moved into position.
- Images are taken immediately, then every 10 minutes for 90 minutes.
- The patient is administered cholecystokinin to stimulate the gallbladder.
- The patient may be administered morphine sulfate to diagnose gallbladder inflammation.
- The patient should drink lots of fluids to flush the tracer from his or her body.
- The patient should flush the toilet quickly after urinating and defecating, since the tracer is excreted in urine and feces in the 2 days following the test.

Teach the Patient

Explain why the procedure is being performed, what the patient will experience during the procedure, and that the patient will not feel any pain during the procedure except for a pinch when the tracer is injected into his vein. The patient must sign a consent form, must not eat or drink for 12 hours before the test, should not take Pepto-Bismol for 48 hours before the test, and should not take anticoagulant medication such as Plavix, coumadin, heparin, or aspirin for 2 weeks prior to the test. The patient should drink lots of fluids to flush the tracer following the test, flush the toilet immediately after urinating and defecating, wash his or her hands thoroughly after urinating and defecating, and apply a warm compress to the injection site if there is swelling. If the patient is breast-feeding, breast milk must be discarded for 2 days after the scan.

Understanding the Results

The procedure takes less than 2 hours. Results are known within 2 days.

- Normal:
  - Gallbladder functions normally
  - Normal shape and size of the gallbladder
- Abnormal:
  - Possible liver disease, if the tracer does not flow into the gallbladder
  - Gallbladder is inflamed or blocked
  - The bile duct is narrowed or blocked

23.5   Kidney Scan

A kidney scan assesses the function of the kidney. A radioactive tracer is injected in the patient's vein. The tracer moves through the blood vessels in the kidneys. A camera takes an image of the tracer as the tracer flows through the kidney, illustrating where blood flows unobstructed and where blood flow is blocked. There are two types of kidney scans:

1. **Function Study**: This measures the time the tracer takes to pass through the kidneys and enter the bladder as part of urine.
2. **Perfusion Study**: This assesses blood flow through the kidneys.

A kidney scan is an alternative to the intravenous pyelogram (IVP) test.

Why the Test Is Performed

The test assesses blood flow through the kidneys and the function of the kidneys.

Before Administering the Test

Assess if the patient:

- Has signed a consent form
- Has drunk three glasses of water before the test
- Can lie still
- Has allergies
- Is pregnant
- Has recently had a barium test performed within 4 days prior to the test
- Has taken anticoagulant medication such as Plavix, coumadin, heparin, or aspirin
- Has taken Pepto-Bismol
- Has taken antihypertensives
- Is breastfeeding. If so, breast milk must be discarded for two days after the scan.

How the Test Is Performed

- The patient signs a consent form.
- The patient removes his or her clothes.
- The patient lies on a table, although the patient may be asked to sit or stand during the test.
- The injection site is cleaned.
- The patient is injected with the radioactive tracer.
- The camera is moved into position.
- Function study:
  - Images are taken every 3 minutes for 30 minutes.
  - The patient may be administered a diuretic to increase kidney function.
- Perfusion study:
  - Movement of the tracer through the kidneys is recorded on a renogram.
- The patient should drink lots of fluid to flush the tracer from his or her body.
- The patient should flush the toilet quickly after urinating and defecating, since the tracer is excreted in urine and feces for 2 days following the test.

Teach the Patient

Explain why the procedure is being performed, what the patient will experience during the procedure, and that the patient will not feel any pain during the procedure except for a pinch when the tracer is injected into his or her vein. The patient must sign a consent form, drink three glasses of water before the test, must not take Pepto-Bismol for 48 hours before the test, and must not take anticoagulant medication such as Plavix, coumadin, heparin, or aspirin for 2 weeks prior to the test. The patient should drink lots of fluids to flush the tracer following the test, flush the toilet immediately after urinating and defecating, wash hands thoroughly after urinating and defecating, and apply a warm compress to the injection site if there is swelling. If the patient is breastfeeding, breast milk must be discarded for 2 days after the scan.

Understanding the Results

The procedure takes less than 2 hours. Preliminary results are known within 2 days.

- Normal:
  - Kidney functions normally
  - Normal kidney size and shape
- Abnormal:
  - Abnormal kidney function
  - Abnormal kidney size and shape
  - There is narrowing or blockage of blood vessels

23.6 Liver and Spleen Scan

A liver and spleen scan assesses the function of the liver and spleen. A radioactive tracer is injected in the patient's vein. The tracer moves through the blood vessels in the liver and spleen. A camera takes an image of the tracer as the tracer flows through the liver and spleen, illustrating where blood flows unobstructed and where blood flow is blocked.

Why the Test Is Performed

The test assesses blood flow through the liver and spleen, if cancer has metastasized to the liver, the spleen after an injury, and the treatment for cancer.

Before Administering the Test

Assess if the patient:

- Has signed a consent form
- Can lie still
- Has allergies
- Is pregnant
- Has recently had a barium test performed within 4 days prior to the test
- Has taken anticoagulant medication such as Plavix, coumadin, heparin, or aspirin
- Has taken Pepto-Bismol
- Has emptied his or her bladder
- Is breastfeeding. Breast milk must be discarded for 2 days after the scan.

How the Test Is Performed

- The patient signs a consent form.
- The patient empties his or her bladder.
- The patient removes his or her clothes.
- The patient lies on a table.
- The injection site is cleaned.
- The patient is injected with the radioactive tracer.
- The camera is moved into position.
- Several images are taken.
- The patient should drink lots of fluid to flush the tracer from his or her body.
- The patient should flush the toilet quickly after urinating and defecating, since the tracer is excreted in urine and feces in the 2 days following the test.

Teach the Patient

Explain why the procedure is being performed, what the patient will experience during the procedure, and that the patient will not feel any pain during the procedure except for a pinch when the tracer is injected into his or her vein. The patient must sign a consent form, must have an empty bladder, should not take Pepto-Bismol for

48 hours before the test because Pepto-Bismol contains aspirin, and should not take anticoagulant medication such as Plavix, coumadin, heparin, or aspirin for 2 weeks prior to the test, since this might decrease coagulation of blood during the test. The patient should drink lots of fluids to flush the tracer following the test, flush the toilet immediately after urinating and defecating, wash hands thoroughly after urinating and defecating, and apply a warm compress to the injection site if there is swelling. If the patient is breastfeeding, breast milk must be discarded for 2 days after the scan.

Understanding the Results

The procedure takes less than 2 hours. Results are known within 2 days.

- Normal:
  - Liver and spleen function normally
  - Normal size and shape of the liver and spleen
- Abnormal:
  - Abnormal liver function
  - Abnormal spleen function
  - Abnormal size and shape of the spleen
  - Abnormal size and shape of the liver

23.7   Urine Analysis

A urine analysis is performed to determine the characteristics of the urine and to determine the existence and amount of substances in the urine. Waste material carried by blood is filtered by kidneys and excreted as urine. Urine characteristics are:

- Clarity: How clear is the urine?
- Color: What color is the urine?
- Specific gravity: The balance between water and substances in the urine.
- Odor: The aroma of urine.
- pH: How acidic or alkaline is the urine?

There are several methods used to capture the urine sample.

- *Clean-catch midstream one-time urine collection*: Urine is collected after the patient begins to urinate.
- *Double voided urine collection*: Urine is collected the second time that the patient voids.
- *24-Hour Urine Collection*: Urine is collected over a 24-hour period.

Why the Test Is Performed

The test assesses for kidney and other disorders.

Before Administering the Test

Assess if the patient:

- Has collected the urine properly
- Has exercised prior to the test
- Is menstruating
- Has eaten blackberries, beets, or foods that might color urine
- Has had usual exposure to sun
- Is on extended bed rest
- Has recently undergone a test that used contrast material
- Has ingested nicotine or caffeine
- Has had a recent illness or is under stress
- Keeps warm during testing, if testing catecholmine levels

- Is pregnant
- Has had severe vomiting
- Has taken Dilantin, Pyridium, vitamin B, diuretics, Rifampin, Trimpex, ascorbic acid, Probalan, Benemid, allopurinol, insulin, lithium, laxatives, steroids, antacids, NSAIDs, antibiotics, potassium supplements, growth hormones or parathyroid hormone, aspirin, antidepressants, nitroglycerin, tetracycline, tricyclic antidepressants, theophylline, and cold and sinus medication
- Has recently taken sodium-based medication

How the Test Is Performed

- The patient washes his or her hands.
- Open the collection cup. Do not touch the inside of the collection cup.
- Clean the urethra area with an antiseptic.
- Do not touch the cup to the urethra or any skin when collecting the sample.
- Do not contaminate the urine sample with feces, pubic hair, or other substances.
- If the sample becomes contaminated, then begin again with a new collection cup.
- Double-voided urine collection:
  - The patient urinates.
  - The patient drinks a lot of water.
  - The patient waits until feeling the need to urinate.
- Urinate for 5 seconds, making sure no skin aside from the urethra touches the urine.
- Move the collection cup into the urine stream.
- Do not touch the collection cup to the urethra or any skin.
- Remove the collection cup and continue urinating.
- Place the lid on the collection cup.
- Refrigerate the collection cup until the sample is sent to the lab.
- Twenty-Four-Hour urine collection:
  - The patient empties the bladder first thing in the morning.
  - The patient collects urine the next and subsequent times that he or she urinates for the 24-hour period.
  - The patient must note the time of urination. This begins the 24-hour period.
  - Urine is kept in a gallon container that must be refrigerated between collections.
  - The patient must note the last time of urination at the end of the 24-hour period.
  - If the patient urinates within the 24-hour period and does not collect the urine, then the patient must begin the 24-hour urine collection again.

Teach the Patient

Explain why the test is being performed, what the patient will experience during the test, that the patient will not feel any pain during the test, and how to perform the test. The patient should not exercise prior to the test and should not take the test if she is menstruating. The patient should avoid eating blackberries, beets, or foods that might color the urine. The patient should not have his or her usual exposure to sun, be on extended bed rest, and ingest nicotine or caffeine. Inform the patient to keep warm during testing, if testing catecholmine levels, and to avoid taking Dilantin, Pyridium, vitamin B, diuretics, Rifampin, Trimpex, ascorbic acid, Probalan, Benemid, allopurinol, insulin, lithium, laxatives, steroids, antacids, NSAIDs, antibiotics, potassium supplements, growth hormones or parathyroid hormone, aspirin, antidepressants, nitroglycerin, tetracycline, tricyclic, theophylline, and cold and sinus medication 2 weeks before the test. The patient should avoid taking sodium-based medication 2 weeks before the test.

Understanding the Results

The collection takes a few seconds, expect for the 24-hour collection. Results are known within 2 days. The laboratory determines normal values based on calibration of testing equipment with a control test. Test results are reported as high, normal, or low based on the laboratory's control test.

- Normal:
  - Color: Pale to dark amber
  - Clarity: Clear
  - Order: Nutty
  - Specific gravity: 1.005 to 1.030
  - pH: 4.6 to 8.0
  - Protein: None
  - Glucose: None
  - Ketones: None
  - Leukocytes: None
  - Erythrocyte: None
  - Casts: None
  - Microorganism: None
  - Crystals: Slight
  - Squamous cells: None
  - Uric acid: 250 to 800 mg (24-hour urine collection)
  - Calcium: 100 to 250 mg (24-hour urine collection)
  - Catecholamines: < 100 mcg (24-hour urine collection)
  - Epinephrine: < 20 mcg (24-hour urine collection)
  - Norepinephrine: < 100 mcg (24-hour urine collection)
  - Dopamine: 65 to 400 mcg (24-hour urine collection)
  - Normetanephrine: 10 to 80 mcg (24-hour urine collection)
  - Metanephrine: < 1.3 mg (24-hour urine collection)
  - Vanillylmandelic acid: < 6.8 mg (24-hour urine collection)
  - Cortisol: < 100 mcg (24-hour urine collection)
  - Phosphate: 0.9 to 1.3 grams (24-hour urine collection)
  - Potassium: 25 to 100 mEq/L (24-hour urine collection)
  - Sodium: 40 to 220 mEq (24-hour urine collection)
  - Microalbumin: < 30 mg (24-hour urine collection)
- Abnormal:
  - Color: Clear (chronic kidney disease, diabetes), dark (dehydration), or red (blood)
  - Clarity: Cloudy (microorganism)
  - Order: Fruity (diabetes), foul (urinary tract infection), maple syrup (maple syrup urine disease)
  - Specific gravity: < 1.005 (over-hydration, kidney disease, diuretics) or > 1.030 (dehydration, hyperglycemia, vomiting, diarrhea)
  - pH: < 4.6 (diabetes, dehydration, excess alcohol, aspirin overdose) or > 8.0 (vomiting, urinary tract infection, kidney disease)
  - Protein: Present (infection, high blood pressure, kidney disorder, glomerulonephritis)
  - Glucose: Present (diabetes, liver disease, kidney disorder, adrenal gland disorder)
  - Ketones: Present (diabetes, starvation, anorexia, bulimia, alcoholism)
  - Leukocytes: Present (urinary tract infection, glomerulonephritis, kidney stones, kidney disorder)
  - Erythrocyte: Present (urinary tract infection, glomerulonephritis, kidney stones, kidney disorder)
  - Casts: Present (inflammation, kidney disorder, lead poisoning, heart failure)
  - Microorganism: Present (urinary tract infection)
  - Crystals: Large amount (kidney stone, kidney disorder)
  - Squamous cells: Present (contaminated urine sample)
  - Uric acid: < 250 or > 800 mg (24-hour urine collection) (kidney stones, gout)
  - Calcium: < 100 or > 250 mg (24-hour urine collection) (hyperparathyroidism, osteoporosis, excess vitamin D, excess dietary calcium, dehydration)
  - Catecholamines: > 100 mcg (24-hour urine collection) (pheochromocytoma)
  - Epinephrine: > 20 mcg (24-hour urine collection) (infection, stress, trauma)
  - Norepinephrine: > 100 mcg (24-hour urine collection) (infection, stress, trauma)
  - Dopamine: < 65 or > 400 mcg (24-hour urine collection) (infection, stress, trauma)
  - Normetanephrine: < 10 or > 80 mcg (24-hour urine collection) (infection, stress, trauma)
  - Metanephrine: > 1.3 mg (24-hour urine collection) (pheochromocytoma)

- Vanillylmandelic acid: > 6.8 mg (24-hour urine collection) (pheochromocytoma)
- Cortisol: > 100 mcg (24-hour urine collection) (Cushing's syndrome)
- Phosphate: < 0.9 or > 1.3 grams (24-hour urine collection) (kidney disorder, hyperparathyroidism, osteomalacia)
- Potassium: < 25 or > 100 mEq/L (24-hour urine collection) (kidney disorder)
- Sodium: < 40 or > 220 mEq (24-hour urine collection) (indicates high blood pressure, heart disease, or kidney disorder)
- Microalbumin: > 30 mg (24-hour urine collection) (kidney disorder or diabetic nephropathy)

23.8   Urine Culture and Sensitivity Test

The urine culture and sensitivity test identifies the presence and type of a microorganism and identifies medication that kills the microorganism. The urine culture and sensitivity test is ordered when the patient is suspected of having a urinary tract infection. A urine collection is placed in an environment conducive to the growth of microorganisms for 3 days. The urine is examined to identify the presence and type of microorganism. The sensitivity test is performed to determine the medication that kills the microorganism.

Why the Test Is Performed

The test assesses the existence and type of microorganism in a patient with a urinary tract infection and the medication to treat the urinary tract infection.

Before Administering the Test

Assess if the patient:

- Has collected the urine properly
- Has taken antibiotics, vitamin C, or diuretics

How the Test Is Performed

- The patient washes his or her hands.
- Open the collection cup. Do not touch the inside of the collection cup.
- Clean the urethra area with an antiseptic.
- Do not touch the cup to the urethra or any skin when collecting the sample.
- Do not contaminate the urine sample with feces, public hair, or other substances.
- If the sample becomes contaminated, then begin again with a new collection cup.
- Urinate for 5 seconds, making sure no skin aside from the urethra touches the urine.
- Move the collection cup into the urine stream.
- Do not touch the collection cup to the urethra or any skin.
- Remove the collection cup and continue urinating.
- Place the lid on the collection cup.
- Refrigerate the collection cup until the sample is sent to the lab.
- A sterile sample may be taken from a Foley catheter.

Teach the Patient

Explain why the test is being performed, what the patient will experience during the test, that the patient will not feel any pain during the test, how to perform the test, and that the patient should not ingest antibiotics, vitamin C, or diuretics before the test.

Understanding the Results

The collection takes a few seconds. Results are known within 3 days.

- Normal (negative):
  - No microorganism present in the urine collection
- Abnormal (positive):
  - Microorganisms are present in the urine collection

23.9   Renin Assay Test

The renin assay test determines the underlying cause of hypertension. The renin assay test is performed with the aldosterone test. Renin is an enzyme produced by the kidneys. Aldosterone is a hormone produced by the adrenal glands. Together, these work to balance the sodium and potassium levels within the patient. A high renin level might indicate a kidney disorder. A low renin level might indicate Conn's syndrome. A low renin level along with a high aldosterone level might indicate an adrenal gland tumor.

Why the Test Is Performed

The test assesses the underlying cause of hypertension.

Before Administering the Test

Assess if the patient:

- Has not taken beta-blockers, ACE inhibitors, diuretics, aspirin, corticosteroids, and estrogen 4 weeks prior to the test
- Has not eaten natural black licorice for 2 weeks prior to the test
- Has not ingested caffeine for 24 hours prior to the test
- Has eaten a low sodium diet for 3 days prior to the test
- Has not eaten or drunk 8 hours prior to the test
- Is pregnant

How the Test Is Performed

A sample of blood is taken from the patient's vein. The patient will experience a tight feeling when the tourniquet is tightened, a pinch or nothing at all when the needle is inserted into the vein, and pressure when a gauze pad is pressed against the insertion site to stop bleeding. It can take up to 10 minutes for bleeding to stop if the patient is taking anticoagulants (aspirin, coumadin). A small bruise might appear at the insertion site, which could become swollen following this test. This is called phlebitis. Applying a warm compress several times a day will reduce the swelling.

Teach the Patient

Explain why the test is being performed, what the patient will experience during the test, that the patient will not feel any pain during the test except a pinch when the blood sample is taken, and that the patient should not take beta-blockers, ACE inhibitors, diuretics, aspirin, corticosteroids, and estrogen 4 weeks prior to the test. The patient should not eat natural black licorice for 2 weeks prior to the test, ingest caffeine 24 hours prior to the test, or eat or drink 8 hours prior to the test. The patient should eat a low sodium diet 3 days prior to the test.

Understanding the Results

Test results are available quickly. The laboratory determines normal values based on calibration of testing equipment with a control test. Test results are reported as high, normal, or low based on the laboratory's control test.

- Normal:
  - Normal level of renin and aldosterone
- Abnormal:
  - High renin level might indicate a kidney disorder
  - Low renin level might indicate Conn's syndrome
  - Low renin level along with a high aldosterone level might indicate an adrenal gland tumor

23.10   Thyroid Scan

A thyroid scan assesses the function of the thyroid gland. There are two types of thyroid scans:

1. *Radioactive Iodine Uptake Test (RAIU)*: This assesses the absorption of a radioactive tracer by the thyroid gland.
2. *Whole-Body Thyroid Scan*: This test assesses whether thyroid cancer has metastasized.

Why the Test Is Performed

The test assesses thyroid function and the treatment for thyroid disease.

Before Administering the Test

Assess if the patient:

- Has signed a consent form
- Has not eaten or drunk 2 hours before the test
- Has not taken antithyroid medication, thyroid hormones, Cordarone, Pacerone, iodine, or kelp a week before the test
- Has eaten a low iodine diet
- Has allergies
- Is pregnant
- Is breast-feeding
- Has recently had a radioactive iodine test performed within 4 weeks prior to the test
- Has taken anticoagulant medication such as Plavix, coumadin, heparin, or aspirin

How the Test Is Performed

- A blood sample is taken to measure the amount of thyroid hormones in the blood.
- The patient signs a consent form.
- The patient removes his or her clothes from above the waist.
- The patient removes dentures.
- The patient removes jewelry from the upper part of the body.
- The patient either swallows the radioactive tracer 24 hours before the test, or is administered technetium 2 hours prior to the test.
- The patient lies on a table.
- The table is tipped backwards.
- The gamma scintillation camera takes images of the thyroid gland.
- Images are also taken 24 hours after the initial images were taken.
- The patient should drink lots of fluid to flush the tracer from his or her body.
- The patient should discard breast milk for 2 days following the test if the patient is breast-feeding.
- The patient should flush the toilet quickly after urinating and defecating, since the tracer is excreted in urine and feces for 2 days following the test.

Teach the Patient

Explain why the test is being performed, what the patient will experience during the test, that the patient will not feel any pain during the procedure except for a pinch when the tracer is injected into the vein, and the patient may feel flushed when technetium is injected, if technetium is administered. The patient swallows the capsule that contains the tracer with water, if the capsule is used. The patient must sign a consent form, must not eat or drink for 2 hours before the test, and should not take anticoagulant medication such as Plavix, coumadin, heparin, or aspirin for 2 weeks prior to the test. Inform the patient to drink lots of fluids to flush the tracer following the test, flush the toilet immediately after urinating and defecating, and wash hands thoroughly after urinating and defecating. If the patient is breastfeeding, breast milk must be discarded for 2 days after the scan. The patient should eat a low iodine diet and should not take antithyroid medication, thyroid hormones, Cordarone, Pacerone, iodine, or kelp a week before the test.

Understanding the Results

The procedure takes less than 1 hour. Results are known within a week.

- Normal:
    - Thyroid functions normally
    - Normal shape and size of the thyroid
- Abnormal:
    - Abnormal shape or size of the thyroid
    - Nodules are found on the thyroid
    - Iodine is in other tissues, indicating that thyroid cancer may have metastasized

23.11   Thyroid and Parathyroid Ultrasound

The thyroid and parathyroid ultrasounds are used to create an image of the thyroid gland and the parathyroid gland. The *thyroid gland* produces *thyroxine* which controls the patient's metabolism. The *parathyroid gland* produces the *parathyroid hormone* (PTH) which controls the patient's calcium and phosphorus balance in the blood. The thyroid and parathyroid ultrasound enables the healthcare provider to assess the size of these glands but not the production of hormones.

Why the Test Is Performed

The test assesses the size of the thyroid gland, size of the parathyroid gland, and for growths. The test also guides the healthcare provider when performing a biopsy.

Before Administering the Test

Assess if the patient:

- Can lie still during the test
- Has removed jewelry and clothes from above the waist
- Signed a consent form, if the ultrasound is used for a biopsy
- Can move his or her head
- Is obese

How the Test Is Performed

- The patient removes all jewelry from the head and neck area.
- The patient may be asked to remove all clothes from above the waist.
- The patient lies on his or her back and a pillow is placed under the patient's shoulders.
- A conductive gel is placed on the neck.
- The healthcare provider may place a bag filled with water or a sponge of gel over the patient's throat to increase conductivity.
- The transducer is placed over and moved around the neck. The patient may be asked to turn his or her head.

Teach the Patient

Explain why the ultrasound is being performed, that the patient will not feel any pain, that the patient must lie still during the test, and that conductive gel is placed on the skin over the neck and that it will be wiped off after the test is completed.

Understanding the Test Results

The test takes 30 minutes and the results are ready immediately.

- Normal:
    - Normal size thyroid
    - Normal size parathyroid
    - No growth

- Abnormal:
  - Unexpected size of thyroid or parathyroid
  - Growths are seen

23.12   Thyroid Hormone Tests

Thyroid hormone tests measure the level of thyroid hormones in the patient's blood. The thyroid produces two hormones: thyroxine (T4) and triiodothyronine (T3). There are three thyroid hormone tests:

1. *Free Thyroxine (FT4)*: This test determines the amount of thyroxine that is not bound to globulin.
2. *Total Thyroxine (T4)*: This test determines the total amount of thyroxine that is attached to globulin and that is not bound to globulin.
3. *Triiodothyronine (T3)*: This test determines the total amount of triiodothyronine that is attached to globulin and not bound to globulin.

Why the Test Is Performed

The test assesses for hyperthyroidism and hypothyroidism, the cause of abnormal thyroid-stimulating hormone (TSH) test results, and treatment of hyperthyroidism and hypothyroidism.

Before Administering the Test

Assess if the patient:

- Has not taken birth control pills, corticosteroids, estrogen, Dilantin, Tegretol, amiodarone, propranolole, and lithium 4 weeks prior to the test
- Has taken anticoagulant medication such as Plavix, coumadin, heparin, or aspirin
- Is pregnant
- Has not undergone a test that used contrast material 4 weeks prior to the test

How the Test Is Performed

A sample of blood is taken from the patient's vein. The patient will experience a tight feeling when the tourniquet is tightened, a pinch or nothing at all when the needle is inserted into the vein, and pressure when a gauze pad is pressed against the insertion site to stop bleeding. It can take up to 10 minutes for bleeding to stop if the patient is taking anticoagulants (aspirin, coumadin). A small bruise might appear at the insertion site, which could become swollen following this test. This is called phlebitis. Applying a warm compress several times a day will reduce the swelling.

Teach the Patient

Explain why the test is being performed, what the patient will experience during the test, and that the patient will not feel any pain during the test except a pinch when the blood sample is taken. The patient should not take birth control pills, corticosteroids, estrogen, Dilantin, Tegretol, amiodarone, propranololir, lithium, or anticoagulant medication such as Plavix, coumadin, heparin, or aspirin 4 weeks prior to the test because these medications increase clotting time.

Understanding the Results

Test results are available quickly. The laboratory determines normal values based on calibration of testing equipment with a control test. Test results are reported as high, normal, or low based on the laboratory's control test.

- Normal:
  - Normal level of thyroxine (T4) and triiodothyronine (T3)

- Abnormal:
  - High level might indicate hyperthyroidism, Graves' disease, goiter, thyroiditis, or excess intake of thyroid medication
  - Low level might indicate hypothyroidism, pituitary gland disorder, or thyroiditis

23.13   Thyroid Stimulating Hormone Test

The thyroid stimulating hormone test determines the underlying cause of thyroid disorder. The hypothalamus produces thyrotropin-releasing hormone (TRH), which causes the pituitary gland to produce the thyroid-stimulating hormone, causing the thyroid to produce thyroid hormones.

Why the Test Is Performed

The test assesses the underlying cause of hyperthyroidism and hypothyroidism.

Before Administering the Test

Assess if the patient:

- Has not taken lithium, Tapazole, prophylthiouracil, and corticosteroids 4 weeks prior to the test
- Has taken anticoagulant medication such as Plavix, coumadin, heparin, or aspirin
- Is pregnant
- Has not undergone a test that used contrast material 4 weeks prior to the test

How the Test Is Performed

A sample of blood is taken from the patient's vein. The patient will experience a tight feeling when the tourniquet is tightened, a pinch or nothing at all when the needle is inserted into the vein, and pressure when a gauze pad is pressed against the insertion site to stop bleeding. It can take up to 10 minutes for bleeding to stop if the patient is taking anticoagulants (aspirin, coumadin). A small bruise might appear at the insertion site, which could become swollen following this test. This is called phlebitis. Applying a warm compress several times a day will reduce the swelling.

Teach the Patient

Explain why the test is being performed, what the patient will experience during the test, that the patient will not feel any pain during the test except a pinch when the blood sample is taken, and that the patient should not take lithium, Tapazole, prophylthiouracil, or corticosteroids 4 weeks prior to the test.

Understanding the Results

Test results are available quickly. The laboratory determines normal values based on calibration of testing equipment with a control test. Test results are reported as high, normal, or low based on the laboratory's control test.

- Normal:
  - Normal level thyroid-stimulating hormone
- Abnormal:
  - High level might indicate hypothyroidism, Hashimoto's thyroiditis, pituitary gland tumor, or insufficient dose of thyroid hormone
  - Low level might indicate hyperthyroidism, Graves' disease, goiter, pituitary gland disorder, or excess dose of thyroid hormone

23.14   Salivary Gland Scan

A salivary gland scan assesses the function of the salivary glands to determine the underlying cause of xerostomia (dry mouth) or swelling.

Why the Test Is Performed

The test assesses the salivary glands' function, underlying cause of swollen salivary glands, and underlying cause of dry mouth.

Before Administering the Test

Assess if the patient:

- Has signed a consent form
- Has allergies
- Is pregnant
- Is breastfeeding
- Has recently had a radioactive iodine test performed within 4 weeks prior to the test
- Has taken anticoagulant medication such as Plavix, coumadin, heparin, or aspirin

How the Test Is Performed

- The patient signs a consent form.
- The patient removes clothes from above the waist.
- The patient removes dentures.
- The patient removes jewelry from the upper part of the body.
- A radioactive tracer is injected into the patient's vein.
- The patient lies on a table.
- The table is tipped backwards.
- The gamma scintillation camera takes images of the salivary glands.
- The patient sucks a lemon, which normally causes the glands to release more saliva.
- The gamma scintillation camera takes images of the salivary glands.
- The patient should drink lots of fluid to flush the tracer from his or her body.
- The patient should discard breast milk for 2 days following the test if the patient is breastfeeding.
- The patient should flush the toilet quickly after urinating and defecating, since the tracer is excreted in urine and feces for 2 days following the test.

Teach the Patient

Explain why the test is being performed, what the patient will experience during the test, that the patient will not feel any pain during the procedure except for a pinch when the tracer is injected into the vein, and that the patient may feel flush when the tracer is injected. Inform the patient that he or she must sign a consent form and should not take anticoagulant medication such as Plavix, coumadin, heparin, or aspirin for two weeks prior to the test. The patient should drink lots of fluids to flush the tracer following the test, flush the toilet immediately after urinating and defecating, and wash hands thoroughly after urinating and defecating. If the patient is breastfeeding, breast milk must be discarded for 2 days after the scan.

Understanding the Results

The procedure takes less than 1 hour. Results are known within a week.

- Normal:
  - Salivary glands function normally
- Abnormal:
  - Abnormal shape or size of the salivary glands
  - Nodules are found on the salivary glands
  - Blockage found on the salivary glands

23.15   D-xylose Absorption Test

The D-xylose absorption test assesses the patient for malabsorption syndrome. Patients with malabsorption syndrome are unable to absorb certain nutrients into their blood from the intestinal tract. This can result in malnutrition and chronic diarrhea. The D-xylose absorption test assesses whether these signs are a result of malabsorption syndrome by asking the patient to drink a solution of D-xylose and then measuring the amount of D-xylose in the patient's blood and urine.

Why the Test Is Performed

The test assesses the intestine's ability to absorb D-xylose.

Before Administering the Test

Assess if the patient:

- Has eaten fruits, jellies, pastries, or other foods high in pentose for 24 hours prior to the test
- Has taken aspirin, indomethacin, cardiac medication, or antibiotics
- Has not eaten or drunk anything except water 12 hours prior the test
- Has emptied the bladder prior to the test
- Does not have an infection
- Has rested prior to and during the test
- Has a digestive disorder that reduces the time it takes the stomach to empty

How the Test Is Performed

- A sample of urine and blood are taken.
- The patient drinks a solution containing D-xylose.
- A blood sample is taken 2 hours after the patient drinks the solution.
- A blood sample is taken 5 hours after the patient drinks the solution.
- A 24-hour urine sample is collected once the patient drinks the solution.
- Urine and blood samples are then sent to the lab for analysis.

Teach the Patient

Explain why the test is administered, how the test is performed, and how to collect a 24-hour urine sample. The patient will not feel pain except a pinch when blood samples are taken, should not eat fruits, jellies, pastries, or other foods high in pentose 24 hours prior to the test, and should not take aspirin, indomethacin, cardiac medication, or antibiotics. In addition, the patient should not eat or drink anything except water 12 hours prior the test, should not empty the bladder prior to the test, and should rest prior to and during the test.

Understanding the Results

The result is available quickly. The laboratory determines normal values based on calibration of testing equipment with a control test. Test results are reported as high, normal, or low based on the laboratory's control test.

- Normal:
  - The patient's intestines absorb D-xylose without a problem
- Low value may indicate:
  - Malabsorption syndrome
  - Celiac disease
  - Whipple's disease
  - Crohn's disease
- High value may indicate:
  - Hodgkin's disease
  - Scleroderma

23.16   Stool Culture

A stool culture identifies microorganisms in a stool sample. A patient may exhibit diarrhea and other signs of an infection. The healthcare provider orders a stool culture to determine if the underlying cause is a microorganism. A sample of the patient's stool is sent to the laboratory where it is placed in an environment that encourages microorganisms to grow. After 3 days, laboratory technicians determine if a microorganism is present and if so, which microorganism. The healthcare provider typically orders a sensitivity test of the sample along with the stool culture. The sensitivity test determines the medication that kills the microorganism.

Why the Test Is Performed

The test assesses if there is a microorganism in the stool sample and identifies the microorganism in the stool sample.

Before Administering the Test

Assess if the patient:

- Has her menstrual period
- Has taken antibiotics or medication to treat an infection
- Has had a test that used contrast material within 10 days of the test
- Has not contaminated the stool sample

How the Test Is Performed

- The patient urinates prior to defecating.
- The patient should not mix urine and stool.
- The patient is asked to defecate in a basin in the toilet or bedpan, not in the toilet, since this might contaminate the sample.
- The patient puts on clean gloves.
- A sample of stool is placed in a clean container. It is critical that the stool sample is not contaminated with hair, toilet paper, and other elements that might produce a false positive test result.
- Cap and label the container.
- Wash hands immediately to prevent the spread of the microorganism.
- The container is immediately sent to the lab.

Teach the Patient

Explain why the test is administered, how the test is performed, how to collect the stool sample, not to take the sample during the patient's menstrual period, not to take antibiotics or medication to treat an infection, and that the patient will not feel pain.

Understanding the Results

The result is available within 3 days.

- Normal:
  - No disease causing microorganism
- Abnormal:
  - Disease causing microorganism identified
- Indeterminate:
  - Insufficient sample size
  - Contaminated sample

23.17   Enterotest (Giardiasis String Test)

The enterotest test determines if the patient has giardiasis. A patient who has severe diarrhea might have giardiasis. Giardiasis is caused by an intestinal parasite called *Giardia intestinalis*, which is found in water, food, or soil which is contaminated with feces. The enterotest test determines if the patient has giardiasis by sampling fluid in the duodenum. The patient swallows a gelatin capsule that is attached to a string. The string is taped to the outside of the patient's mouth while the capsule dissolves in the stomach and the duodenum. The string is then removed and examined under a microscope.

Why the Test Is Performed

The test assesses the presence of *Giardia intestinalis*.

Before Administering the Test

Assess if the patient can swallow and is able to have the string attached to the outside of the mouth.

How the Test Is Performed

- The patient swallows a gelatin capsule attached to a string.
- The string is taped to the outside of the patient's cheek.
- The patient waits 6 hours.
- The string is removed and sent to the lab for microscopic analysis to determine the presence of *Giardia intestinalis*.

Teach the Patient

Explain why the test is administered, how the test is performed, how to collect the stool sample, not to take antibiotics or medication to treat an infection, and that the patient will not feel pain, although the string might feel uncomfortable.

Understanding the Results

The result is available within 3 days.

- Normal:
  - No *Giardia intestinalis* is present
- Abnormal:
  - *Giardia intestinalis* is present

23.18   Stool Analysis

A stool analysis is the examination of the patient's feces to identify digestive tract disorders. The patient's stool sample is examined for: color, volume, consistency, odor, and presence of blood, fat, mucus, fiber, bile, and glucose.

Why the Test Is Performed

The test assesses for digestive tract disorder, liver disorder, pancreas disorder, colon cancer, and absorption disorder.

Before Administering the Test

Assess if the patient:

- Has her menstrual period
- Has taken aspirin, Aleve, ibuprofen, antacids, NSAIDs, laxatives, antidiarrheal medication, antibiotics, or medication to treat an infection for 2 weeks prior to the test

- Has had a test that used contrast material within 10 days of the test
- Has not contaminated the stool sample
- Has not eaten cauliflower, bananas, red meat, cantaloupe, parsnips, turnips, or beets prior to the test
- Has not taken vitamin C prior to the test
- Has not drunk alcohol prior to the test
- Has not had an enema prior to the test

How the Test Is Performed

- The patient urinates prior to defecating.
- The patient should not mix urine and stool.
- The patient is asked to defecate in a basin in the toilet or bedpan, not in the toilet, since this might contaminate the sample.
- The patient puts on clean gloves.
- A sample of stool is placed in a clean container. It is critical that the stool sample is not contaminated with hair, toilet paper, and other elements that might produce a false positive test result.
- Cap and label the container.
- Wash hands immediately to prevent the spread of the microorganism.
- The container is immediately sent to the lab.

Understanding the Results

Explain why the test is administered, how the test is performed, and how to collect the stool sample. The patient should not take the sample during her menstrual period, take aspirin, Aleve, ibuprofen, antacids, NSAIDs, laxatives, antidiarrheal medication, antibiotics, or medication to treat an infection for 2 weeks prior to the test, and not eat cauliflower, bananas, red meat, cantaloupe, parsnips, turnips, or beets prior to the test. In addition, the patient should not take vitamin C, drink alcohol, or have an enema prior to the test, and will not feel pain.

Test Results

The result is available within 3 days.

- Normal:
  - Stool is well-formed, soft, and brown
  - No mucus or blood in the stool
  - Minimum amount of glucose
- Abnormal:
  - Stool is loose, hard, or a color other than brown
  - Mucus or blood in the stool
  - Significant amount of glucose, fat, trypsin, or elastase in stool

23.19   Fecal Occult Blood Test (FOBT)

The fecal occult blood test examines stool for blood that is not visible to the naked eye. Blood in stool is not always visible. Blood in stool that is not visible is referred to as *occult blood*. Although the presence of occult blood is linked to colon cancer, there are many other causes of occult blood in stool.

Why the Test Is Performed

The test assesses for blood in the stool.

Before Administering the Test

Assess if the patient:

- Has her menstrual period
- Has not contaminated the stool sample
- Has been taking anticoagulant medication Plavix, coumadin, aspirin, or heparin

How the Test Is Performed

- The patient urinates prior to defecating.
- The patient should not mix urine and stool.
- The patient is asked to defecate in a basin in the toilet or bedpan, not in the toilet, since this might contaminate the sample.
- The patient puts on clean gloves.
- A sample of stool is placed on a card that is chemically treated. It is critical that the stool sample is not contaminated with hair, toilet paper, and other elements that might produce a false positive test result.
- A reaction agent is placed on the stool sample. If the sample turns blue there is blood in the stool sample.
- Wash hands immediately.
- The healthcare provider may collect a stool sample during a digital rectum examination rather than asking the patient to defecate.

Teach the Patient

Explain why the test is administered, how the test is performed, and how to collect the stool sample. The patient should not take the sample during her menstrual period, should stop taking anticoagulant medication, Plavix, coumadin, aspirin, or heparin, and will not feel pain.

Understanding the Results

The result is available immediately.

- Normal:
  - No blood in the stool sample
- Abnormal:
  - Anal fissures
  - Peptic ulcer
  - Polyps
  - Hemorrhoids
  - Gastroesophageal reflux disease (GERD)
  - Ulcerative colitis
  - Use of anticoagulation medication
  - Crohn's disease

23.20   Overnight Dexamethasone Suppression Test

The overnight dexamethasone suppression test is used to assess if the patient has Cushing's syndrome. The pituitary glands secrete adrenocorticotropic hormone (ACTH) based on the amount of cortisol in the patient's blood. Adrenocorticotropic hormone signals the adrenal glands to secrete cortisol. In Cushing's syndrome, cortisol is secreted regardless of the secretion of the adrenocorticotropic hormone level. The overnight dexamethasone suppression test requires the patient to take dexamethasone, which is a corticosteroid. This increases the cortisol level in the patient's blood and therefore signals the pituitary glands not to secrete adrenocorticotropic hormone. As a result, the adrenal glands should not secrete cortisol. In the morning, the patient's cortisol level should be relatively low. If not, then the patient might have Cushing's syndrome.

Why the Test Is Performed

The test assesses for Cushing's syndrome.

Before Administering the Test

Assess if the patient:

- Has not eaten or drunk 12 hours prior to drawing the blood sample
- Has taken methadone, aspirin, MAOIs, lithium, and diuretics 48 hours before the blood sample is drawn

How the Test Is Performed

- At 11 p.m. the patient is administered dexamethasone by mouth with milk or antacid.
- A blood sample is taken at 8 a.m.
- The level of cortisol in the blood sample is measured.

Teach the Patient

Explain why and how the test is performed. The patient should not eat or drink 12 hours prior to drawing the blood sample and should not take methadone, aspirin, MAOI, lithium, or diuretics 48 hours before the blood sample is drawn.

Understanding the Results

The result is available quickly. The laboratory determines normal values based on calibration of testing equipment with a control test. Test results are reported as high, normal, or low based on the laboratory's control test.

- Normal:
  - A relatively low level of cortisol in the blood sample
- High value may indicate:
  - Cushing Syndrome
  - Cancer
  - Diabetes
  - Hyperthyroidism

Solved Problems

Upper Gastrointestinal (UGI) Series

23.1 Why might the healthcare provider order a UGI series?

The UGI series assesses the cause of stomach pain and indigestion and the cause of malabsorption syndrome.

23.2 What should you assess before the UGI series is administered?

Assess if the patient:
- Has signed a consent form
- Has any allergies
- Has taken anticoagulant medication such as Plavix, coumadin, heparin, or aspirin
- Can lie on his or her back or stomach
- Is able to lie still
- Is able to follow instructions
- Has eaten a lower fiber diet for 3 days before the test
- Has not eaten or drunk 12 hours before the test
- Has taken a laxative 12 hours before the test
- Has removed dentures before the test
- Is able to swallow the barium contrast material

23.3 The patient who is undergoing a UGI series asks about swallowing the barium contrast material. How would you respond?

The patient will be swallowing the barium contrast material several times during the test. Barium contrast material is sweet flavored.

Gallbladder Scan

23.4 The patient asks how the gallbladder scan works. How would you respond?

- The patient signs a consent form.
- The patient removes his or her clothes.
- The patient lies on a table.
- The injection site is cleaned.
- The patient is injected with the radioactive tracer.
- The camera is moved into position.
- Images are taken immediately, then every 10 minutes for 90 minutes.
- The patient is administered cholecystokinin to stimulate the gallbladder.
- The patient may be administered morphine sulfate to diagnose gallbladder inflammation.

23.5 What instructions would you give the patient following a gallbladder scan?

The patient should drink lots of fluid to flush the tracer from his or her body. The patient should flush the toilet quickly after urinating and defecating, since the tracer is excreted in urine and feces in the 2 days following the test.

23.6 What instructions would you give a patient before the gallbladder scan?

Explain why the procedure is being performed, what the patient will experience during the procedure, and that the patient will not feel any pain during the procedure except a pinch when the tracer is injected into the vein. The patient must sign a consent form, must not eat or drink for 12 hours before the test, should not take Pepto-Bismol for 48 hours before the test, and should not take anticoagulant medication such as Plavix, coumadin, heparin, or aspirin for 2 weeks prior to the test. In addition, the patient should drink lots of fluids to flush the tracer following the test, flush the toilet immediately after urinating and defecating, wash hands thoroughly after urinating and defecating, and apply a warm compress to the injection site if there is swelling. If the patient is breast-feeding, breast milk must be discarded for 2 days after the scan.

Kidney Scan

23.7 What is a kidney function study?

A kidney function study measures the time that the tracer takes to pass through the kidneys and enter the bladder as a part of urine.

23.8 What is a kidney perfusion study?

A kidney perfusion study assesses blood flow through the kidneys.

23.9 Why might a healthcare provider order a kidney scan?

A kidney scan assesses blood flow through the kidneys and the function of the kidneys.

23.10 What must you assess before the patient is administered a kidney scan?

Assess if the patient:
- Has signed a consent form
- Has drunk 3 glasses of water before the test
- Can lie still
- Has allergies
- Is pregnant
- Has recently had a barium test performed within 4 days prior to the test
- Has taken anticoagulant medication such as Plavix, coumadin, heparin, or aspirin
- Has taken Pepto-Bismol
- Has taken antihypertensives
- If the patient is breast-feeding, breast milk must be discarded for 2 days after the scan

23.11   How is the kidney scan performed?
- The patient signs a consent form.
- The patient removes his or her clothes.
- The patient lies on a table, although the patient may be asked to sit or stand during the test.
- The injection site is cleaned.
- The patient is injected with the radioactive tracer.
- The camera is moved into position.
- Function study:
  ○ Images are taken every 3 minutes for 30 minutes.
  ○ The patient may be administered a diuretic to increase kidney function.
- Perfusion study:
  ○ Movement of the tracer through the kidneys is recorded on a renogram.
- The patient should drink lots of fluid to flush the tracer from the body.
- The patient should flush the toilet quickly after urinating and defecating, since the tracer is excreted in urine and feces for 2 days following the test.

23.12   What should you tell a patient who is about to undergo a kidney scan?

Explain why the procedure is being performed, what the patient will experience during the procedure, and that the patient will not feel any pain during the procedure except for a pinch when the tracer is injected into the vein. The patient must sign a consent form, drink three glasses of water before the test, should not take Pepto-Bismol for 48 hours before the test, and should not take anticoagulant medication such as Plavix, coumadin, heparin, or aspirin for 2 weeks prior to the test. In addition, the patient should drink lots of fluids to flush the tracer following the test, flush the toilet immediately after urinating and defecating, wash hands thoroughly after urinating and defecating, and apply a warm compress to the injection site if there is swelling. If the patient is breast-feeding, breast milk must be discarded for 2 days after the scan.

Urine Analysis

23.13   What are the characteristics of urine that are examined in a urine analysis?

The urine characteristics which are examined are:
- Clarity: How clear is the urine?
- Color: What color is the urine?
- Specific gravity: The balance between water and substances in the urine.
- Odor: The aroma of urine.
- pH: How acidic or alkaline is the urine?

23.14   What is the clean-catch midstream one-time urine collection?

Clean-catch midstream one-time urine collection is urine collected after the patient begins to urinate.

23.15   What is a double voided urine collection?

Double voided urine collection is urine collected the second time the patient voids.

23.16   What should you assess before administering the urine analysis test?

Assess if the patient:
- Has collected the urine properly
- Has exercised prior to the test
- Is menstruating
- Has eaten blackberries, beets, or foods that might color urine
- Has had the usual amount of exposure to the sun
- Is on extended bed rest
- Has recently undergone a test that used contrast material
- Has ingested nicotine or caffeine
- Has had a recent illness or is under stress
- Keeps warm during testing, if testing catecholmine levels
- Is pregnant

- Has had severe vomiting
- Has taken Dilantin, Pyridium, vitamin B, diuretics, Rifampin, Trimpex, ascorbic acid, Probalan, Benemid, allopurinol, insulin, lithium, laxatives, steroids, antacids, NSAIDs, antibiotics, potassium supplements, growth hormones or parathyroid hormone, aspirin, antidepressants, nitroglycerin, tetracycline, tricyclic, theophylline, and cold and sinus medication
- Has recently taken sodium-based medication

23.17   What instructions would you give to the patient who is undergoing urine analysis?

- The patient washes his or her hands.
- Open the collection cup. Do not touch the inside of the collection cup.
- Clean the urethra area with an antiseptic.
- Do not touch the cup to the urethra or any skin when collecting the sample.
- Do not contaminate the urine sample with feces, pubic hair, or other substances.
- If the sample becomes contaminated, then begin again with a new collection cup.
- Double-voided urine collection:
  - The patient urinates.
  - The patient drinks a lot of water.
  - The patient waits until he or she has the feeling to urinate.
- Urinate for 5 seconds, making sure no skin aside from the urethra touches the urine.
- Move the collection cup into the urine stream.
- Do not touch the collection cup to the urethra or any skin.
- Remove the collection cup and continue urinating.
- Place the lid on the collection cup.
- Refrigerate the collection cup until the sample is sent to the lab.
- Twenty-four-hour urine collection:
  - The patient empties the bladder the first thing in the morning.
  - The patient collects urine the next and subsequent times that he or she urinates for the 24-hour period.
  - The patient must note the time of urination. This begins the 24-hour period.
  - Urine is kept in a gallon container that must be refrigerated between collections.
  - The patient must note the last time of urination at the end of the 24-hour period.
  - If the patient urinates within the 24-hour period and does not collect the urine, the patient must begin the 24-hour urine collection again.

Urine Culture and Sensitivity Test

23.18   Why might the healthcare provider order a urine culture and sensitivity test?

A urine culture and sensitivity test assesses the existence and type of microorganism in a patient with a urinary tract infection and the medication to treat the urinary tract infection.

23.19   What should you assess before the urine culture and sensitivity test is administered?

Assess if the patient:
- Has collected the urine properly
- Has taken antibiotics, vitamin C, or diuretics

23.20   What is the objective of the urine culture and sensitivity test?

The urine culture and sensitivity test identifies the presences and type of a microorganism and identifies medication that kills the microorganism.

Renin Assay Test

23.21   Why might the healthcare provider order the renin assay test?

The renin assay test determines the underlying cause of hypertension.

23.22 The patient who is undergoing the renin assay test asks you the rationale for the test. How would you respond?

"The renin assay test is performed with the aldosterone test. Renin is an enzyme produced by the kidneys. Aldosterone is a hormone produced by the adrenal glands. Together these work to balance the sodium and potassium levels within the patient. A high renin level might indicate a kidney disorder. A low renin level might indicate Conn's syndrome. A low renin level along with a high aldosterone level might indicate an adrenal gland tumor."

23.23 What should you assess before the patient undergoes the renin assay test?

Assess if the patient:
- Has not taken beta-blockers, ACE inhibitors, diuretics, aspirin, corticosteroids, and estrogen 4 weeks prior to the test
- Has not eaten natural black licorice for 2 weeks prior to the test
- Has not ingested caffeine 24 hours prior to the test
- Has eaten a low sodium diet 3 days prior to the test
- Has not eaten or drunk 8 hours prior to the test
- Is pregnant

23.24 What are abnormal results of the renin assay test?

A high renin level might indicate a kidney disorder. A low renin level might indicate Conn's syndrome. A low renin level along with a high aldosterone level might indicate an adrenal gland tumor.

23.25 Following the renin assay test the patient reports that the insertion site is swollen. How would you respond?

"The insertion site may become swollen following this test. This is called phlebitis. Applying a warm compress several times a day will reduce the swelling."

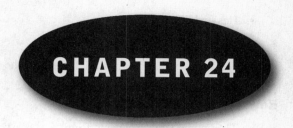

CHAPTER 24

Bone Tests

24.1   Definition

Bones tests assess the cause of a patient's complaints about discomfort or pain in bones. Healthcare providers have an assortment of tests and procedures that are used to investigate signs of a disorder. An image of the bone can be taken using a bone scan, in which a radioactive tracer highlights the structure of the bone. A bone mineral density test is ordered to determine the thickness of bone, looking for the first sign of osteoporosis. When X-ray, ultrasound, and other imaging technologies indicate something is abnormal, the healthcare provider may perform arthroscopy to look directly into the joint, or a bone biopsy or bone marrow aspiration to take samples of suspicious tissue.

24.2   Bone Mineral Density (BMD) Test

The bone mineral density (BMD) test measures the density of bone to assess if the patient has osteopenia or osteoporosis. A low bone density might result in an increased risk of fracture. There are five ways to measure bone mineral density:

1. **Ultrasound**: This test uses sound waves to determine the density of bone. However, this method does not assess the hip and the spine, which are bones that commonly fracture because of low bone mineral density.
2. **Dual Photo Absorptiometry (DPA)**: This method uses a low-dose radioactive tracer to measure bone density in all bones, including the hip and spine.
3. **Quantitative Computed Tomography (QCT)**: This method measures the density of the vertebra. However, this test is less accurate than the DPA, DEXA, and PDEXA methods.
4. **Dual-Energy X-Ray Absorptiometry (DEXA)**: This method uses two X-ray beams to measure bone density and can measure up to 2% bone loss, making it the most accurate way to measure bone mineral density.
5. **Peripheral Dual-Energy X-Ray Absorptiometry (P-DEXA)**: This method measures bone density in the arms and legs but cannot be used to measure the bone density of the hip or spine.

Why the Test Is Performed

The test assesses for osteoporosis, the progression of osteoporosis, and the impact of long-term treatment with corticosteroids.

Before Administering the Test

Assess if the patient:

- Has signed a consent form
- Is pregnant
- Is able to lie still

- Has had broken bones
- Has arthritis
- Has had a bone replacement
- Has had a barium test within 2 weeks of the test

How the Test Is Performed

- The patient signs a consent form.
- The patient lies on a table.
- The ultrasound, CT, or X-ray device scans the site.
- The insertion site is cleaned with an anesthetic.

Teach the Patient

Explain why the procedure is being performed, what the patient will experience during the procedure, and that the patient will not feel any pain.

Understanding the Results

The procedure takes less than 1 hour. Results are ready within 2 weeks of the procedure.

- The patient is given a T-score.
  - The T-score compares the patient's bone mineral density with the average healthy 30-year-old's T-score.
  - A negative T-score indicates that the patient's bone mineral density is less than the T-score of the average healthy 30-year-old.
  - A positive T-score indicates that the patient's bone mineral density is greater than the T-score of the average healthy 30-year-old.
- The patient is given a Z-score.
  - The Z-score compares the patient to patients of the same age, sex, and race.
  - A negative Z-score indicates that the patient's bone mineral density is less than the Z-score of the average person of his or her age, sex, and race.
  - A positive Z-score indicates that the patient's bone mineral density is greater than the Z-score of the average person of his or her age, sex, and race.
- Normal:
  - T-Score
    - Normal is within +/− 1 of the T-score of the average healthy 30-year-old's T-score.
  - Z-Score
    - Normal is within +/− 1 of the Z-score of the average person of the patient's age, sex, and race.
- Abnormal:
  - T-Score
    - 2.5 or less than the T-score of the average healthy 30-year-old's T-score indicates osteoporosis.
  - Z-Score
    - 2.5 or less than the Z-score of the average person of the patient's age, sex, and race.

24.3 Bone Scan

A bone scan assesses the infection, trauma, and metastasized cancer growth to the bone. A radioactive tracer is injected in the patient's vein. The tracer is removed from the blood into the bone. A gamma camera takes an image of the tracer as the tracer is absorbed. Lack of absorption indicates bone infarction and possibly cancer. Areas of high absorption might indicate an infection, tumor, or fracture.

Why the Test Is Performed

The test determines if cancer has metastasized and assesses for bone infection.

Before Administering the Test

Assess if the patient:

- Has signed a consent form
- Has emptied his or her bladder
- Has allergies
- Is pregnant
- Is breast-feeding
- Has recently had a barium test performed within 4 days prior to the test
- Has taken anticoagulant medication such as Plavix, coumadin, heparin, or aspirin
- Has taken Pepto-Bismol

How the Test Is Performed

- The patient signs a consent form.
- The patient removes his or her clothes.
- The patient lies on a table.
- The injection site is cleaned.
- The patient is injected with the radioactive tracer.
- The gamma camera is moved into position.
- Images are taken immediately, then periodically for up to 5 hours.
- The patient should drink lots of fluid to flush the tracer from his or her body.
- The patient should flush the toilet quickly after urinating and defecating, since the tracer is excreted in urine and feces in the 2 days following the test.

Teach the Patient

Explain why the procedure is being performed, what the patient will experience during the procedure, and that the patient will not feel any pain during the procedure except for a pinch when the tracer is injected into his or her vein. The patient must sign a consent form, should not take Pepto-Bismol for 48 hours before the test, and should not take anticoagulant medication such as Plavix, coumadin, heparin, or aspirin for 2 weeks prior to the test. In addition, the patient must empty his or her bladder before the test, drink lots of fluids to flush the tracer following the test, flush the toilet immediately after urinating and defecating, wash hands thoroughly after urinating and defecating, and apply a warm compress to the injection site if there is swelling. If the patient is breast-feeding, breast milk must be discarded during the 2 days after the scan.

Understanding the Results

The test takes less than 1 hour. Results are known within 2 days.

- Normal:
  - The bone is normal
- Abnormal:
  - Cancer has metastasized to the bone
  - The bone is inflamed
  - A bone infarction is identified

Solved Problems

Bone Mineral Density

24.1 What does the BMD test measure?

The bone mineral density (BMD) test measures the density of bone to assess if the patient has osteopenia or osteoporosis.

24.2   What is a dual photo absorptiometry test?

A dual photo absorptiometry (DPA) test uses a low-dose radioactive tracer to measure bone density in all bones, including the hip and spine.

24.3   What is a dual-energy X-Ray absorptiometry test?

A dual-energy X-Ray absorptiometry (DEXA) test uses two X-ray beams to measure bone density and can measure up to 2% bone loss, making it the most accurate way to measure bone mineral density.

24.4   What is a peripheral dual-energy X-Ray absorptiometry test?

A peripheral dual-energy X-Ray absorptiometry (P-DEXA) test measures the bone density in arms and legs but cannot be used to measure the bone density of the hip or spine.

24.5   What is the drawback of using an ultrasound test to measure bone mineral density?

An ultrasound test uses sound waves to determine the density of bone. However, this method does not assess the hip and the spine, which are bones that commonly fracture because of low bone mineral density.

24.6   Why might a healthcare provider order a bone density test?

The test assesses for osteoporosis, the progression of osteoporosis, and the impact of long-term treatment with corticosteroids.

24.7   What should you assess before the bone density test is administered?

Assess if the patient:
- Has signed a consent form
- Is pregnant
- Is able to lie still
- Has had broken bones
- Has arthritis
- Has had bone replacements
- Has had a barium test within 2 weeks of the test

24.8   What is a T-score?

The patient is given a T-score following a bone density test.
- The T-score compares the patient's bone mineral density with the average healthy 30-year-old's T-score.
- A negative T-score indicates that the patient's bone mineral density is less than the T-score of the average healthy 30-year-old.
- A positive T-score indicates that the patient's bone mineral density is greater than the T-score of the average healthy 30-year-old.

24.9   What is a Z-score?

The patient is given a Z-score following a bone density test.
- The Z-score compares the patient to patients of the same age, sex, and race.
- A negative Z-score indicates that the patient's bone mineral density is less than the Z-score of the average person of his or her age, sex, and race.
- A positive Z-score indicates that the patient's bone mineral density is greater than the Z-score of the average person of his or her age, sex, and race.

24.10   What are abnormal T-scores and Z-scores?

An abnormal T-score is 2.5 or less than the T-score of the average healthy 30-year-old's T-score, indicating osteoporosis. An abnormal Z-score is 2.5 or less than the Z-score of the average person of the patient's age, sex, and race.

Bone Scan

24.11   What is a bone scan?

A bone scan assesses the infection, trauma, and metastasized cancer growth to the bone.

24.12 What should you assess before the patient undergoes a bone scan?

Assess if the patient:
- Has signed a consent form
- Has emptied his bladder
- Has allergies
- Is pregnant
- Is breast-feeding
- Has recently had a barium test performed within 4 days prior to the test
- Has taken anticoagulant medication such as Plavix, coumadin, heparin, or aspirin
- Has taken Pepto-Bismol

24.13 How is a bone scan performed?

- The patient signs a consent form.
- The patient removes his or her clothes.
- The patient lies on a table.
- The injection site is cleaned.
- The patient is injected with the radioactive tracer.
- The gamma camera is moved into position.
- Images are taken immediately, then periodically for up to 5 hours.

24.14 What should you tell a patient following a bone scan?

The patient should drink lots of fluid to flush the tracer from his or her body. The patient should flush the toilet quickly after urinating and defecating, since the tracer is excreted in urine and feces in the 2 days following the test.

24.15 What should you teach the patient who is about to undergo a bone scan?

Explain why the procedure is being performed, what the patient will experience during the procedure, and that the patient will not feel any pain during the procedure except for a pinch when the tracer is injected into his or her vein. The patient must sign a consent form, should not take Pepto-Bismol for 48 hours before the test, and should not take anticoagulant medication such as Plavix, coumadin, heparin, or aspirin for 2 weeks prior to the test. In addition, the patient must empty his or her bladder before the test, drink lots of fluids to flush the tracer following the test, flush the toilet immediately after urinating and defecating, and wash hands thoroughly after urinating and defecating.

24.16 What should you tell a patient who is breast-feeding and who is about to undergo a bone scan?

If the patient is breastfeeding, breast milk must be discarded during the 2 days after the scan.

24.17 What should you tell the patient who reports that the injection site following a bone scan is swollen?

Apply a warm compress to the injection site if there is swelling.

24.18 What are possible abnormal findings in a bone scan?

Possible abnormal findings in a bone scan are that cancer has metastasized to the bone, the bone is inflamed, and a bone infarction is identified.

24.19 How would you respond if the patient asks you how long a bone scan will take?

The test takes less than 1 hour.

24.20 How long does it take to learn the results of a bone scan?

Results are known within 2 days.

24.21 Why should the patient avoid taking anticoagulant medication such as Plavix, coumadin, heparin, or aspirin for 2 weeks prior to the test?

The test requires that the tracer be injected into the patient's vein. Anticoagulants might increase the clotting time of blood following the injection.

24.22 How would you respond if the patient raises concerns about having a radioactive tracer injected into his or her vein?

Only a very small amount of radioactive tracer is injected. The side effects are minimal and the patient is in no danger.

24.23 What would you say if the patient asks why the tracer is injected into the patient's vein and not into the bone?

A radioactive tracer is injected in the patient's vein because the tracer is removed from the blood into the bone.

24.24 What might be indicated by the lack of absorption of the tracer by bone?

Lack of absorption indicates bone infarction and possibly cancer.

24.25 What might high absorption of the tracer by the bone indicate?

Areas of high absorption might indicate an infection, tumor, or fracture.

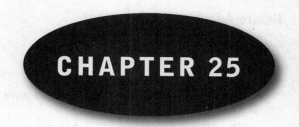

CHAPTER 25

Tests of Male Sexual Functioning

25.1 Definition

There are a number of medical tests and procedures that are specifically designed to diagnose and treat disorders that affect men. When a man is unable to impregnate a woman, the healthcare provider orders tests to assess if there is an underlying problem with the man's reproductive organs. The initial test is a semen analysis that assesses the man's semen and sperm. Depending on the results, a testicular scan or testicular ultrasound is ordered to determine if there is a structural disorder. One such structural disorder is *varicoceles*, which is a large vein that blocks blood flow to the testicles. This is relieved by performing a varicoceles repair.

The healthcare provider may follow up with a testicular examination or an erectile dysfunction test. If the erectile dysfunction test returns positive results, the healthcare provider may perform a penile implant procedure where a device is inserted to cause an erection. Some men desire to become infertile by having their vas deferens cut or blocked by a vasectomy. This prevents sperm from mixing with semen, resulting in no sperm in the ejaculate. In some instances a vasectomy can be reversed by performing a vasovasostomy.

Men are susceptible to developing an enlarged prostate gland, which could be caused by prostate cancer. Prostatic cancer cells are in part fueled by testosterone, which is produced by the testicles. The healthcare provider might perform an *orchiectomy*, which is the surgical removal of one or both testicles. This reduces the level of testosterone in the patient's body. Alternatively, the healthcare provider may perform a *prostatectomy*, which is the removal of the prostate gland. However, this procedure may leave the patient with erectile dysfunction and urinary incontinence.

25.2 Erectile Dysfunction Tests

Erectile dysfunction is commonly caused by psychological, blood vessel, and nerve disorders. There are three tests that are commonly ordered to assess erectile dysfunction:

1. **Color Duplex Doppler**: This test assesses blood flow through the penis using an ultrasound.
2. **Nocturnal Penile Tumescence (NPT)**: This test assesses if the patient has erections during sleep.
3. **Intracavernosal Injection**: This test injects prostaglandin E1 into the base of the penis to cause an erection.

Why the Test Is Performed

The test assesses the underlying cause of erectile dysfunction.

Before Administering the Test

Assess if the patient:

- Has signed a consent form
- Is stressed or depressed
- Has not taken Cialis, Levitra, or Viagra prior to the test
- Has any allergies
- Has not taken sleeping pills 2 days before the test, if the patient is undergoing the nocturnal penile tumescence test
- Has not ingested alcohol 2 days before the test, if the patient is undergoing the nocturnal penile tumescence test
- Has not had an erection lasting more than 4 hours
- Has not ingested nicotine within 2 hours of the test
- Has taken anticoagulant medication such as Plavix, coumadin, heparin, or aspirin
- Can lie still

How the Test Is Performed

- The patient signs a consent form.
- The patient removes his clothes below the waist.
- The patient lies on a table.
- Color duplex Doppler:
  - Conductive gel is placed on the penis.
  - The Doppler ultrasound transducer is moved across the penis.
  - An image on a video screen shows the direction and velocity of blood flowing through the penis.
- Nocturnal penile tumescence:
  - A snap gauge is placed around the penis when the patient goes to sleep.
  - An erection during sleep will snap the film, indicating that the patient had an erection while sleeping.
  - Alternatively, a transducer is placed on the penis when the patient goes to sleep and it records the number of erections, the length of time of the erection, and how rigid the erection was during sleep.
- Intracavernosal injection:
  - Prostaglandin E1 is injected into the base of the penis, causing an erection.
  - A measurement is taken of the erection's duration and how rigid the erection is.

Teach the Patient

Explain why the procedure is being performed, what the patient will experience during the procedure, and that the patient will not feel any pain during the procedure except for a pinch from the needle if an intracavernosal injection is performed. The patient will have to sign a consent form, must not take Cialis, Levitra, or Viagra prior to the test, and must not take sleeping pills 2 days before the test (if the patient is undergoing the nocturnal penile tumescence test). In addition, the patient must not ingest alcohol 2 days before the test (if the patient is undergoing the nocturnal penile tumescence test), must not ingest nicotine within 2 hours of the test, and must stop taking anticoagulant medication such as Plavix, coumadin, heparin, or aspirin until after the test is completed.

Understanding the Results

The procedure takes less than 1 hour except for the nocturnal penile tumescence test, which is performed overnight. Results are immediate.

- Normal:
  - Normal blood flow in the penis
  - Normal erection immediately and overnight

- Abnormal:
  - Abnormal blood flow in the penis
  - Abnormal or no erection

25.3   Testicular Ultrasound

A testicular ultrasound is a procedure used to produce an image of the testicles, scrotum, epididymis, and vas deferens to detect if there is any structural dysfunction.

Why the Test Is Performed

The test assesses a mass on the testicles, the underlying cause of pain in the scrotum, and structures within the scrotum.

Before Administering the Test

Assess if the patient:

- Can lie still

How the Test Is Performed

- The patient removes his clothes below the waist.
- The patient lies on a table.
- Conductive gel is placed on the scrotum.
- A transducer is moved across the scrotum.
- An image of the testicles, scrotum, epididymis, and vas deferens appears on a video screen.

Teach the Patient

Explain why the procedure is being performed, what the patient will experience during the procedure, and that the patient will not feel any pain during the procedure.

Understanding the Results

The procedure takes less than 1 hour. Results are known within 2 days.

- Normal:
  - Normal structures in the scrotum
- Abnormal:
  - Inflammation
  - Twisted spermatic cord
  - Growth
  - Pyocele, spermatocele, or hematocele in the scrotum
  - Hernia is present

25.4   Testicular Scan

A testicular scan assesses the function of the testicles and is used to identify blockages. A radioactive tracer is injected in the patient's vein. The tracer flows into the testicles. A camera takes an image of the tracer as the tracer flows through the testicles.

Why the Test Is Performed

The test assesses the testicles.

Before Administering the Test

Assess if the patient:

- Has signed a consent form
- Has allergies
- Has had a barium test performed within 4 days prior to the test
- Has taken aspirin

How the Test Is Performed

- The patient signs a consent form.
- The patient removes his clothes from below the waist.
- The patient lies on a table.
- The penis is taped to the abdomen.
- The testicles are supported by a towel.
- The injection site is cleaned.
- The patient is injected with the radioactive tracer.
- The camera is moved into position.
- Two images are taken, one every 15 minutes.

Teach the Patient

Explain why the procedure is being performed, what the patient will experience during the procedure, and that the patient will not feel any pain during the procedure except for a pinch when the tracer is injected into his vein. The patient must sign a consent form and should not take anticoagulant medication such as Plavix, coumadin, heparin, or aspirin for 2 weeks prior to the test. In addition, the patient should drink lots of fluids to flush the tracer following the test, flush the toilet immediately after urinating and defecating, wash hands thoroughly after urinating and defecating, and apply a warm compress to the injection site if there is swelling.

Understanding the Results

The procedure takes less than 1 hour. Results are known within 2 days.

- Normal:
  - No blockages in the testicles
  - Normal shape and size of the testicles
- Abnormal:
  - Abnormal shape and size of the testicles
  - Testicles are inflamed or blocked

25.5 Testicular Examination

A testicular examination is performed to assess the patient's testicles, scrotum, and penis for testicular atrophy, growths, and abnormalities.

Why the Test Is Performed

The test assesses the testicles, scrotum, and penis.

Before Administering the Test

Assess if the patient:

- Can lie still
- Can stand

How the Test Is Performed

- The patient should empty his bladder prior to the examination.
- The patient removes his clothes from below the waist.
- The patient lies on a table and then stands during the examination.
- The scrotum and testicles are palpated.
- Transillumination is performed to highlight any growth found during palpation. A light is placed behind the testicles, making the outline of a growth visible.
- The healthcare provider assesses the testicles for consistency, weight, size, and texture.
- Lymph nodes in the groin and thigh are palpated.

Teach the Patient

Explain why the examination is being performed, what the patient will experience during the examination, that the patient will not feel any pain during the examination, and that the patient should empty his bladder before the examination.

Understanding the Results

The procedure takes less than 1 hour. Results are known immediately.

- Normal:
  - Normal shape and size of the testicles, scrotum, and penis
  - Normal shape and size of the lymph nodes
- Abnormal:
  - Abnormal shape and size of the testicles, scrotum, and penis
  - Abnormal shape and size of the lymph nodes

25.6   Semen Analysis

Semen analysis is performed to assess the volume of semen and number of quality sperm that are produced in an ejaculation to determine the underlying cause of infertility. There are eight factors that are analyzed:

1. **Semen Volume**: This is the amount of semen in an ejaculation.
2. **Liquefaction Time**: This is the time it takes for the semen to liquefy.
3. **Sperm Morphology**: This is the number of normally shaped sperm.
4. **Sperm Motility**: This is the percentage of sperm that show forward movement.
5. **Sperm Count**: This is the number of sperm in a milliliter of semen in one ejaculation.
6. **Fructose Level**: This is the amount of fructose in semen. Fructose provides energy for sperm.
7. **pH**: This measures the pH level of the semen.
8. **White Blood Cell Count**: This measures the number of white blood cells in semen, which is normally zero.

Why the Test Is Performed

Assesses the underlying cause of infertility, and the success of a vasectomy, and vasovasectomy.

Before Administering the Test

Assess if the patient:

- Has not taken tagament, sulfasalazine, testosterone, estrogen, or nitrofurantoin
- Has not taken Echinacea, St. John's Wort, caffeine, cocaine, alcohol, marijuana or tobacco
- Has not ejaculated for 2 days before the semen sample is taken
- Has ejaculated within 5 days before the semen sample is taken
- Has urinated before the semen sample was taken

- Washed his hands and penis before the semen sample was taken
- Did not use lubricants or condoms when collecting the semen sample
- Did not collect a semen sample after withdrawing from intercourse
- Placed the semen sample in a sterile cup
- Kept the sample at body temperature
- Kept the sample from direct sunlight
- Delivered the sample to the lab immediately
- Has signed a consent form

How the Test Is Performed

- The patient signs a consent form.
- Ejaculation should not occur for 2 days before the semen sample is taken.
- Ejaculation should occur within 5 days before the semen sample is taken.
- Before the semen sample is taken, the patient should urinate.
- The patient's hands and penis should be washed.
- The patient should not use lubricants or condoms when collecting the sample.
- The patient should not collect a semen sample after withdrawing from intercourse.
- The patient places the semen sample in a sterile cup.
- The patient keeps the sample at body temperature.
- The patient keeps the sample from direct sunlight.
- The patient delivers the sample to the lab immediately.

Teach the Patient

Explain why the procedure is being performed, what the patient will experience during the procedure, how to collect the semen sample, and that the patient will not feel any pain during the procedure. The patient must sign a consent form, must not take tagament, sulfasalazine, testosterone, estrogen, or nitrofurantoin, and must not take Echinacea, St. John's Wort, caffeine, cocaine, alcohol, marijuana, or tobacco.

Understanding the Results

The procedure takes less than 1 hour. Results are known within 2 days.

- Normal:
  - Normal semen volume
  - Liquefaction time is less than 60 minutes
  - 70% of sperm have normal shape
  - 70% of sperm show forward mobility
  - Sperm count is more than 20 million sperm per milliliter of semen, or zero if a vasectomy was performed
  - Semen pH is between 7.1 and 8.0
  - 300 milligrams of fructose in 100 milliliter of semen
  - No white blood cells in the semen
- Abnormal:
  - Low semen volume
  - Liquefaction time is 60 minutes or greater
  - Less than 70% of sperm have normal shape
  - Less than 70% of sperm show forward mobility
  - Sperm count is less than 20 million sperm per milliliter of semen, or greater than zero if a vasectomy was performed
  - Semen pH is less than 7.1 or greater than 8.0
  - Less than 300 milligrams of fructose in 100 milliliter of semen
  - White blood cells present in the semen

Solved Problems

Erectile Dysfunction Tests

25.1 What is a color duplex Doppler test?

A color duplex Doppler test assesses blood flow through the penis using an ultrasound.

25.2 What is a nocturnal penile tumescence test?

A nocturnal penile tumescence (NPT) test assesses if the patient has erections during sleep.

25.3 What is the intracavernosal injection test?

The intracavernosal injection test injects prostaglandin E1 into the base of the penis to cause an erection.

25.4 What should be assessed before the erectile dysfunction test is administered?

Assess if the patient:
- Has signed a consent form
- Is stressed or depressed
- Has not taken Cialis, Levitra, or Viagra prior to the test
- Has any allergies
- Has not taken sleeping pills 2 days before the test, if the patient is undergoing the nocturnal penile tumescence test
- Has not ingested alcohol 2 days before the test, if the patient is undergoing the nocturnal penile tumescence test
- Has not had an erection lasting more than 4 hours
- Has not ingested nicotine within 2 hours of the test
- Has taken anticoagulant medication such as Plavix, coumadin, heparin, or aspirin
- Can lie still

25.5 How is the color duplex Doppler test performed?

- Conductive gel is placed on the penis.
- The Doppler ultrasound transducer is moved across the penis.
- An image on a video screen shows the direction and velocity of blood flowing through the penis.

25.6 How is the nocturnal penile tumescence test performed?

- A snap gauge is placed around the penis when the patient goes to sleep.
- An erection during sleep will snap the film, indicating that the patient had an erection while sleeping.
- Alternatively, a transducer is placed on the penis when the patient goes to sleep and it records the number of erections, the length of time of the erection, and how rigid the erection was during sleep.

25.7 How is the intracavernosal injection test performed?

- Prostaglandin E1 is injected into the base of the penis, causing an erection.
- A measurement is taken of the duration of the erection and how rigid the erection is.

25.8 What should you teach a patient who is undergoing an erectile dysfunction test?

Explain why the procedure is being performed, what the patient will experience during the procedure, and that the patient will not feel any pain during the procedure except for a pinch from the needle if an intracavernosal injection is performed. The patient will have to sign a consent form, must not take Cialis, Levitra, or Viagra prior to the test, and must not take sleeping pills 2 days before the test, if the patient is undergoing the nocturnal penile tumescence test. In addition, the patient must not ingest alcohol 2 days before the test (if the patient is undergoing the nocturnal penile tumescence test), must not ingest nicotine within 2 hours of the test, and must stop taking anticoagulant medication such as Plavix, coumadin, heparin, or aspirin until after the test is completed.

Testicular Ultrasound Tests

25.9   Why is a testicular ultrasound test ordered?

The test assesses a mass on the testicles, the underlying cause of pain in the scrotum, and structures within the scrotum.

25.10   What structures are viewed using a testicular ultrasound?

A testicular ultrasound is a procedure used to produce an image of the testicles, scrotum, epididymis, and vas deferens.

25.11   How is the testicular ultrasound performed?

- The patient removes his clothes below the waist.
- The patient lies on a table.
- Conductive gel is placed on the scrotum.
- A transducer is moved across the scrotum.
- An image of the testicles, scrotum, epididymis, and vas deferens appears on a video screen.

25.12   What should you teach the patient who is scheduled to undergo a testicular ultrasound?

Explain why the procedure is being performed, what the patient will experience during the procedure, and that the patient will not feel any pain during the procedure.

25.13   What are abnormal findings of a testicular ultrasound?

Abnormal findings of a testicular ultrasound are inflammation, twisted spermatic cord, growth, hernia, and pyocele, spermatocele, or hematocele in the scrotum.

Testicular Scan

25.14   Why is a testicular scan ordered by the healthcare provider?

A testicular scan assesses the function of the testicles and is used to identify blockages.

25.15   How is the testicular scan performed?

- The patient signs a consent form.
- The patient removes his clothes from below the waist.
- The patient lies on a table.
- The penis is taped to the abdomen.
- The testicles are supported by a towel.
- The injection site is cleaned.
- The patient is injected with the radioactive tracer.
- The camera is moved into position.
- Two images are taken, one every 15 minutes.

25.16   What should you assess before the patient undergoes a testicular scan?

Assess if the patient:
- Has signed a consent form
- Has allergies
- Has recently had a barium test performed within the 4 days prior to the test
- Has taken aspirin

25.17   What should you teach the patient who is scheduled to undergo a testicular scan?

Explain why the procedure is being performed, what the patient will experience during the procedure, and that the patient will not feel any pain during the procedure except for a pinch when the tracer is injected into his vein. The patient must sign a consent form and should not take anticoagulant medication such as Plavix, coumadin, heparin, or aspirin 2 weeks prior to the test.

25.18   What should the patient do following the testicular scan?

Following the testicular scan, the patient should drink lots of fluids to flush the tracer, flush the toilet immediately after urinating and defecating, and wash his hands thoroughly after urinating and defecating.

25.19   What would be an abnormal finding of a testicular scan?

An abnormal finding of a testicular scan would be an abnormal shape and size of the testicles, or the testicles are inflamed or blocked.

Testicular Examination

25.20   Why would a healthcare provider examine a patient's testicles?

A testicular examination is performed to assess the patient's testicles, scrotum, and penis for testicular atrophy, growths, and abnormalities.

25.21   What would you assess before the patient undergoes a testicular examination?

Assess if the patient can lie still and stand.

25.22   How is transillumination performed?

Transillumination is performed to highlight any growth found during palpation. A light is placed behind the testicles, making the outline of a growth visible.

25.23   What does the healthcare provider assess during a testicular examination?

The healthcare provider assesses the testicles for consistency, weight, size, and texture. Lymph nodes in the groin and thigh are palpated.

25.24   What would you explain to a patient who is scheduled to undergo a testicular examination?

Explain why the examination is being performed, what the patient will experience during the examination, that the patient will not feel any pain during the examination, and that the patient should empty his bladder before the examination.

Semen Analysis

25.25   What are the factors analyzed in a semen analysis?

There are eight factors that are analyzed:
1. **Semen Volume**: This is the amount of semen in an ejaculation.
2. **Liquefaction Time**: This is the time it takes for the semen to liquefy.
3. **Sperm Morphology**: This is the number of normally shaped sperm.
4. **Sperm Motility**: This is the percentage of sperm that show forward movement.
5. **Sperm Count**: This is the number of sperm in a milliliter of semen in one ejaculation.
6. **Fructose Level**: This is the amount of fructose in semen. Fructose provides energy for sperm.
7. **pH**: This measures the pH level of the semen.
8. **White Blood Cell Count**: This measures the number of white blood cells in semen, which is normally zero.

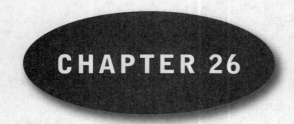

CHAPTER 26

Skin Tests

26.1 Definition

Healthcare providers perform an assortment of tests and procedures to diagnose and treat skin conditions. Lesions, warts, and blemishes that make skin unsightly and unhealthy can be removed by performing one of a number of procedures. Undesired tissue can be frozen with cryosurgery and removed or layers of skin can be peeled away using chemicals or micrographic surgery. Layers can also be removed using curettage, electrosurgery, or the dermabrasion procedure, where a rotating burr scrapes scars and aging skin to encourage new skin growth. Melanoma and nonmelanoma skin cancer affects many patients. The healthcare provider can cure or minimize discomfort of this condition by performing a skin excision where the tumor is surgically removed. Infected skin can be treated once the microorganism that causes the infection is identified. The healthcare provider is able to identify the microorganism by performing a wound culture where a sample of the infected tissue is placed in an environment that is favorable for the growth of the microorganism (culture), and then identified.

Once the lab determines which medication will fight the microorganism, then the medication is administered to the microorganism to determine which medication kills the microorganism. Skin is also a perfect site for testing allergic reactions. There are several tests that healthcare providers administer to the skin to identify allergens that cause the patient to develop an allergic reaction. The skin is also the site of the Mantoux skin test to determine if the patient has ever been exposed to *Mycobacterium tuberculosis*.

26.2 Chemical Peel

A chemical peel is a procedure that exfoliates injured or dead skin, enabling new skin to replace it. There are three types of chemical peels:

1. *Superficial*: This procedure removes the surface layer of the skin for a smoother, brighter appearance, and uses glycolic acid or dry ice for the peel.
2. *Medium*: This procedure is commonly used to smooth fine wrinkles, remove blemishes, and treat pigment problems. It uses trichloroacetic acid (TCA) for the peel.
3. *Deep*: This procedure is commonly used to correct coarse wrinkles and blotches on the face only, and uses phenol for the peel. New skin might be lighter in tone because the skin loses some ability to produce pigment.

A chemical peel might change the patient's skin tone and result in scarring and cold sores. A chemical peel might cause flaking and dryness.

Why the Procedure Is Performed

The procedure enables cosmetic improvement to the skin.

Before Administering the Procedure

Assess if the patient:

- Has signed a consent form
- Has taken anticoagulant medication such as Plavix, coumadin, heparin, or aspirin
- Can lie still
- Has moisturized his or her skin twice a day for 3 weeks prior to the procedure
- Has administered acyclovir 2 weeks prior to the procedure to prevent a viral infection

How the Procedure Is Performed

- The patient will moisturize his or her skin twice a day for 3 weeks prior to the procedure.
- The patient is administered acyclovir 2 weeks prior to the procedure to prevent a viral infection.
- The patient signs a consent form.
- The patient removes clothes in the affected area.
- The patient will lie on a table.
- The healthcare provider may test the peel on skin in a less visible location.
- The site is cleaned with an antiseptic.
- Superficial peel:
  - The chemical is applied to the site using an applicator.
  - The chemical remains on the site for several minutes.
  - Alcohol or water is applied to the site to neutralize the chemical.
  - The chemical is removed by wiping the skin.
  - Discomfort is relieved by using a fan.
- Medium peel:
  - The patient is administered a sedative.
  - The chemical is applied to the site using an applicator.
  - The chemical remains on the site for several minutes longer than in a superficial peel.
  - Alcohol or water is applied to the site to neutralize the chemical.
  - The chemical is removed by wiping the skin.
  - Discomfort is relieved by using a cool compress.
- Deep peel:
  - The patient is administered a general anesthetic.
  - The patient is connected to an EKG to monitor his or her heart.
  - The patient is connected to a pulse oximeter to monitor the oxygen level in the blood.
  - A breathing tube is inserted into the patient's mouth.
  - The chemical is applied to a small area of the site using an applicator.
  - The chemical remains on the site for several minutes.
  - Alcohol or water is applied to the site to neutralize the chemical.
  - The chemical is removed by wiping the skin.
  - The healthcare provider waits 15 minutes before repeating treatment to another small area of the site in order to prevent the buildup of chemical on the skin.
  - The healthcare provider may cover the area with an ointment or tape. The ointment is removed with water 24 hours following the procedure. The tape is removed 2 days following the procedure.
- After the peel the patient might be told to administer Retin-A on the site to speed healing.

Teach the Patient

Explain why the procedure is being performed, what the patient will experience during the procedure, that the patient will not feel any pain during the procedure, and that the patient must moisturize the skin twice a day for 3 weeks prior to the procedure. The patient must administer acyclovir 2 weeks prior to the procedure to prevent a viral infection, might have to administer Retin-A on the site to encourage healing, and must apply tretinoin cream every night on the site beginning 3 weeks following the procedure. In addition, the patient must clean the site frequently following the procedure, avoid exposure to the sun until the site heals, and use sunblock every day, since new skin can be damaged by the sun.

For the superficial peel, the skin is pink but eventually fades to the patient's natural skin tone. Normal activities can resume immediately. For the medium peel, it takes 7 days to heal, during which the site is swollen and reddish. A crust forms over the site, which will fall off within 10 days following the procedure. Normal activities can resume in 1 week. For the deep peel, it takes 2 weeks for regrowth to occur. The skin is reddened for 2 months. Healing takes less than 6 months. The patient will be prescribed pain medication for discomfort, antibiotics for infection, and corticosteroids for swelling. The patient can reduce crusting at the site by showering several times a day. Normal activities can resume in 2 weeks.

The patient should call the healthcare provider if he or she has fever and drainage from the site following the procedure, or if the site remains reddened longer than 2 months following the procedure.

Understanding the Results

The procedure takes less than 2 hours. Result is realized in 6 months following the procedure.

- Normal:
  - The wrinkle or blemish is removed
- Abnormal:
  - Scarring occurs

26.3   Allergy Skin Testing

Allergy skin testing is performed to identify allergens. An allergen is a substance that causes an immune reaction. There are 3 types of skin tests for allergens:

1. **Skin Patch Test**: This test is used to identify allergens that cause contact dermatitis and requires the placement of a pad that contains an allergen solution on the skin for 72 hours. An allergic reaction occurs if the patient is allergic to the allergen.
2. **Skin Prick Test**: This test requires that a drop of an allergen solution is placed on the patient's skin. The skin is scratched, allowing the allergen solution to penetrate the skin. A wheal occurs if the patient is allergic to the allergen.
3. **Intradermal Test**: This test requires that a small amount of an allergen solution be injected into the dermal layer of the skin. A wheal occurs if the patient is allergic to the allergen.

Why the Test Is Performed

The test identifies a source of a patient's allergic reaction.

Before Administering the Test

Assess if the patient:

- Has signed a consent form
- Has taken anticoagulant medication such as Plavix, coumadin, heparin, or aspirin
- Can lie still
- Develops an itch at the site
- Has been taking antihistamines
- Has been taking antidepressants

How the Test Is Performed

- The patient signs a consent form.
- The patient removes clothes in the affected area.
- The patient lies on a table.

- The site is cleaned with an antiseptic.
- Skin prick test and intradermal test:
  - The allergen is introduced into the skin.
  - The healthcare provider examines the site for wheals in 15 minutes.
- Skin patch test:
  - The allergen-containing pad is applied to the site.
  - The pad is removed in 72 hours.
  - The site is assessed for redness and wheals.

Teach the Patient

Explain why the procedure is being performed, what the patient will experience during the procedure, and that the patient will not feel any pain during the procedure except a pinch if the intradermal test or the skin prick test are performed. Inform the patient that he/she must keep the site clean and dry until the site is assessed by the healthcare provider. The patient should not scratch the site, take antihistamines 2 weeks prior to the test, or take antidepressants 2 weeks prior to the test. The patient should call his or her healthcare provider if he or she experiences itchiness while the skin patch test is being performed.

Understanding the Results

The procedure takes less than 1 hour. Result is immediate except for the skin patch test, which takes 72 hours.

- Normal (negative):
  - No change to the site
- Abnormal (positive):
  - Wheals appear at the site

26.4 Dermabrasion

Dermabrasion is a procedure that removes the upper layers of damaged skin caused by scars and aging to encourage new skin growth. The procedure is performed by using a rotating burr to remove damaged tissue.

Why the Procedure Is Performed

The procedure removes scars, wrinkles, and growths from the upper layer of the skin.

Before Administering the Procedure

Assess if the patient:

- Has signed a consent form
- Has taken anticoagulant medication such as Plavix, coumadin, heparin, or aspirin
- Can lie still
- Has not used isotretinoin
- Has not had a face lift
- Has active herpes
- Has an immune disorder

How the Procedure Is Performed

- The patient signs a consent form.
- The patient removes clothes in the affected area.
- The patient lies on a table.
- The site is cleaned with an antiseptic.

- A local anesthetic is administered to the patient.
- The skin is then hardened by using liquid nitrogen or ice packs.
- A rotating burr is used to scrape the skin.
- An antibiotic-treated dressing is applied to the site.

Teach the Patient

Explain why the procedure is being performed, what the patient will experience during the procedure, and that the patient will not feel any pain during the procedure except a pinch when the local anesthetic is administered. The patient must keep the site clean and dry until it heals and should not scratch or remove the scab that forms over the site. The site will heal within 6 weeks following the procedure, there might be a scar or skin tone change to the site, and the procedure may not produce the desired result. The patient should apply sunscreen every day and call his or her healthcare provider if he or she has fever and drainage from the site following the procedure.

Understanding the Results

The procedure takes less than 1 hour. Result is immediate.

- Normal:
  - The skin is removed
- Abnormal:
  - Not all of the skin is removed

26.5   Mantoux Skin Test

The Mantoux skin test determines if the patient has ever been exposed to *Mycobacterium tuberculosis*. The healthcare provider injects the purified protein derivative (PPD), which is *Mycobacterium tuberculosis* antigen, into the patient's forearm. If the patient develops a wheal within 48 hours, it indicates a positive immune response. The patient either is or was infected with *Mycobacterium tuberculosis*. A chest X-ray is taken to diagnose a current infection of *Mycobacterium tuberculosis,* should there be a positive immune response to the test.

Why the Test Is Performed

The test identifies if the patient is or was ever exposed to *Mycobacterium tuberculosis.*

Before Administering the Test

Assess if the patient:

- Has signed a consent form.
- Has taken anticoagulant medication such as Plavix, coumadin, heparin, or aspirin.
- Has had the bacilli Calmette-Guerin (BCG) vaccination. Patients who have had this vaccination will likely test positive.
- Has taken corticosteroids.
- Has an immune-compromise disease.
- Has not had measles, mumps, rubella, chickenpox, or polio vaccines 6 weeks prior to the test.
- Is older than 3 months of age.
- Has had a prior positive PPD and should not have another PPD.

How the Test Is Performed

- The patient signs a consent form.
- The patient exposes his or her forearm.
- The site is cleaned with an antiseptic.
- A needle is inserted slightly under the upper layer of the skin.

- Purified protein derivative is injected.
- The site remains uncovered.

Teach the Patient

Explain why the procedure is being performed, what the patient will experience during the procedure, and that the patient will not feel any pain during the procedure except a pinch when the needle is inserted beneath the skin. The patient must keep the site clean and dry, should not scratch the site, and must return in 48 hours to have the healthcare provider assess the test results.

Understanding the Results

The procedure takes less than 10 minutes. The result is known in 48 hours. A negative test result does not mean that the patient is not infected with *Mycobacterium tuberculosis*. It can take up to 10 weeks following the infection for the immune system to develop antibodies.

- Normal (negative):
  - No change to the site
- Abnormal (positive):
  - Wheals appear at the site

26.6   Wound Culture

A wound culture is ordered when the patient is suspected of having a skin infection. A tissue sample of the infected area is taken and placed in an environment conducive to the growth of microorganisms for 3 days. The tissue sample is then examined to identify the presence and type of the microorganism. Once the microorganism is identified, a sensitivity test is usually performed to determine the medication that kills the microorganism.

Why the Test Is Performed

The test assesses the existence and type of a microorganism in a patient with a skin infection, and the medication to treat the skin infection.

Before Administering the Test

Assess if the patient:

- Has taken antibiotics or applied an antiseptic to the wound prior to the test

How the Test Is Performed

- The healthcare provider swabs the wound with a sterile swab to collect a tissue sample.
- More than one sample might be taken if the healthcare provider suspects that the microorganism may be aerobic (grows in the present of oxygen) or anaerobic (grows without oxygen present) bacteria.
- The sterile swab is placed in either an aerobic or anaerobic culture tube and sent to the lab.
- The sample(s) is then placed in a culture dish in an environment conducive to growing microorganisms.
- After 3 days, tests are performed to identify the microorganism.
- Medication is applied to a portion of the culture to determine which medication kills the microorganism.
- Preliminary results are known quickly, but final results can take 72 hours or longer.

Teach the Patient

Explain why the test is being performed, what the patient will experience during the test, that the patient will not feel any pain during the test, and that the patient should not use antibiotics or apply antiseptic to the wound before the test.

Understanding the Results

The collection takes a few seconds. Results are known within 3 days.

- Normal (negative):
  - No microorganism present in the tissue sample
- Abnormal (positive):
  - Microorganisms are present in the tissue sample

Solved Problems

Chemical Peel

26.1 What is a chemical peel?

A chemical peel is a procedure that exfoliates injured or dead skin, enabling new skin to replace it.

26.2 What is a superficial chemical peel?

A superficial chemical peel removes the surface layer of the skin for a smoother, brighter appearance, and uses glycolic acid or dry ice for the peel.

26.3 What is a medium chemical peel?

A medium chemical peel is commonly used to smooth fine wrinkles, remove blemishes, and treat pigment problems. It uses trichloroacetic acid (TCA) for the peel.

26.4 What is a deep chemical peel?

A deep chemical peel is commonly used to correct coarse wrinkles and blotches on the face only, and uses phenol for the peel. New skin might be lighter in tone because the skin loses some ability to produce pigment.

26.5 What are 2 risks of a chemical peel?

A chemical peel might change the patient's skin tone and result in scarring and cold sores. A chemical peel might cause flaking and dryness.

26.6 What should be assessed before the patient undergoes a chemical peel?

Assess if the patient:
- Has signed a consent form
- Has taken anticoagulant medication such as Plavix, coumadin, heparin, or aspirin
- Can lie still
- Has moisturized his or her skin twice a day for 3 weeks prior to the procedure
- Has administered acyclovir 2 weeks prior to the procedure to prevent a viral infection

26.7 How is a superficial chemical peel performed?

- The chemical is applied to the site using an applicator.
- The chemical remains on the site for several minutes.
- Alcohol or water is applied to the site to neutralize the chemical.
- The chemical is removed by wiping the skin.
- Discomfort is relieved by using a fan.

26.8 How is a deep chemical peel performed?

- The patient is administered a general anesthetic.
- The patient is connected to an EKG to monitor his or her heart.
- The patient is connected to a pulse oximeter to monitor the oxygen level in the blood.
- A breathing tube is inserted into the patient's mouth.
- The chemical is applied to a small area of the site using an applicator.
- The chemical remains on the site for several minutes.
- Alcohol or water is applied to the site to neutralize the chemical.
- The chemical is removed by wiping the skin.
- The healthcare provider waits 15 minutes before repeating treatment to another small area of the site in order to prevent the building of chemical on the skin.

* The healthcare provider may cover the area with an ointment or tape. The ointment is removed with water 24 hours following the procedure. The tape is removed 2 days following the procedure.

26.9   How is a medium chemical peel performed?
* The patient is administered a sedative.
* The chemical is applied to the site using an applicator.
* The chemical remains on the site for several minutes longer than a superficial peel.
* Alcohol or water is applied to the site to neutralize the chemical.
* The chemical is removed by wiping the skin.
* Discomfort is relieved by using a cool compress.

26.10 How can the patient speed healing following a chemical peel?

After the peel the patient might be told to administer Retin-A on the site to speed healing.

26.11 What should you teach the patient who is scheduled to undergo a chemical peel?

Explain why the procedure is being performed, what the patient will experience during the procedure, and that the patient will not feel any pain during the procedure. The patient must moisturize his or her skin twice a day for 3 weeks prior to the procedure, must administer acyclovir 2 weeks prior to the procedure to prevent a viral infection, and might have to administer Retin-A to the site to encourage healing. In addition, the patient must apply tretinoin cream every night on the site beginning 3 weeks following the procedure, must clean the site frequently following the procedure, must avoid exposure to the sun until the site heals, and must use sunblock every day since new skin can be damaged by the sun.

For a superficial peel, the skin is pink but eventually fades to the patient's natural skin tone. Normal activities can resume immediately. For a medium peel, it takes 7 days to heal, during which the site is swollen and reddish. A crust forms over the site, which will fall off within 10 days following the procedure. Normal activities can resume in a week. For a deep peel, it takes 2 weeks for regrowth to occur. The skin is reddened for 2 months. Healing takes less than 6 months. The patient will be prescribed pain medication for discomfort, antibiotics for infection, and corticosteroids for swelling. The patient can reduce crusting at the site by showing several times a day. Normal activities can resume in 2 weeks.

The patient should call his or her healthcare provider if she or he has fever and drainage from the site following the procedure or if the site remains reddened longer than 2 months following the procedure.

Allergy Skin Testing

26.12 What is an allergen?

An allergen is a substance that causes an immune reaction.

26.13 What is the skin patch test?

A skin patch test is used to identify allergens that cause contact dermatitis and requires the placement of a pad that contains an allergen solution on the skin for 72 hours. An allergic reaction occurs if the patient is allergic to the allergen.

26.14 What is the skin prick test?

A skin prick test requires that a drop of an allergen solution is placed on the patient's skin. The skin is scratched, allowing the allergen solution to penetrate the skin. A wheal occurs if the patient is allergic to the allergen.

26.15 What is the intradermal test?

The intradermal test requires that a small amount of an allergen solution be injected into the dermal layer of the skin. A wheal occurs if the patient is allergic to the allergen.

26.16 Why are allergy tests performed?

Allergy tests are performed to identify a source of a patient's allergic reaction.

26.17 What should be assessed before an allergy test is performed?

Assess if the patient:
* Has signed a consent form
* Has taken anticoagulant medication such as Plavix, coumadin, heparin, or aspirin

- Can lie still
- Develops an itch at the site
- Has been taking antihistamines
- Has been taking antidepressants

26.18 What should be taught to the patient who is scheduled to undergo an allergy test?

Explain why the procedure is being performed, what the patient will experience during the procedure, and that the patient will not feel any pain during the procedure except for a pinch if the intradermal test or the skin prick test are performed. The patient must keep the site clean and dry until the site is assessed by the healthcare provider. The patient should not scratch the site, take antihistamines 2 weeks prior to the test, or take antidepressants 2 weeks prior to the test. The patient should call his or her healthcare provider if he or she experiences itchiness while the skin patch test is being performed.

26.19 What is an abnormal result of an allergy test?

An abnormal result of an allergy test is wheals appearing at the site.

Dermabrasion

26.20 What is dermabrasion?

Dermabrasion is a procedure that removes the upper layers of damaged skin caused by scars and aging to encourage new skin growth.

26.21 How is dermabrasion performed?

The dermabrasion procedure is performed by using a rotating burr to remove damaged tissue.

26.22 Why might a healthcare provider order dermabrasion?

A healthcare provider might order dermabrasion to remove scars, wrinkles, or growths from the upper layer of the skin.

26.23 What should you assess before the patient undergoes dermabrasion?

Assess if the patient:
- Has signed a consent form
- Has taken anticoagulant medication such as Plavix, coumadin, heparin, or aspirin
- Can lie still
- Has not used isotretinoin
- Has not had a face lift
- Has active herpes
- Has an immune disorder

26.24 What should you teach the patient about dermabrasion?

Explain why the procedure is being performed, what the patient will experience during the procedure, and that the patient will not feel any pain during the procedure except a pinch when the local anesthetic is administered. The patient must keep the site clean and dry until it heals and should not scratch or remove the scab that forms over the site. The site will heal within 6 weeks following the procedure, there might be a scar or skin tone change to the site, and the procedure may not produce the desired result. The patient should apply sunscreen every day and call his or her healthcare provider if he or she has fever and drainage from the site following the procedure.

Mantoux Skin Test

26.25 What would you expect the healthcare provider to do if the Mantoux skin test is positive?

A chest X-ray is taken to diagnose a current infection of *Mycobacterium tuberculosis* should there be a positive immune response to the test.

CHAPTER 27

Ears, Nose, and Throat (ENT) Tests

27.1 Definition

Ear, nose, and throat tests are used to assess the underlying problems that might impair the patient's hearing, nasal function, and throat. The healthcare provider might order a throat culture, sputum culture, or sputum cytology study to identify the cause of the infection and the medication that will kill the infecting microorganism. Decreased hearing can be caused by a number of factors including a buildup of cerumen (ear wax) in the ear canal, disorders of the eardrum, or a neurological problem. The healthcare provider can perform tympanometry and audiometric tests to determine the cause of hearing loss.

27.2 Throat Culture

A throat culture is ordered when the patient has a throat infection. A tissue sample of the infected area is taken and placed in an environment conducive to the growth of microorganisms for 3 days. The tissue sample is then examined to identify the presence and the type of microorganism. Once the microorganism is identified, a sensitivity test is usually performed to determine the medication that kills the microorganism.

Why the Test Is Performed

The test assesses the existence and type of microorganism in a patient with a throat infection and the medication to treat the throat infection.

Before Administering the Test

Assess if the patient:

- Has taken antibiotics or applied an antiseptic to the throat prior to the test

How the Test Is Performed

- The healthcare provider swabs the throat with a sterile swab to collect a tissue sample. More than one sample might be taken.
- The sterile swab is placed in a culture tube and sent to the lab.
- The sample(s) is then placed in a culture dish in an environment conducive to growing microorganisms.
- After 3 days, tests are performed to identify the microorganism.
- Medication is applied to a portion of the culture to determine which medication kills the microorganism.

Teach the Patient

Explain why the test is being performed, what the patient will experience during the test, that the patient will not feel any pain during the test, and that the patient should not use antibiotics or apply antiseptic to the throat before the test.

Understanding the Test Results

The collection takes a few seconds. Results are known within 3 days.

- Normal (negative):
  - No microorganism present in the sample
- Abnormal (positive):
  - Microorganisms are present in the sample

27.3   Sputum Culture

A sputum culture is ordered when the patient has a respiratory infection. Sputum is not saliva. Sputum is produced in the respiratory system. A sample of sputum is collected in a sterile container and taken to the lab where the sample is placed in an environment conducive to the growth of microorganisms for 3 days. The sample is then examined to identify the presence and the type of microorganism. Once the microorganism is identified, a sensitivity test is usually performed to determine the medication that kills the microorganism.

Why the Test Is Performed

The test assesses the existence and type of microorganism in a patient with a respiratory infection and the medication to treat the respiratory infection.

Before Administering the Test

Assess if the patient:

- Has used mouthwash prior to collecting the sample
- Has taken antibiotics prior to collecting the sample
- Has eaten or drunk 6 hours prior to collecting the sample, if the healthcare provider is using a bronchoscope to collect the sample

How the Test Is Performed

- The sample is taken immediately after the patient awakens from sleeping.
- The patient removes dentures.
- The patient rinses his or her mouth with water.
- The patient coughs deeply to produce the sputum.
- If the patient is unable to produce the sputum, the healthcare provider may loosen sputum in the lungs by using a mist inhaler.
- If this does not produce the sputum, then the healthcare provider collects the sputum using a bronchoscope that is inserted into the patient's airway.
- The sample(s) is then placed in a culture dish in an environment conductive to growing microorganisms.
- After 3 days, tests are performed to identify the microorganism.
- Medication is applied to a portion of the culture to determine which medication kills the microorganism.

Teach the Patient

Explain why the test is being performed, what the patient will experience during the test, and that the patient will not feel any pain during the test. The patient should not use antibiotics prior to the test and should not use mouthwash prior to collecting the sample. The patient should cough deeply prior to taking the sample, take the sample the first thing in the morning upon awakening from sleep, and make sure the sample is delivered to the lab immediately after the sample is collected. The sputum is different than saliva.

Understanding the Test Results

The collection takes a few seconds. Results are known within 3 days.

- Normal (negative):
  - No microorganism present in the sample
- Abnormal (positive):
  - Microorganisms are present in the sample

27.4 Sputum Cytology

Sputum cytology is a procedure that examines cells contained in a sputum sample. Sputum cytology assesses for asbestosis, pneumonia, respiratory infection, tuberculosis, and lung cancer.

Why the Test Is Performed

The test assesses for lung cancer, pneumonia, and asbestosis.

Before Administering the Test

Assess if the patient:

- Has used mouthwash prior to collecting the sample
- Has taken antibiotics prior to collecting the sample
- Has eaten or drunk 6 hours prior to collecting the sample, if the healthcare provider is using a bronchoscope to collect the sample

How the Test Is Performed

- The sample is taken immediately after the patient awakens from sleeping.
- The patient removes dentures.
- The patient rinses his or her mouth with water.
- The patient coughs deeply to produce the sputum.
- If the patient is unable to produce the sputum, the healthcare provider may loosen sputum in the lungs by using a mist inhaler.
- If this does not produce the sputum, then the healthcare provider collects the sputum using a bronchoscope that is inserted into the patient's airway.
- The sample(s) is then viewed with a microscope to identify cells contained in the sputum.

Teach the Patient

Explain why the test is being performed, what the patient will experience during the test, and that the patient will not feel any pain during the test. The patient should not use antibiotics prior to the test and should not use mouthwash prior to collecting the sample. The patient should cough deeply prior to taking the sample, take the sample the first thing in the morning after awakening from sleep, and make sure the sample is delivered to the lab immediately after the sample is collected. The sputum is different than saliva.

Understanding the Test Results

The collection takes a few seconds. Results are known within 3 days.

- Normal (negative):
  - Normal cells in the sample
- Abnormal (positive):
  - None respiratory cells in the sample

27.5   Sinus X-ray

An X-ray of the sinus is ordered if the healthcare provider suspects that the patient has sinusitis or other conditions that might cause similar symptoms. The healthcare provider may also order a CT scan of the head, which provides clearer images of the sinus than an X-ray.

Why the Test Is Performed

The test identifies blockages in the sinus and diagnoses sinusitis.

Before Administering the Test

Assess if the patient:

- Has signed a consent form
- Can sit still

How the Test Is Performed

- The patient signs a consent form.
- The patient sits in front of the X-ray machine.
- Several X-rays are taken, each at a different angle.

Teach the Patient

Explain why the test is being performed, what the patient will experience during the test, and that the patient will not feel any pain during the test.

Understanding the Test Results

The procedure takes less than 30 minutes. Results are immediate.

- Normal:
  - Normal sinuses
- Abnormal:
  - A blockage is identified
  - The patient has sinusitis

27.6   Tympanometry

The tympanometry test measures the eardrum's response to pressure and sound, and assesses if there is fluid behind the eardrum. Tympanometry is ordered when the patient is suspected of having otitis media, hearing loss, fluid behind the eardrum, or a blocked eustachian tube. This test is frequently performed in children.

Why the Test Is Performed

The test identifies fluid behind the eardrum and blockage of the eustachian tube. It also assesses for otitis media and hearing loss.

Before Administering the Test

Assess if the patient:

- Can lie still

How the Test Is Performed

- The tympanometer is placed into the ear canal.
- A tone that causes pressure change in the ear is played.
- The tympanometer measures the pressure change.

Teach the Patient

Explain why the test is being performed, what the patient will experience during the test, and that the patient will not feel any pain during the procedure.

Understanding the Test Results

The procedure takes less than 5 minutes. Results are known immediately.

- Normal:
  - Normal pressure
- Abnormal:
  - Abnormal pressure

27.7   Audiometic Testing

Audiometric testing determines the degree with which a patient can hear. Hearing loss is the patient's inability to hear or understand a range of sound frequencies due to either structural problems with the ear or neural problems, preventing the brain from receiving impulses from the ear or properly interpreting those impulses. There are 8 types of audiometic tests:

1. **Pure Tone Audiometry**: This test determines sound frequencies that can be heard by the patient.
2. **Whispered Speech Test**: This test determines if the patient can hear low volume sounds spoken behind him or her.
3. **Speech Reception/Word Recognition**: This test is used to identify sensorineural hearing loss.
4. **Tuning Fork Test**: This test determines if a hearing problem is caused by sound being received by nerves in the ear or nerve problems.
5. **Auditory Brain Stem Response (ABR)**: This test is used to detect sensorineural hearing problems.
6. **Otoacoustic Emissions (OAE)**: This test identifies hearing problems in newborns.
7. **Vestibular Test**: This test identifies problems with the inner ear.
8. **Acoustic Immitance**: This test assesses the middle ear's ability to conduct sound.

Why the Test Is Performed

The test assesses the patient's hearing and the underlying cause of hearing loss.

Before Administering the Test

Assess if the patient:

- Has signed a consent form
- Can sit still
- Can respond to instructions
- Can indicate if a sound is heard

How the Test Is Performed

- The patient signs a consent form.
- Pure tone audiometry:
  - The patient wears headphones that are connected to an audiometer.
  - The audiometer produces a series of tones.
  - The patient indicates which tones are heard.

- Whispered speech test:
  - The patient places his or her finger in the ear canal of one ear.
  - The healthcare provider stands 2 feet behind the patient.
  - The healthcare provider whispers words.
  - The patient indicates if he or she can hear those words.
  - The test is repeated using the opposite ear.
- Speech reception/word recognition:
  - The healthcare provider speaks familiar two-syllable words at various degrees of loudness.
  - The patient is asked to repeat those words.
  - The results are measured as the patient's spondee threshold.
- Tuning fork test:
  - The healthcare provider places a vibrating tuning fork either behind the ear or on the patient's head.
  - The patient indicates when he or she hears the tuning fork.
- Auditory brain stem response (ABR):
  - Electrodes are placed on the patient's ear lobe and scalp.
  - Earphones are placed in the patient's ears.
  - A clicking noise is sounded through the earphones.
  - The electrodes detect neural responses to the clicking noise and record the response on a graph.
- Otoacoustic emissions (OAE):
  - A microphone is placed in a newborn's ear.
  - A flexible probe is also placed in the baby's ear.
  - Sound is passed through the probe.
  - The microphone detects the response of the inner ear to the sound.
- Vestibular test:
  - The patient moves arms and legs, stands on one foot, walks heel-to-toe with his or her eyes open, and then closed.
  - The patient's ability to keep his or her balance is assessed.
- Acoustic immitance:
  - The ear canal is sealed closed using a soft-tip instrument.
  - Sound and air is directed toward the ear at different pressures.
  - A measurement is taken that registers how the middle ear relays sound.

Teach the Patient

Explain why the procedure is being performed, what the patient will experience during the procedure, and that the patient will not feel any pain during the procedure.

Understanding the Test Results

The procedure takes less than 1 hour. Results are immediate.

- Normal:
  - Normal hearing
- Abnormal:
  - Structural or neurological problems cause reduced hearing ability

Solved Problems

Throat Culture

27.1 Why might the healthcare provider order a throat culture?

A throat culture is ordered when the patient has a throat infection. The tissue sample is then examined to identify the presence and type of microorganism. Once the microorganism is identified, a sensitivity test is usually performed to determine the medication that kills the microorganism.

27.2   What should be assessed before the throat culture is performed?

Assess if the patient has taken antibiotics or applied an antiseptic to the throat prior to the test.

27.3   How is a throat culture performed?
- The healthcare provider swabs the throat with a sterile swab to collect a tissue sample. More than one sample might be taken.
- The sterile swab is placed in a culture tube and sent to the lab.
- The sample(s) is then placed in a culture dish in an environment conducive to growing microorganisms.
- After 3 days, tests are performed to identify the microorganism.
- Medication is applied to a portion of the culture to determine which medication kills the microorganism.

27.4   What should you teach a patient who is scheduled to undergo a throat culture?

Explain why the test is being performed, what the patient will experience during the test, that the patient will not feel any pain during the test, and that the patient should not use antibiotics or apply antiseptic to the throat before the test.

Sputum Culture

27.5   What is sputum?

Sputum is not saliva. It is produced in the respiratory system.

27.6   Why is a sputum culture ordered by the healthcare provider?

The test assesses the existence and type of microorganisms in a patient with a respiratory infection and the medication to use to treat the respiratory infection.

27.7   What should be assessed prior to administering the sputum culture?

Assess if the patient:
- Has used mouthwash prior to collecting the sample
- Has taken antibiotics prior to collecting the sample
- Has eaten or drunk 6 hours prior to collecting the sample, if the healthcare provider is using a bronchoscope to collect the sample

27.8   What happens if the patient is unable to produce the sputum?

If the patient is unable to produce the sputum, the healthcare provider may loosen sputum in the lungs by using a mist inhaler. The healthcare provider collects the sputum using a bronchoscope that is inserted into the patient's airway.

27.9   How would you instruct a patient to produce a sputum sample?

The sample is taken immediately after the patient awakens from sleeping. The patient removes dentures. The patient rinses his or her mouth with water. The patient coughs deeply to produce the sputum.

Sputum Cytology

27.10   What is sputum cytology?

Sputum cytology is a procedure that examines cells contained in a sputum sample.

27.11   Why is the sputum cytology test ordered by the healthcare provider?

The sputum cytology test is ordered to assess for lung cancer, pneumonia, and asbestosis.

27.12   What must you assess before the sputum sample is taken from the patient?

Assess if the patient:
- Has used mouthwash prior to collecting the sample
- Has taken antibiotics prior to collecting the sample
- Has eaten or drunk 6 hours prior to collecting the sample, if the healthcare provider is using a bronchoscope to collect the sample

27.13   What should you teach the patient before the sputum sample is obtained?

Explain why the test is being performed, what the patient will experience during the test, and that the patient will not feel any pain during the test. The patient should not use antibiotics prior to the test and should not use mouthwash prior to collecting the sample. The patient should cough deeply prior to taking the sample, take the sample first thing in the morning after awakening from sleep, and make sure the sample is delivered to the lab immediately after the sample is collected. Sputum is different than saliva.

Sinus X-ray

27.14   Why might a healthcare provider order a sinus X-ray?

An X-ray of the sinus is ordered if the healthcare provider suspects that the patient has sinusitis or other conditions that might cause similar symptoms.

27.15   What might be an abnormal finding of a sinus X-ray?

An abnormal finding of a sinus X-ray is a blockage or sinusitis.

Tympanometry

27.16   How is the tympanometry test performed?

The tympanometer is placed into the ear canal. A tone that causes pressure change in the ear is played. The tympanometer measures the pressure change.

27.17   Why is the tympanometry test ordered?

The tympanometry test is ordered to identify fluid behind the eardrum and blockage of the eustachian tube. It also assesses for otitis media and hearing loss.

27.18   What kind of patient is frequently administered the tympanometry test?

This test is frequently performed in children.

27.19   What should you teach the patient who is scheduled to be administered the tympanometry test?

Explain why the test is being performed, what the patient will experience during the test, and that the patient will not feel any pain during the procedure.

Audiometic Testing

27.20   What is pure tone audiometry?

Pure tone audiometry is a test that determines sound frequencies that can be heard by the patient.

27.21   What is the speech reception/word recognition test?

The speech reception/word recognition test is used to identify sensorineural hearing loss.

27.22   What is the auditory brain stem response test?

The auditory brain stem response (ABR) test is used to detect sensorineural hearing problems.

27.23   What is the acoustic immitance test?

The acoustic immitance test assesses the middle ear's ability to conduct sound.

27.24   What should you teach the patient about audiometric testing?

Explain why the procedure is being performed, what the patient will experience during the procedure, and that the patient will not feel any pain during the procedure.

27.25   How is the vestibular test performed?

The patient moves arms and legs, stands on one foot, walks heel-to-toe with his or her eyes open, and then closed. The patient's ability to keep his or her balance is assessed.

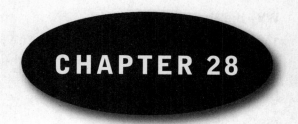

CHAPTER 28

Vision Tests and Procedures

28.1 Definition

Vision tests are used to diagnose problems with sight and disorders that can lead to loss of vision. Light rays pass through the cornea, the pupil, and lenses that focus the ray of light onto the retina located at the back of the eye. When light rays are not properly focused on the retina, the patient is unable to see clearly. Light rays focused in front of the retina cause myopia (nearsightedness), enabling patients to see things better near them than at a distance. Light rays focused behind the retina causes hyperopia (farsightedness), enabling patients to see things better at a distance than up close. When light rays are irregularly bent, images are blurred, resulting in astigmatism.

A standard vision test is used to assess the patient's ability to see up close and at a distance. A standard vision test determines if the patient is experiencing peripheral vision difficulty or might have macular degeneration. A standard vision test determines the refractive error of the patient's eye, which determines the corrective lenses needed to restore the patient's eyesight. Patients who have myopia might be able to have this condition fixed by having corneal ring implants or by reshaping the cornea using photorefractive keratectomy. Glaucoma is caused by increased intraocular pressure. The healthcare provider assesses intraocular pressure by performing tonometry. If intraocular pressure is elevated, the healthcare provider may perform one of several procedures to relieve the pressure. Blood flow in the eye can be assessed by performing an eye angiogram, which detects a vitreous hemorrhage.

28.2 Vision Tests

The healthcare provider examines the patient's peripheral vision and ability to see near distances and far distances along with the patient's ability to distinguish colors by performing nine vision tests:

1. **Confrontation Test**: This test assesses the patient's peripheral vision by gazing at the healthcare provider's nose.
2. **Amsler Grid Test**: This test assesses for macular degeneration.
3. **Perimetry Test**: This test assesses the patient's peripheral vision by flashing lights randomly in a perimeter.
4. **Tangent Screen Test**: This test assesses the patient's peripheral vision by gazing at a concentric circle image.
5. **Snellen Test**: This test assesses the patient's ability to see distances.
6. **E Chart Test**: This test assesses the patient's ability to see distances when the patient is unable to read.
7. **Near Test**: This test assesses the patient's ability to see near distances.
8. **Color Vision Test**: This test assesses the patient's ability to distinguish colors.
9. **Refraction Test**: This test measures the refractive error of the patient's eyes to determine the lens that corrects the patient's eyesight.

Why the Test Is Performed

The test assesses if the patient is color blind, if the patient's vision should be corrected with glasses or contact lenses, if the patient is losing his or her peripheral vision, and if the patient has macular degeneration.

Before Administering the Test

Assess if the patient:

- Has signed a consent form
- Can sit still
- Can read
- Wears glasses or contact lenses
- Has an eye infection
- Can follow instructions
- Has his or her glasses or contact lenses with him or her

How the Test Is Performed

- Confrontation test:
  - The healthcare provider sits 3 feet from where the patient is sitting.
  - The patient covers one eye.
  - The patient stares at the healthcare provider's nose with the other eye.
  - The healthcare provider moves his or her finger from outside the visual field to the center of the visual field.
  - The healthcare provider moves his or her finger from the center of the visual field to opposite outside visual field.
  - The patient signals when he or she first sees the healthcare provider's finger.
  - The test is repeated using the other eye.
- Amsler grid test:
  - The patient covers one eye.
  - A 4-inch square chart containing straight lines and a grid with a black dot at the center is held 14 inches from the patient.
  - The patient focuses his or her eye on the black dot on the chart.
  - The patient tells the healthcare provider if he or she can see the black dot, a dark spot other than the black dot, and the straight lines.
  - The patient should see the black dot and the straight lines.
- Perimetry test:
  - The patient looks into the perimeter focusing on a dot in the center of the perimeter screen.
  - Lights randomly flash at various locations on the perimeter screen.
  - The patient presses a button each time he or she sees a light on the screen.
  - The perimeter generates a printout showing areas in the patient's peripheral vision where he or she did not see the light.
- Tangent screen test:
  - The patient sits 6 feet away from the black screen that contains concentric circles and lines.
  - The patient covers one eye.
  - The patient focuses the other eye on a center of the circle.
  - A wand containing an object is moved from outside the circle to inside the circle.
  - The patient signals the healthcare provider when he or she sees the object.
  - The test is repeated using different sized objects on the wand.
  - The test is repeated for the other eye.
- Snellen test:
  - The patient is positioned 20 feet from the Snellen chart.
  - The patient covers one eye.
  - The patient reads the smallest row of letters on the chart.

- ○ Each row is designated with a visual acuity value.
- ○ A row designated as 20/20 visual acuity means a person with normal vision can read this line at a distance of 20 feet.
- ○ A row designated as 20/40 visual acuity means a person with normal vision can read this line at a distance of 40 feet.
- E chart test:
  - ○ The patient covers one eye.
  - ○ The patient reads the smallest E on the chart.
  - ○ Each row is designated with a visual acuity value the same as the Snellen test.
- Near test:
  - ○ The patient is given a card that contains text.
  - ○ The patient holds the card 14 inches from his or her eyes.
  - ○ The patient reads the text on the card.
  - ○ The test is repeated with cards that have progressively smaller type size.
- Color vision test:
  - ○ The patient views pages that contain numbers, symbols, and paths that appear on a background of colored dots.
  - ○ The patient is asked to say out loud the number, symbol, or path.
  - ○ The patient may have problems differentiating colors if he or she is unable to identify the number, symbol, or path correctly.
- Refraction test:
  - ○ The patient views the Snellen chart or E chart and the cards used for the near test while looking through corrective lenses.
  - ○ The patient then notifies the healthcare provider when he or she can clearly read the chart and cards.
  - ○ The healthcare provider then writes a prescription for those lenses.

Teach the Patient

Explain why the procedure is being performed, what the patient will experience during the procedure, that the patient will not feel any pain during the procedure, and that the patient should bring his or her glasses or contact lenses to the test.

Understanding the Test Results

The procedure takes less than 1 hour. Results are immediate.

- Normal:
  - ○ Normal eyesight
  - ○ Normal peripheral vision
  - ○ No macular degeneration
  - ○ Can see all colors
- Abnormal:
  - ○ Nearsighted (can see near distances)
  - ○ Farsighted (can see far distances)
  - ○ Restricted peripheral vision
  - ○ Possible macular degeneration
  - ○ Color blind

28.3 Tonometry

Tonometry is a test for glaucoma that measures the intraocular pressure of the patient's eye. The healthcare provider assesses the amount of pressure necessary to flatten the cornea. There are four methods used to perform tonometry:

1. **Pneumotonometry**: This method uses a puff of air to measure intraocular pressure. No direct contact is made with the eye.
2. **Applanation Tonometry**: This method uses a tonometer to measure intraocular pressure.

3. **Electronic Indentation Tonometry**: This method uses a tonometer that is connected to a computer to measure intraocular pressure.
4. **Schiotz Tonometry**: This method uses a plunger to measure intraocular pressure.

Why the Test Is Performed

The test assesses for glaucoma.

Before Administering the Test

Assess if the patient:

- Has not drunk alcohol 12 hours before the test
- Has not drunk anything for 4 hours before the test
- Can sit still
- Has not smoked marijuana 24 hours before the test
- Can respond to direction during the procedure
- Can withstand a probe being directed at his or her eye
- Has removed his or her contact lenses
- Signed a consent form

How the Test Is Performed

- The patient removes his or her contact lenses.
- Pneumotonometry:
  - The patient sits.
  - The patient places his or her chin on a chin rest and forehead against a stabilizing bar of the slit lamp.
  - A light is shone into the eye.
  - A puff of air is blown into the eye.
  - The tonometer measures the change in the reflection of the light off the cornea when the puff of air strikes the eye.
  - Intraocular pressure is read from the tonometer.
- Applanation tonometry:
  - The patient sits.
  - A local anesthetic is placed in the eye.
  - Fluorescein is administered to the eye to make the cornea visible.
  - The patient places his chin on a chin rest and forehead against a stabilizing bar of the slit lamp.
  - A tonometer is pressed against the cornea.
  - The tension dial on the tonometer records the intraocular pressure.
- Electronic indentation tonometry:
  - The patient sits.
  - A local anesthetic is placed in the eye.
  - The patient places his or her chin on a chin rest and forehead against a stabilizing bar of the slit lamp.
  - A tonometer is pressed against the cornea.
  - A click sounds when a reading is taken.
  - Four readings are taken.
  - Intraocular pressure is displayed on the computer screen.
- Schiotz tonometry:
  - The patient lies on a table.
  - A local anesthetic is placed in the eye.
  - The patient stares at a fixed point on the ceiling.
  - A tonometer is pressed against the cornea.
  - Intraocular pressure is displayed on the tonometer.

Teach the Patient

Explain why the procedure is being performed, how the procedure is performed, and that the patient will not feel any pain during the procedure. The patient should not insert contact lenses for 2 hours following the test, drink alcohol 12 hours before the test, drink anything for 4 hours before the test, smoke marijuana 24 hours before the test, or rub his/her eyes for 30 minutes following the test.

Understanding the Test Results

The procedure takes less than 30 minutes. Results are immediate.

- Normal:
  - Normal intraocular pressure
- Abnormal:
  - High intraocular pressure
  - Low intraocular pressure

28.4   Electronystagmogram (ENG)

Electronystagmogram is a test that measures eye movement, both voluntary eye movement and nystagmus, to assess the patient's balance and the underlying cause of vertigo.

Why the Test Is Performed

The test assesses the underlying cause of loss of balance and vertigo, and the inner ear.

Before Administering the Test

Assess if the patient:

- Has not taken tranquilizers 5 days before the test
- Has not drunk alcohol 5 days before the test
- Has not ingested caffeine 5 days before the test
- Has not eaten 4 hours before the test
- Is not wearing facial makeup
- Has a back or neck disorder

How the Test Is Performed

- The patient signs a consent form.
- Any obstruction in the ear canal is removed.
- Five electrodes are pasted on the patient's face.
- The room is darkened.
- During each of the following, electrical activities from the electrodes are recorded.
- The patient follows a moving light with his or her eyes while holding his or her head still.
- The patient closes his or her eyes and is asked to perform mental arithmetic.
- The patient opens his or her eyes and follows the back and forth movement of a moving pendulum.
- The patient is asked to look at objects that are moved in front of him or her.
- The patient is asked to move his or her head up and down and side to side.
- Cool water is placed in the patient's ear.
- Warm water is placed in the patient's ear.

Teach the Patient

Explain why the procedure is being performed, how the procedure is performed, and that the patient will not feel any pain during the procedure. The patient should not take tranquilizers 5 days before the test, drink alcohol 5 days before the test, ingest caffeine 5 days before the test, eat 4 hours before the test, or wear facial makeup during the test.

Understanding the Test Results

The procedure takes less than 2 hours. Results are known within a week.

- Normal:
  - Normal voluntary and involuntary eye movement
- Abnormal:
  - Abnormal involuntary eye movement

Solved Problems

Vision Test

28.1 Why would a healthcare provider order an Amsler grid test?

The Amsler grid test assesses for macular degeneration.

28.2 What is assessed by the tangent screen test?

The tangent screen test assesses the patient's peripheral vision by having the patient gaze at a concentric circle image.

28.3 What is the confrontation test?

The confrontation test assesses the patient's peripheral vision by gazing at the healthcare provider's nose.

28.4 What would you expect the healthcare provider to order to assess the patient's vision if the patient is unable to read?

The E chart vision test assesses the patient's ability to see distances when the patient is unable to read.

28.5 What is measured by the refraction test?

The refraction test measures the refractive error of the patient's eyes to determine lenses that correct the patient's eyesight.

28.6 What should you assess before the patient undergoes a vision test?

Assess if the patient:

- Has signed a consent form
- Can sit still
- Can read
- Wears glasses or contact lenses
- Has an eye infection
- Can follow instructions
- Has his or her glasses or contact lenses with him or her

28.7 How is the Amsler grid test performed?

- The patient covers one eye.
- A 4-inch square chart containing straight lines and a grid with a black dot at the center is held 14 inches from the patient.
- The patient focuses his or her eyes on the black dot on the chart.
- The patient tells the healthcare provider if he or she can see the black dot, a dark spot other than the black dot, or straight lines.
- The patient should see the black dot and the straight lines

28.8 How is the tangent screen test performed?

- The patient sits six feet away from the black screen that contains concentric circles and lines.
- The patient covers one eye.
- The patient focuses the other eye on the center of the circle.
- A wand containing an object is moved from outside the circle to inside the circle.
- The patient signals the healthcare provider when he or she sees the object.
- The test is repeated, using different sized objects on the wand.
- The test is repeated for the other eye.

28.9   How is the Snellen test performed?

- The patient is positioned 20 feet from the Snellen chart.
- The patient covers one eye.
- The patient reads the smallest row of letters on the chart.
- Each row is designated with a visual acuity value.
- A row designated as 20/20 visual acuity means a person with normal vision can read this line at a distance of 20 feet.
- A row designated as 20/40 visual acuity means a person with normal vision can read this line at a distance of 40 feet.

28.10   How is the near test vision test performed?

- The patient is given a card that contains text.
- The patient holds the card 14 inches from the eyes.
- The patient reads the text on the card.
- The test is repeated with cards that have progressively smaller type size.

28.11   What should you teach the patient about the vision test?

Explain why the procedure is being performed, what the patient will experience during the procedure, that the patient will not feel any pain during the procedure, and that the patient should bring his or her glasses or contact lenses to the test.

28.12   The patient asks the difference between being near- or farsighted. How would you respond?

Nearsighted means the patient can see near distances. Farsighted means the patient can see far distances.

Tonometry

28.13   Why would the healthcare provider order a tonometry test?

A tonometry test assesses for glaucoma.

28.14   What is pneumotonometry?

Pneumotonometry is a test that uses a puff of air to measure intraocular pressure. No direct contact is made with the eye.

28.15   What is electronic indentation tonometry?

Electronic indentation tonometry is a test that uses a tonometer that is connected to a computer to measure intraocular pressure.

28.16   What test uses a plunger to measure intraocular pressure?

Schiotz tonometry uses a plunger to measure intraocular pressure.

28.17   What should you assess before the patient undergoes tonometry testing?

Assess if the patient:
- Has not drunk alcohol 12 hours before the test
- Has not drunk anything for 4 hours before the test
- Can sit still
- Has not smoked marijuana 24 hours before the test
- Can respond to direction during the procedure
- Can withstand a probe being directed at his or her eye
- Has removed his or her contact lenses
- Signed a consent form

28.18   How is the pneumotonmetry test performed?

- The patient sits.
- The patient places his or her chin on a chin rest and his or her forehead against a stabilizing bar of the slit lamp.
- A light is shone into the eye.

- A puff of air is blown into the eye.
- The tonometer measures the change in the reflection of the light off the cornea when the puff of air strikes the eye.
- Intraocular pressure is read from the tonometer.

28.19 How is the applanation tonometry test performed?

- The patient sits.
- A local anesthetic is placed in the eye.
- Fluorescein is administered to the eye to make the cornea visible.
- The patient places his or her chin on a chin rest and forehead against a stabilizing bar of the slit lamp.
- A tonometer is pressed against the cornea.
- The tension dial on the tonometer records the intraocular pressure.

Electronystagmogram

28.20 What is the electronystagmogram?

Electronystagmongram is a test that measures eye movement, both voluntary eye movement and nystagmus, to assess the patient's balance and to assess the underlying cause of vertigo.

28.21 What should you assess before the patient undergoes an electronystagmogram?

Assess if the patient:
- Has not taken tranquilizers 5 days before the test
- Has not drunk alcohol 5 days before the test
- Has not ingested caffeine 5 days before the test
- Has not eaten 4 hours before the test
- Is not wearing facial makeup
- Has a back or neck disorder

28.22 How is the electronystagmogram performed?

- The patient signs a consent form.
- Any obstruction in the ear cannel is removed.
- Five electrodes are pasted on the patient's face.
- The room is darkened.
- During each of the following, electrical activities from the electrodes are recorded.
- The patient follows a moving light with his or her eyes while holding his or her head still.
- The patient closes his or her eyes and is asked to perform mental arithmetic.
- The patient opens his or her eyes and follows the back and forth movement of a moving pendulum.
- The patient is asked to look at objects that are moved in front of him or her.
- The patient is asked to move his or her head up and down and side to side.
- Cool water is placed in the patient's ear.
- Warm water is placed in the patient's ear.

28.23 What instructions should a patient receive before undergoing an electronystagmogram?

Explain why the procedure is being performed, how the procedure is performed, and that the patient will not feel any pain during the procedure. The patient should not take tranquilizers 5 days before the test, drink alcohol 5 days before the test, ingest caffeine 5 days before the test, eat 4 hours before the test, or wear facial makeup during the test.

28.24 What might be an abnormal result of an electronystagmongram?

Abnormal involuntary eye movement might be an abnormal result of an electronystagmongram.

28.25 What is assessed by an electronystagmongram?

An electronystagmongram assesses the underlying cause of loss of balance and vertigo, and the inner ear.

INDEX